SAUNDERS REVIEW FOR PRACTICAL NURSES

Third Edition

CLAIRE BRACKMAN KEANE

R.N., B.S. in Nursing Education, M.Ed.
Formerly Director, Athens General Hospital
School of Practical Nursing, Athens, Georgia

With a contribution by

VERNA JANE MUHL

R.N., B.S.N., M.Ed.
Director, Practical Nurse Program,
Mitchell Area Vocational-Technical School
Mitchell, South Dakota

W. B. SAUNDERS COMPANY
PHILADELPHIA • LONDON • TORONTO

W. B. Saunders Company: West Washington Square
                         Philadelphia, PA 19105

                         1 St. Anne's Road
                         Eastbourne, East Sussex BN21 3UN, England

                         1 Goldthorne Avenue
                         Toronto, Ontario M8Z 5T9, Canada

Library of Congress Cataloging in Publication Data

Keane, Claire Brackman.

Saunders review for practical nurses.

Bibliography: p.

Includes index.

1. Practical nursing—Outlines, syllabi, etc.   2. Practical
   nursing—Examinations, questions, etc.   I. Muhl,
   Verna Jane, joint author.   II. Title.   III. Title:
   Review for practical nurses.

RT62.K37 1977   610.73'076   76–41537

ISBN 0–7216–5327–8

Saunders Review for Practical Nurses   ISBN 0-7216-5327-8

Last digit is the print number: 9   8   7   6   5   4   3

PREFACE

This third edition of *Saunders Review for Practical Nurses* is designed to give the reader an opportunity to study basic information in outline form and then to actively answer questions related to the material studied. It would be very difficult, if not impossible, to include in a book of this type all the scientific principles and nursing techniques utilized by today's practical nurse. The reader is encouraged to supplement the outlines with additional information that is considered pertinent and useful. The bibliography on page 380 may serve as a guide to the reader seeking references for further study.

It is best to read the text and answer the questions in the sequences in which they have been presented. Many of the basic principles covered in the first units will be incorporated in later units. Throughout this revised edition an effort has been made to stimulate critical thinking and encourage intelligent decision making in realistic nursing situations. Some of the wrong answers presented as possible choices are from actual events witnessed by the author in the classroom and clinical area. The NOTE TO THE STUDENT was written to familiarize students and graduates with some of the proper techniques as well as the common pitfalls of "test taking."

It is a pleasure to acknowledge the help of Verna Jane Muhl, R.N., M.Ed., in the revision of Part XI, Nursing the Mother and Her Newborn Infant.

The author wishes to express her sincere thanks to all instructors, students, and graduates who have taken time to offer constructive criticisms of the first edition of this review and suggestions for its revision. Their assistance has been invaluable in helping determine the real needs of those using the text.

Athens, Georgia   CLAIRE BRACKMAN KEANE

CONTENTS

NOTE TO THE STUDENT

The content of this review is divided so that one entire part or one unit of a part can usually be completed in a single study period. It should be possible for you to cover the outline and then immediately answer the questions related to the material reviewed. If, however, you cannot complete one section at a sitting, the questions follow almost exactly the same order as do the headings and outlined material in the unit. The material has been presented in such a manner that you should be able to proceed from beginning to end without difficulty and at your own rate of speed, but you must take an active part and do more than just read the material.

Most persons have some fears and misgivings whenever they take a test. If an individual is very apprehensive, his fear can affect his mental processes and prevent him from thinking clearly. A good way to overcome this fear is by practice in taking tests. Psychiatrists often help a patient overcome extreme anxiety about a future event by having him act out the situation he fears well in advance of the reality. Your experience in using the answer sheets provided to answer the questions in this review can help you gain confidence and overcome some of the feelings of inadequacy and dread with which you may face an examination or test.

Answering the Question Asked. Read each question very carefully and be sure that you know exactly what is being asked. As you read the question look for key words such as *first, most important, chief, primary.* If you are asked, for example, "What is the first thing the nurse must do," in a given situation, don't choose the answer that describes the most important action, or the one with which you are most familiar. The correct answer will be the one that tells what the nurse must do *first* in a series of steps.

Try this question:

The first thing you should do for a victim requiring mouth-to-mouth resuscitation is:
1. tilt the head back and extend the neck
2. pinch the nose and place your mouth directly over the victim's mouth
3. check the mouth and throat for obstruction of the air passage
4. breath into the victim's mouth at the rate of 16 per minute

When you learned mouth-to-mouth resuscitation, you were taught that tilting the head backward to lift the tongue away from the back of the throat might be the only maneuver needed for the victim to begin breathing on his own. All of the answers given above are part of the resuscitation procedure, but the first step is tilting the head of the victim backward. The correct answer, therefore, is #1.

Reading the Question. It is hard to believe the number of incorrect answers that are given simply because the person answering the questions did not really know what was being asked. No one who is sincerely interested in testing knowledge and ability will deliberately set out to write "tricky" questions and answers. But sometimes the reader tricks himself because he does not read each word of the question or he answers the question too hurriedly. Here are five sample questions that are designed to make you stop and think before you answer.

1. How many of each species of animal did Moses take aboard the ark?
2. Why is it against the law in North Carolina for a man to marry his widow's sister?

3. Is this statement true or false? All household poisons should be kept in the locked medicine cabinet when there are small children in the house.
4. A coin collector claimed that he had a gold coin dated 776 B.C. Do you think the coin was authentic? If not, why not?
5. If a physician gave you three tablets with instructions to take them 30 minutes apart, how long would it take to consume all three tablets?

Answers:
1. None. It was Noah, not Moses, who built the ark.
2. A man who has a widow is no longer living.
3. False. Poisons are *never* kept in the medicine cabinet.
4. No, it was not authentic. Persons minting coins before Christ had no way of knowing how many years it would be before the birth of Christ.
5. One hour. If you missed this, think about it for a while and imagine the time at which each tablet will be taken.

Making "Educated Guesses."   Making wild guesses can at times cost you more points than leaving the answer unmarked, if the marking procedure is to subtract the incorrect answers from the correct answers. There are times, however, when you can use what you already know to correctly answer a question you are not too sure about. Let us suppose, for example, that you are asked about the location of the trachea. You know that it is a part of the respiratory tract but you are undecided as to exactly where it is located. Here are the choices offered:
1. above the larynx
2. in front of the esophagus
3. above the thyroid cartilage
4. below the esophagus

Now you have had experience caring for a patient with a tracheotomy and you know that the patient could not make vocal sounds when the tracheotomy tube was open. The larynx is the voice box and air must pass through the larynx to produce sound. If the trachea were above the larynx, the patient could make vocal sounds as his exhaled air passed through the vocal cords on its way to the trachea. You can conclude, then, that #1 is incorrect. Since a patient with a tracheotomy does not have an incision in his esophagus (he could not eat or drink if he did), the trachea must be in front of the esophagus. So #2 seems to be the correct answer. Number 3 mentions the thyroid cartilage and you know that this is the Adam's apple, which is above the site for a tracheotomy. Number 3, then, is incorrect. Number 4 again mentions the esophagus, but this organ is a part of the digestive tract and does not normally connect with the respiratory tree.

Many times when you are looking over the choices provided you will instantly decide that one answer is obviously wrong. Your first impression is usually correct, so avoid changing your mind unless you have a very good reason for doing so. The same is true for a correct answer. Students often do very poorly on a test because they go back and erase the correct answer and mark an incorrect one!

Reading into a Question Facts That Are Not There.   This mistake is frequently made by persons who feel insecure and want to demonstrate how much they *do* know about a subject. It is also a common pitfall for those who have a good bit of information in their heads but have it very poorly organized. An example is the reader who sees a question about a nursing measure that should be taken while a semiconscious patient is vomiting. The correct answer is to turn the patient's head to the side to prevent aspiration of vomitus. This choice is among those given but other choices include checking the vital signs, withholding oral fluids, and protecting the bed linens. Now the reader goes off on a tangent of "suppose the patient is dehydrated and has an elevated temperature?" In this case she decides that the vital signs should be taken. She also reasons that oral fluids must be withheld when a patient is semiconscious. On and on her thoughts run, gathering up all the possibilities of nursing measures that can be used for a patient with nausea and vomiting. If she would reread the question, however, she would see that she is simply asked what to do *while* the patient is vomiting.

Another common mistake is trying to fit the situation given on a test to one in which you have had experience. This is fine as long as you do not alter the facts that are given in the situation and subsequent questions. Remember that each patient is an individual, and the treatment and nursing care required by one patient with a thyroidectomy will not be identical in every detail to that required by another patient with the same diagnosis.

Allotting Time Wisely. There probably will be some questions that you cannot answer immediately even though you have the nagging feeling that you should be able to answer them. Don't linger too long on questions of this kind. Make a note of the number of each of the troublesome questions on a corner of your scratch pad and come back to them later. Subsequent questions may give you a clue to help you remember a fact you could not immediately recall. Or, you may be fortunate enough to have a helpful subconscious mind that works on one problem while your conscious mind is grappling with another.

Perhaps the information you need may not come to you at all and you are forced to leave an answer blank. At least you have not squandered precious time at the expense of other questions that you can answer correctly. At best you will be able to complete the test and then return to ponder the questions you have omitted.

As you work your way through this review make every effort to take an active part in the learning process. Use the answer sheets and "grade" your own work. If you have missed some questions, go back and try to determine why you missed them. Don't get discouraged if you have more wrong answers than you anticipated. Remember that even wrong answers can be a learning experience if you know why they are wrong.

Part I

PERSONAL HYGIENE AND COMMUNITY HEALTH

I. **Personal Hygiene**
   A. Definition—maintenance of health in an individual.
   B. Good health habits include
      1. Adequate sleep and rest.
      2. Recreation and relaxation.
      3. Balanced diet.
      4. Exercise and physical fitness activities.
      5. Preservation of eyesight.
      6. Care of teeth.
   C. Mental health and emotional stability have a direct effect on physical well-being.
      1. Definition—mental health means peace of mind, happiness, and the enjoyment and satisfaction derived from living.
      2. Characteristics of mental health
         a. Feeling comfortable about one's self and environment.
         b. Having self-respect.
         c. Knowing one's own limitations and capabilities.
         d. Ability to control the emotions.
         e. Ability to get along with others.
         f. Ability to make decisions and live with our decisions.
         g. Having realistic goals in life.
      3. Mental health promoted by
         a. Healthful physical and social environment.
         b. Occupational, social, and economic successes.
         c. Well-grounded religious beliefs and consistent moral behavior.
         d. Respect and friendship of others.

II. **Community Health**
   A. The family is the basic unit of society and the home is the central social unit of the community.
   B. Family is composed of husband and wife and any children they may have.
   C. The community provides many services for the health and welfare of its citizens.
      1. Water purification.
      2. Protection of milk supplies.
      3. Disposal of garbage and sewage.
   D. Facilities provided by the community may include

1. Hospitals.
2. Clinics.
   a. Well-baby clinics.
   b. Maternal and infant care.
   c. Specialized care, e.g., cancer clinic, mental health center
3. Nursing homes.
4. Convalescent homes.
5. Home-care programs for aged or chronically ill.
   E. There are two general types of health services provided by the community
      1. Governmental or official agencies.
      2. Voluntary or nonofficial agencies.
   F. Governmental agencies
      1. May be on a national, state, or local level. The trend is toward more local responsibility.
      2. Supported by taxes.
      3. Functions include
         a. Measures to control communicable diseases.
         b. Infant and maternal care.
         c. Child health and school programs.
         d. Recording of births, deaths, and causes of illness (vital statistics).
         e. Education and counseling in the prevention of disease and the care of the chronically ill.
         f. United States Public Health Service is a part of the federal Department of Health, Education, and Welfare (HEW) under the direction of the federal government. This service includes
            1. Office of the Surgeon General.
            2. National Institutes of Health.
            3. Bureaus of State Services and Medical Services.
      4. World Health Organization (WHO)—one of the specialized agencies of the United Nations.
         a. Concerned with raising the level of health throughout the entire world.
         b. More than 100 countries are involved.
         c. Provides a means of exchanging knowledge and experience among public health officials and members of

1

the health team from participating
countries.

d. Function is to help control and
eradicate diseases that are potential
dangers to all citizens of the world.

G. Voluntary or nonofficial agencies
   1. Usually concerned with specific diseases.
   2. Often are national organizations with local chapters.
   3. Examples of this type of agency
      a. American Heart Association.
      b. American Cancer Society.
      c. American Lung Association.

d. National Association for Mental Health.
e. Visiting Nurse Associations.

H. Disaster in the community
   1. Disaster defined as a sudden major emergency in which a large number of people are killed or injured or left homeless.
   2. American Red Cross has been authorized by a congressional charter to act in any type of disaster.
   3. Each local community should have some plan for civil defense and some organized method for helping its citizens when a disaster occurs.

Questions

1. The term personal hygiene means:
   1. cleanliness and good grooming
   2. prevention of disease
   3. maintenance of physical and mental health in an individual
   4. treatment of disease
2. A person who is healthy is one who is:
   1. free from disease
   2. in a state of physical, mental, and social well-being
   3. able to perform the necessary activities of daily living
   4. physically strong and able to resist disease
3. The physical well-being of an individual may be affected by his:
   a. environment
   b. mental outlook
   c. emotional stability
   d. personal habits
   1. all of these
   2. a and b
   3. a, b, and c
   4. d only
4. Good physical health depends on many factors. Adequate sleep and rest are necessary to allow the body time to rebuild tissues. The amount of sleep needed for each 24 hour period:
   1. is 8 to 10 hours
   2. is 4 to 6 hours
   3. depends on the individual needs of each person
   4. is increased by the amount of physical activity during the day
5. A balanced diet is also necessary for maintenance of health. A good diet is best defined as one that:
   1. includes at least 1 quart of milk per day
   2. contains all the necessary vitamins
   3. contains essential minerals such as iron and calcium
   4. supplies all the substances the body needs
6. It is not difficult to eat a well-balanced diet if:
   1. a large variety of foods is eaten
   2. emphasis is placed on animal products such as meat and eggs
   3. sweets and starches are eliminated from the diet
   4. fried foods are avoided
7. The food we eat will be of more benefit if:
   a. mealtime is a pleasant and relaxed time
   b. food is eaten slowly
   c. we eat only one large meal a day and fill in with small "snacks"
   d. we eat only when we are hungry
   1. all of these
   2. a and b
   3. b, c, and d
   4. a only

8. It is important for the nurse to "practice what she preaches" about good food habits because she:
    a. serves as an example to others
    b. will tire easily and become less efficient if she does not eat well
    c. does not have time to eat properly while on duty and must make up for it while at home
    d. is more likely to gain weight than others who are more active while working

    1. all of these
    2. all but d
    3. b and c
    4. a and b

9. When choosing the kind of shoes to be worn on duty the nurse should remember that:
    1. shoes that are too tight will usually stretch and adjust to the foot after they are worn a few days
    2. it is better to have shoes that are too big than too small
    3. shoes that do not fit can cause fatigue and poor posture
    4. the more expensive a shoe, the better it will fit the foot

10. Since nurses are on their feet a good part of the day their shoes should:
    a. have a broad heel for adequate support
    b. be wide enough at the toe so the toes are not cramped
    c. fit snugly at the heel to prevent rubbing and blistering
    d. have a sole thick enough to cushion the foot

    1. a, b, and c
    2. all of these
    3. b and d
    4. a and c

11. Recreation is important to health chiefly because:
    1. it provides the physical exercise needed to keep good muscle tone
    2. everyone should have a hobby
    3. a change of activities helps a person to relax
    4. very few people enjoy working for a living

12. The term good posture means:
    1. keeping the body straight and the muscles tensed
    2. straightening the spine so that there are no curves in the spinal column
    3. standing straight with the shoulders back and the head held high
    4. positioning the body so that the trunk and extremities are in balance and properly arranged

13. Good posture is important because:
    a. it improves one's appearance
    b. it helps promote normal functioning of the body organs
    c. it enables the muscles to work most effectively
    d. it minimizes fatigue

    1. all of these
    2. all but d
    3. b and c
    4. a and b

14. Good dental care is necessary to one's physical health. Regular visits should be made to the dentist:
    1. at least once every 2 years
    2. every 6 months
    3. whenever it is necessary to have teeth pulled or cavities filled
    4. every other month

15. Tooth decay can be kept at a minimum by:
    a. brushing the teeth regularly and correctly
    b. eating a high fat diet
    c. avoiding an abundance of sweets and starches in the diet
    d. taking calcium tablets regularly

    1. all of these
    2. all but c
    3. c and d
    4. a and c

16. The term *dental caries* means:
    1. an infection of the gums
    2. dentures or false teeth
    3. bad breath
    4. cavities due to decay of the teeth

17. Mental health means:
    1. the enjoyment and satisfaction of living
    2. freedom from worries
    3. absence of problems in daily living
    4. resignation to one's lot in life

18. No single characteristic can indicate mental health; however, a person who is mentally healthy is usually one who is:
    1. very religious
    2. able to adjust to his environment without losing his individuality
    3. able to suppress his true feelings in order to get along with others
    4. never satisfied with his accomplishments and always striving to be perfect

19. An emotionally mature individual should be able to:
    1. find fault with others and have the courage to remind them of their imperfections
    2. show a willingness to admit that he is not perfect, and welcome constructive criticism
    3. ignore the problems of others and avoid becoming involved
    4. display his emotions whenever he feels like it

20. We consider attitude to be extremely important in nursing because:
    1. nursing instructors and supervisors always consider attitude when they evaluate nurses' performance
    2. patients will be impressed with the nurse's sincerity if she pretends to like her work even though she may not enjoy nursing
    3. everyone expects nurses to be unemotional and aloof in any situation
    4. the nurse's feelings toward her vocation will be reflected in everything she does for her patients

21. One of the best ways to maintain your self-respect and enjoy a feeling of satisfaction in your work is to:
    1. be sure that others notice how hard you work
    2. inform your co-workers that you take orders from your immediate supervisor and no one else
    3. try to please your supervisors because they will be evaluating your work
    4. do your own work to the best of your ability and let your co-workers accept responsibility for their actions

22. The word family can have many different meanings depending on the way in which the word is used. Sociologists describe the modern family as one that is:
    a. composed of all persons living under one roof
    b. composed of husband and wife and any children they may have
    c. an important group that is the basic unit of society
    d. no longer considered important in the welfare of the community in general

    1. a and d
    2. b and d
    3. a and c
    4. b and c

23. Many aspects of family life have been changed in recent years because of a shift of population from rural living to urban living. This means that families have:
    1. moved from the cities to large subdivisions in the country
    2. become less dependent on their communities for help in matters of health and welfare
    3. moved from farming communities into large industrial areas in cities
    4. accepted more responsibility for the welfare of the members of their families and community

24. Which of the following statements most accurately describes the role of the family in modern society?
    1. The family is no longer responsible for the health and welfare of its members.
    2. The physical, mental, and social well-being of the family as a group is of great importance to the community and the nation.
    3. Increased facilities and services provided by the government have eliminated the need for the family to concern itself with the health and well-being of its individual members.
    4. Family life has little effect on the development of the individual or the welfare of the community.

25. When we speak of a community we mean:
   1. the outstanding citizens of a town
   2. a very small group of people living together
   3. a group of families and individuals who live in the same area under the same laws and rules
   4. a group of people who have the same cultural background

26. Some of the services usually provided by a community include:
   a. water purification
   b. protection of milk supplies
   c. sewage and garbage disposal
   d. recreation facilities

   1. all of these
   2. a and c
   3. b and d
   4. b and c

27. When a practical nurse knows something about the community in which her patients live and work she will:
   a. be better able to help them take advantage of the services and facilities available
   b. understand her patients better
   c. realize that most communities are not interested in the welfare of their citizens
   d. find it easier to recognize the patient as an individual who is influenced by the community in which he lives

   1. all of these
   2. c only
   3. all but c
   4. b and d

28. The two general types of health services available to citizens of a community are:
   a. government or official agencies
   b. local and state agencies
   c. voluntary or nonofficial agencies
   d. federal or county agencies

   1. a and c
   2. b and c
   3. b and d
   4. c and d

29. Governmental agencies are supported by:
   1. contributions and private funds
   2. money obtained through taxes
   3. fees paid by the persons receiving help from these agencies
   4. the community chest

30. Which of the following statements best describes the organization and operation of the public health departments?
   1. All local health departments are under the direct supervision and control of the U.S. Public Health Service.
   2. The local health departments operate independently of the national organization.
   3. The basic responsibility for community health rests with the local health department, and the U.S. Public Health Service gives assistance through financial aid and technical services.
   4. The federal government controls all the functions of the state and local health departments.

31. The U.S. Public Health Service is a part of the:
   1. National Institutes of Health
   2. Department of Health, Education, and Welfare
   3. Federal Bureau of Health
   4. Bureau of Medical Services

32. Most local health departments have a division of vital statistics. The function of this division is to record and analyze:
   1. information about communicable diseases
   2. available clinics in the area and the services they offer
   3. data concerning births, deaths, and causes of illness in the area
   4. health needs of the citizens of the community

33. The initials WHO stand for an organization that is primarily concerned with:
   1. improving the health of individuals in developing countries
   2. controlling and eradicating health hazards potentially dangerous to all citizens of the world.
   3. establishing schools that will improve the medical care of all citizens of the world.
   4. setting up standards of health that can be used as a guide by public health officials throughout the world.

34. The WHO is a specialized agency of the:
    1. U.S. Public Health Service
    2. Department of Health, Education and Welfare
    3. National Institutes of Health
    4. United Nations

35. Some of the functions of the public health nurse would include:
    a. assisting in clinics for maternal and child health
    b. educating the public in prevention of disease
    c. nursing in homes in which a member of the family is chronically ill and in need of professional care constantly
    d. assisting in inspection of nursing homes, nursery schools, and other facilities of this type in the community

    1. all of these
    2. a and b
    3. c and d
    4. all but c

36. Most communities have agencies other than governmental ones concerned with health. These nongovernmental agencies are called:
    1. special agencies
    2. civil defense programs
    3. private agencies
    4. voluntary or nonofficial agencies

37. The nongovernmental agencies are supported by:
    1. subsidies from the government
    2. contributions and private funds
    3. local citizens in each community
    4. taxes

38. Which of the following are examples of nongovernmental agencies?
    a. American Heart Association
    b. National Association for Mental Health
    c. Visiting Nurse Association
    d. National Institutes of Health

    1. all of these
    2. a and c
    3. b and d
    4. all but d

39. Disaster nursing has recently been recognized as an important aspect of nursing. The term disaster is best defined as:
    1. destruction of a community during wartime
    2. loss of life and property due to floods and fires
    3. an epidemic or sudden occurrence of illness throughout a community
    4. a sudden major emergency in which a large number of persons in an area are killed or injured or left homeless

40. The organization that is legally authorized by Congress to move into a community at a time of disaster is the:
    1. Public Health Department
    2. Visiting Nurse Association
    3. American Red Cross
    4. Community Health Services

41. Another organization that is responsible for planning defense of a community against disaster and care of the citizens when a disaster occurs is the:
    1. Office of Civil Defense and Mobilization
    2. Disaster Planning Committee
    3. National Guard
    4. Office of the Surgeon General

42. The Visiting Nurse Associations are:
    1. under the direction of the Public Health Department
    2. governmental agencies
    3. local groups of private duty nurses
    4. voluntary or nongovernmental agencies

Part II

PERSONAL AND VOCATIONAL RELATIONSHIPS

I. **Nursing As a Career**
  A. Nursing may be defined as caring for and helping those who cannot help themselves.
  B. History of nursing
    1. As old as mankind.
    2. *Organized* nursing has developed gradually through the centuries. Was given impetus by various religious organizations which applied the ideals of Christianity to nursing.
    3. First real school of nursing was begun at Kaiserswerth, Germany.
    4. Florence Nightingale is considered to be the founder of modern nursing.
      a. Many of the principles and ideals set forth by Miss Nightingale are still used in the education of nurses today.
      b. Her work in the Crimean War earned her the title "Lady with the Lamp."

II. **Practical Nursing**
  A. Schools of practical nursing began as short courses of a few weeks. Were concerned with training in simple skills used in home nursing.
  B. Early schools of practical nursing
    1. Ballard School in New York, sponsored by YWCA, in 1893.
    2. Thompson School in Brattleboro, Vermont, 1907.
    3. Boston City Hospital School, 1918.
  C. Licensure of practical nurses
    1. All 50 states, the Commonwealth of Puerto Rico, and the District of Columbia legally permit the licensure of practical nurses.
    2. Type of licensure may depend on state law.
      a. Permissive licensure means that a person may practice in the state without a license but cannot use LPN or LVN after her name.
      b. Mandatory licensure means that all persons practicing as practical nurses must have a license from the state.
    3. Mandatory licensure and formal education of the practical nurse have done much to elevate the status of the practical nurse.
    4. The licensed graduate practical nurse has graduated from an approved school of practical nursing and is trained and legally qualified to participate in nursing care.
    5. The licensed practical nurse receiving her license by waiver is not a graduate of a school of practical nursing.
    6. The licensed practical nurse must always work under the supervision of a licensed physician, dentist, or registered professional nurse.

III. **Nursing Organizations**
  A. Every licensed practical nurse has the privilege and responsibility of belonging to and working for the organizations that represent her and the other members of her group.
    1. National organizations
      a. National Association of Practical Nurse Education and Services (NAPNES). Founded in 1941 to improve the standards of practical nurse education and raise the quality of care rendered by practical nurses.
      b. National Federation of Licensed Practical Nurses. Founded in 1949 as the official organization for licensed practical nurses in the U.S. Its purposes are to improve the working conditions of LPN's and promote a better understanding of practical nursing.
      c. National League for Nursing. In 1952 three national organizations and four national committees united to form the NLN. This organization is concerned with improving nursing education and nursing service *at all levels.* Membership includes professional

and practical nurses, allied professional persons, and other interested citizens.
2. State organizations
   a. Each state has a state association for practical nurses.
   b. Help coordinate all vocational activities of the licensed practical nurses practicing within each state.
3. District associations
   a. Each state divided into smaller districts similar to counties.
   b. Local organizations composed of practical nurses working in a certain area.
   c. Keep members informed of new legislation and new developments in practical nursing. Keep them in touch with the activities of the state and national association.
B. The state board of nursing
1. A special board set up under state government.
2. May be another department of state government or may be a committee acting under the secretary of state.
3. Carries out state laws and recommendations of the state legislature which apply to nursing practice.
C. American Nurses' Association—official organization for registered nurses:
1. First formed as the Nurses Associated Alumnae of the United States and Canada in 1896.
2. Was named A.N.A. in 1911.
3. Official organ—*the American Journal of Nursing*

IV. Responsibilities of the Practical Nurse
A. Ethical responsibilities
1. Are made known through a code of ethics.
2. A code of ethics is a list of rules dictating good conduct and reflecting the highest ideals of the group.
3. Ethical responsibilities include
   a. The basic responsibility of the nurse is to conserve life and promote health.
   b. Continued study and reading to keep abreast of latest developments in nursing.
   c. Faithfulness toward any and all patients entrusted to her care.
   d. Loyalty toward her patient, other members of the nursing team, the medical profession, and her employers.
   e. Maintenance of high standards of personal and moral behavior in her private life.
   f. Acceptance of responsibility for the health and welfare of others in her community and exercising her privileges as a citizen.
   g. Active participation in nursing organizations.
B. Legal responsibilities
1. The nurse must always be aware of the laws governing the functions of nursing. "Ignorance of the law is no excuse."
2. Illegal actions:
   a. *Crime*—a wrongful act against society.
   b. *Tort*—a wrongful act against an individual, usually compensated for in the form of money.
3. Some common legal problems encountered in nursing
   a. Negligence—failure to exercise good judgment or use knowledge and skills expected of a person.
   b. Assault and battery—a threat or attempt to carry out a threat of physical injury to the body of another person.
   c. False imprisonment—the unnecessary restriction of the freedom of another.
   d. Invasion of privacy—unnecessary exposure of a patient or divulging personal information obtained while caring for a patient.
   e. Libel and slander—written or spoken word that may subject another to contempt or ridicule.
4. Last will and testament
   a. A will is a written declaration for disposition of a person's possessions after his death.
   b. Nurse should draft a will only if no one else is available.
   c. Nurses should avoid witnessing patients' wills whenever possible.
   d. Wills must be witnessed by two or three persons, depending on state law.
5. Narcotic controls
   a. Harrison Narcotic Law regulates interstate commerce and enforces laws regarding narcotics for the purpose of taxation.
   b. Uniform Narcotic Drug Act requires a state license for prescribing narcotics. Also requires a detailed record for narcotics administered to patients.
   c. Practical nurse is obligated to observe hospital rules and policies in regard to administering narcotics and accounting for all those wasted by accident.
   d. The Harrison Narcotic Law defines narcotics as: opium and any of its derivatives, and drugs made from coca leaves (example, cocaine).

V. Securing and Resigning from a Position

A. Letter of application
1. Neat and legible, not written on lined paper.
2. Addressed to a particular person if possible.
3. Content of letter
   a. Position desired.
   b. Qualifications and experience.
   c. Date available for employment.
   d. Request for personal interview at time and place to be specified.
B. Interview
1. Be prompt.
2. Dress conservatively and give neat and dignified appearance.
3. Answer questions briefly and to the point.
4. Ask questions concerning the position.
5. Avoid making a hasty decision.
C. Letter of resignation
1. Give ample notice, 2 weeks usually enough.
2. Do not air your grievances in the letter; you may need to work there again.
3. Give plausible reason for leaving the position.
4. Remember that the letter will be kept as part of your record in the institution.

Questions

1. Which of the following do you consider to be the *best* reason for becoming a practical nurse?
    1. The job opportunities and regular pay are good.
    2. Most people respect nurses.
    3. There is much personal satisfaction to be gained from helping others.
    4. There is a shortage of nurses in this country and a nurse can always find a job.
2. Practical nursing dates back to the earliest records of mankind. One change that has greatly improved the status of the practical nurse is:
    1. the requirement that all practical nurses should wear white uniforms
    2. formal education of practical nurses and their licensure by the states
    3. increases in pay and improved working conditions
    4. allowing practical nurses to work in hospitals as well as in private homes
3. Florence Nightingale was an English gentlewoman who:
    a. became known as the first public health nurse
    b. cared for soldiers during the Civil War
    c. wrote a code of ethics for nurses that served as a guide for all nurses
    d. provided the ideals and ethical standards which are the basis of nursing education today

    1. all of these
    2. all but b
    3. c and d
    4. all but a
4. The earliest school of practical nursing in the United States was:
    a. the Ballard school in New York City
    b. the Louis J. Goldberg school in Detroit
    c. a school sponsored by the YWCA
    d. opened in 1893

    1. a and c
    2. all but c
    3. all but b
    4. a and d
5. There are several different types of licensure for practical nurses. The type of licensure a practical nurse may obtain depends on:
    1. the federal law governing licensure of all nurses
    2. the state law governing licensure of practical nurses
    3. the decision of the state board
    4. the amount of experience she has had in nursing
6. When a license to practice as a practical nurse is issued by waiver this means that:
    1. the nurse has graduated from an approved school of practical nursing
    2. any person making application to the state may obtain a license
    3. the requirements for formal education in practical nursing have been set aside and the applicant is issued a license on the basis of her experience in practical nursing

4. a nurse who has a license in one state may transfer her license to another state without permission from the state board of nursing

7. Mandatory licensure laws are laws that:
    1. permit the licensing of all persons working in a hospital
    2. allow only graduates of approved schools to obtain a license in practical nursing
    3. require all practical nurses to have current licenses in the state in order to practice
    4. demand payment of required fees before a license can be issued

8. Permissive licensure means that:
    1. only a certain quota of practical nurses are permitted to have licenses
    2. licensure of practical nurses is recommended but not required or enforced as a law
    3. practical nurses are granted permits rather than official licenses
    4. the state allows schools of practical nursing to issue licenses to their graduates

9. There are some schools that offer courses in practical nursing by correspondence. A graduate of such a school:
    1. must complete clinical experience in a hospital before applying for state board examination
    2. is not eligible for examination or licensure as a practical nurse
    3. may take a state board examination only after paying the required fee
    4. has about the same privileges as a graduate of an approved school of practical nursing

10. If a nurse plans to move from one state to another and wishes to obtain a license to practice in her new location she can obtain a license:
    1. by passing the state's examination for nurses
    2. by filling out an application and paying the required fee
    3. automatically, simply by writing for it
    4. only by meeting the individual requirements of the state board of nursing issuing the license

11. The practical nurse works under the supervision of a registered nurse because:
    1. registered nurses have college degrees
    2. practical nurses do not know as much as registered nurses
    3. the registered nurse has more formal education and is qualified to accept full responsibility for nursing care
    4. the practical nurse is limited in the things she can do for a patient because of her lack of experience

12. In 1941 an organization was formed for the specific purpose of extending and improving the education of practical nurses. This organization is still very active and is called the:
    1. National Association of Practical Nurses
    2. National Federation of Practical Nurses
    3. National Association for Practical Nurse Education and Services
    4. National Board of Nurse Examiners

13. Another national organization, formed in 1949, to promote high standards in practical nursing is the:
    1. National League for Nurses
    2. American Nurses' Association
    3. National Association for Practical Nurse Education and Services
    4. National Federation of Licensed Practical Nurses

14. Practical nurses may belong to all but one of the following organizations:
    1. NAPNES
    2. National Federation of Licensed Practical Nurses
    3. American Nurses' Association
    4. National League for Nurses

15. All practical nurses who are licensed and practicing in the state should belong to the state association of practical nurses because:
    1. it will improve their social life
    2. it will help them keep abreast of the changes and have some voice in the affairs of practical nurses in the state

3. most hospitals require this membership before they hire a practical nurse
4. it is not possible to obtain a license from the state unless you are a member of this organization

16. Each state of the union has a board of nursing. The main function of this board is to:
1. accredit schools of nursing
2. issue all licenses throughout the state
3. carry out laws and legislative recommendations pertaining to nursing
4. establish schools of nursing wherever needed

17. Whenever you wear your nurse's uniform you must be especially careful of your conduct because:
1. you are representing all nurses when you are in uniform
2. someone may report you to your employer
3. actions speak louder than words
4. if you get caught misbehaving you may lose your license

18. A code of ethics means:
1. a list of rules of behavior in social situations
2. the legal rules governing behavior
3. a list of rules of conduct which reflects the ideals of a certain group
4. secret rules of behavior known only to the members of a certain group

19. The basic responsibility of any nurse is to:
1. earn a living for herself
2. diagnose and treat illness
3. conduct herself with dignity
4. promote health and conserve life

20. If, in an emergency, the practical nurse is asked by a physician to administer a medication intravenously it would be best for her to:
1. give the medication but record it as given by the doctor
2. administer the medication only if the agency in which she works has a written policy allowing LPN's to give I.V. medications
3. refuse to assist with this particular patient
4. insert the needle into the vein but ask the physician to give the medication

21. A practical nurse should not wear strong perfume while on duty because:

a. most persons are easily offended by strong odors when they are ill	1. all but c
	2. c only
b. the patient may be offended by her choice of perfume	3. b and c
	4. a and b
c. perfumes should be used only on special occasions	
d. cleanliness is preferable to covering up body odor with strong perfume	

22. When a patient confides in you and wishes to discuss a personal problem with you it is best to:
1. change the subject and tell the patient that you would rather not listen to his problems
2. discuss the patient's problem with your co-workers and enlist their aid in finding a solution to the patient's problem
3. listen to the patient but respect his confidence in you
4. tell the patient's family about his problem even though he may have asked you not to tell them

23. Nurses frequently find themselves in the midst of very emotional situations. In order to cope with these situations the nurse should:
1. avoid becoming involved whenever possible
2. develop an attitude of indifference so that she can function more efficiently
3. demonstrate her warmth and sympathy by freely showing her emotions
4. learn to show sympathy and kindness but keep her emotions under control

24. The practical nurse has legal obligations toward her patients. She may be held legally responsible if she:

a. fails to perform certain acts required of her as a practical nurse	1. all of these
	2. a and b
b. causes injury to a patient by negligence or ignorance of procedures she would be	3. c and d
	4. all but c

expected to perform as a practical nurse
  c. refuses to perform some acts that are considered to be above the level of practical nursing
  d. threatens or carries out a threat to the patient's personal safety or freedom

25. A tort may best be defined as:
  1. a wrong committed against an individual
  2. a crime committed against society
  3. an unethical action that does not involve any transgression of the law
  4. an act contrary to the mores of a group

26. If a nurse divulges personal information obtained while caring for a patient she may be sued for:
  1. negligence
  2. assault and battery
  3. malpractice
  4. invasion of privacy

27. Slander is best defined as:
  1. a written defamation of another's character
  2. gossip or rumor-mongering
  3. the utterance of statements that will leave another person open to contempt and ridicule
  4. telling lies about another person

28. A nurse may be sued for negligence if she is responsible for injury to a patient due to:
  a. administration of the wrong dosage of medication
  b. failing to raise the side rails on the patient's bed before leaving his room
  c. using a piece of equipment that is obviously defective
  d. applying a hot water bottle that is too hot

  1. all of these
  2. a and b
  3. b and d
  4. c and d

29. Suppose you were asked to nurse a member of your family who is seriously ill in the hospital. Before you can accept any responsibility for the nursing care of this person you must:
  a. secure permission from the physician in charge
  b. secure permission from the director of nurses at the hospital to function as a practical nurse in the hospital
  c. wear your uniform if you intend to function as a private duty nurse for this patient
  d. bear in mind that your relationship to the patient does not change the amount of responsibility you may assume as a practical nurse

  1. all of these
  2. all but b
  3. a and c
  4. all but d

30. For a will to be valid it must be made:
  a. in the presence of at least two witnesses (in most states)
  b. by a person of sound mind
  c. in the presence of a lawyer
  d. with the assistance of a nurse if the patient is under sedation

  1. all but c
  2. c and d
  3. a and b
  4. all of these

31. If a patient asks a nurse to witness his will she should:
  1. do so only if no one else is available
  2. refuse to do so because she cannot be a legal witness
  3. inform the patient that he must have a lawyer to help him with his will
  4. call a member of the family to witness the will

32. Whenever a practical nurse administers a narcotic she will be held legally responsible for:
    a. administering the narcotic only under the direction and written order of a licensed physician or dentist
    b. keeping a record of all narcotics administered, lost, or discarded
    c. having knowledge of all laws concerned with the proper handling of narcotics
    d. accepting the responsibility for preventing the patient from becoming a narcotics addict

    1. a only
    2. b and c
    3. all but a
    4. all but d

33. The Harrison Narcotic Act is concerned with:
    1. correct labeling of drugs
    2. revenue from the sale of narcotics and taxation of that revenue
    3. the correct dosage of narcotics
    4. all medications prepared by a pharmacist in the United States

34. Any person who administers narcotics in a hospital must:
    1. sign his name in the narcotic book and account for each narcotic he takes from the cabinet
    2. lock the cabinet and return the keys to the supervisor immediately
    3. pay for the narcotics he misplaces
    4. return to the pharmacy any unused portions left in an ampule

35. According to the Harrison Narcotic Act, the following drugs are to be considered narcotics:
    1. opium or its derivatives
    2. barbiturates
    3. all analgesics
    4. any drug that produces sleep

36. A letter of application for a job should be:
    a. written on lined paper and in pencil so that you can write neatly and erase mistakes easily
    b. addressed to a specific person whenever possible
    c. a friendly letter giving many personal details so that the employer can decide from the letter whether or not he wishes to hire you
    d. explicit in the type of work you desire, your reasons for wanting the job, and your qualifications

    1. all but c
    2. b and d
    3. a and c
    4. all of these

37. When you have a personal interview with a prospective employer you should:
    a. dress neatly and simply
    b. ask questions concerning the job and what will be expected of you
    c. answer all questions briefly and to the point
    d. be prepared to give a definite answer whether or not you will accept the position without further consideration

    1. all of these
    2. all but d
    3. a and c
    4. b and d

38. Once you have accepted a position as a licensed practical nurse you should:
    a. report on duty on time and in full uniform
    b. be willing to accept the full responsibility for conducting yourself with dignity and refinement
    c. realize that you cannot walk off duty when things don't go your way

    1. all but b
    2. a and c
    3. all of these
    4. all but d

d. always give ample notice when you cannot report for duty so that someone can be called in to assume your duties

39. Changing jobs frequently is:
1. stimulating and keeps one from getting in a rut
2. considered a poor practice because it gives one a reputation for being unreliable
3. the best thing to do if you have trouble getting along with others
4. better than sticking with the job and trying to find out why you are unhappy with the work

40. When you resign from a position you should:
a. give ample notice
b. give your resignation in writing
c. be perfectly frank in your letter of resignation giving your reasons for leaving, and airing your grievances, if any
d. tell your co-workers why you have been unhappy with the work and make some suggestions for improving the situation

1. all of these
2. a and b
3. all but d
4. c and d

Part III

BASIC SCIENCES

UNIT 1 CHEMISTRY AND PHYSICS

I. Introduction

A. Chemistry—the study of the composition of matter and the changes which substances may undergo under certain conditions.

B. Digestion of foods, action of hormones, chemical changes in the cells of the body, maintenance of acid-base balance, and many other bodily functions are chemical in nature.

C. Basic principles of chemistry are applicable to many nursing procedures, pharmacology, laboratory tests for diagnosis, and almost all aspects of medicine and nursing.

II. Matter and Energy

A. Matter—anything which occupies space and possesses weight or mass. May be visible or invisible. The "stuff" of which everything in our world is made.

 1. Three forms of matter
  a. Solids—have definite shape and boundaries; particles tightly packed with little space between.
  b. Liquids—have no definite shape of their own, take the shape of their container; particles are less tightly packed.
  c. Gases—have no shape or boundaries; particles move about freely.

 2. Kinds of matter: There are three kinds of of matter: elements, compounds, and mixtures.
  a. We recognize different substances (or matter) by their properties.
   1. *Physical properties* are those characteristics that are ascertained or observed without chemical action.
   2. *Chemical properties* are those characteristics which relate to the action, or lack of action, with other substances.
   3. An example would be oxygen, which is recognized by its physical

properties; i.e., a colorless gas that is heavier than air and only slightly soluble in water. Its chemical properties would include its ability to support combustion and its reaction with certain elements to form oxides.

 3. Elements—the simplest form of matter; substances that cannot be broken down by any ordinary chemical change into simpler substances.
  a. All elements are composed of invisible particles called *atoms.*
  b. John Dalton's atomic theory states that: All atoms of the same element have the same properties and the same weight, and they are different from the atoms of all other elements in these respects. Atoms of most elements are able to combine with atoms of other elements. When atoms enter into chemical combination, they do not change.
  c. Oxygen is the most abundant of all the elements. Carbon and hydrogen are elements present in large amounts in plant and animal tissues.
  d. Carbon, hydrogen, and oxygen are the only elements in carbohydrates and fats. Proteins contain these three plus nitrogen.
  e. Only six elements make up 99 per cent of the human body; they are oxygen, carbon, hydrogen, nitrogen, calcium, and phosphorus.

 4. Compounds—formed when the atoms of two or more elements unite. Table salt is a compound formed from the union of atoms of the elements sodium and chlorine.

 5. Molecule—the smallest unit of a compound. Usually formed by the chemical union of two or more different atoms.
  a. All molecules of the same chemical

substance contain the same number and kind of atoms.

  b. Examples of molecules
   1. A molecule of sodium chloride (table salt) is composed of one atom of sodium and one atom of chlorine.
   2. A molecule of water is composed of two atoms of hydrogen and one atom of oxygen — H_2O.
  c. All molecules of all substances are in constant motion, even those of solid substances.
 6. Mixtures — two or more elements or compounds that are chemically combined and that are put together in any proportion.
B. Electron theory — a description of the structure of an atom as a miniature solar system with a small, compact nucleus surrounded by revolving orbital or planetary electrons.
 1. *Electrons* are negatively charged particles orbiting around the nucleus. *Protons* are positively charged particles within the nucleus. The nucleus also contains neutral particles called *neutrons.*
 2. *Atoms* contain an equal number of electrons and protons; that is, the number of electrons revolving around the nucleus is equal to the number of protons in the nucleus. The nitrogen atom, for example, has seven electrons and, therefore, seven protons.
 3. The *atomic number* of each element is defined as the number of electrons (or protons) in each of its atoms. If the atomic number of oxygen is 8, then we can conclude that each atom of oxygen has eight revolving electrons, and eight protons in its nucleus.
 4. Since an element is composed of two or three different kinds of atoms, its *atomic weight* is best defined as the average weight of its atoms compared to carbon.
 5. *Isotopes* are atoms that are alike except for their atomic weight. For example, chlorine has two isotopes: Cl 35 and Cl 37.
 6. *Unstable or radioactive elements.* Some elements are classified as stable; that is, they have a balanced number of protons and neutrons. Other elements do not have this stability and, apparently in an effort to achieve some kind of balance, they emit (give off) "undesirable" particles. These elements are said to be unstable or radioactive because as their nuclei disintegrate they emit rays — *alpha, beta,* and *gamma* rays. These rays are useful in diagnosis and treatment of a variety of illnesses.

C. Energy and matter
 1. Energy is the ability to do work — the power to produce motion or bring about physical change in matter.
 2. Physics is concerned with matter in general and energy in particular.
 3. Matter and energy can neither be created nor destroyed. It is possible, however, to convert energy into matter and matter into energy.
 4. Every chemical change is accompanied by a change in energy. Muscles are provided energy to move because of the chemical change that takes place when glucose is oxidized in the muscle cells.

III. **Heat**
 A. A form of energy
  1. Fahrenheit scale — freezing point of water = 32 degrees; boiling point of water = 212 degrees.
  2. Celsius (Centigrade) scale — freezing point of water = 0 degrees; boiling point of water = 100 degrees. Called centigrade because the scale has 100 gradations (steps of degrees).
  3. Equivalents:

F degrees	C degrees
90	32.2
95	35
96	35.5
97	36.1
98	36.6
98.6	37
99	37.2
100	37.7
101	38.3
102	38.8
103	39.4
104	40

 C. Quantity — not the same as temperature
  1. Calories — the quantity of heat required to raise the temperature of 1 Gm. of water 1 degree C.
 D. Vaporization — when a liquid evaporates, it absorbs heat from the surrounding area.

IV. **Physical and Chemical Changes**
 A. Physical change — a temporary alteration in the physical properties without the formation of any new substance.
  1. In a physical change the original substance does not cease to exist.
  2. Examples of physical change — freezing water to form ice; chewing food into smaller pieces.
 B. Chemical change — a permanent change in the composition of substances. Results in the formation of new and different sub-

stances, and the original substances cease to exist.

  1. In a chemical change there is no loss or gain in weight, but there is a change in energy.

  2. Examples of chemical changes—rusting of iron, digestion of food, oxidation of nutrients, and the release of energy.

C. Catalyst—a substance that can speed up or slow down a chemical reaction without being changed itself.

  1. Water is a common catalyst, possibly because of its ability to bring into closer contact the atoms of the substance undergoing chemical change.

  2. Bacteria, yeasts, and molds all secrete enzymes that are catalysts.

  3. Enzymes are complex proteins that act in a very specific manner, choosing only the particular substance to which they are attracted. Most of the chemical reactions that are vital to life are catalyzed by enzymes. For example, it is the enzymes in digestive juices that facilitate the chemical breakdown of food so its elements can be utilized by the body's cells.

V. Acids, Bases, and Salts

A. Acids—compounds containing hydrogen and a nonmetal, and sometimes oxygen.

  1. Properties of acids in solution in water

    a. Have sour taste.

    b. React with certain metals to release hydrogen.

    c. React with carbonates to release carbon dioxide.

    d. React with bases to form salts and water.

  2. Examples of acids

    a. Hydrochloric acid in gastric juice.

    b. Acetic acid—the acid in vinegar.

    c. Boric acid—used frequently as a mild antiseptic.

B. Bases—compounds of a metal, oxygen, and hydrogen.

  1. Properties of bases in solution in water

    a. Slimy or soapy feeling.

    b. Bitter taste.

    c. React with acids to form salts and water.

  2. Examples of bases

    a. Caustic soda or potash (lye).

    b. Ammonia water.

    c. Milk of magnesia.

C. pH—the power of hydrogen ion concentration; a convenient way to express the degree to which a solution is an acid or a base (acidic or basic).

  1. Many biological processes depend on the pH of their environment. All body fluids have very definite pH values that must be maintained within relatively narrow range in order for the body to function normally.

  2. A neutral solution has a pH of 7. A pH of less than 7 indicates an acid solution; a pH of more than 7 is alkaline.

  3. The pH of blood is normally between 7.35 and 7.45. Gastric juice has a pH of 1.6 to 1.8. Saliva is nearly neutral (pH 7).

  4. If the pH of blood falls below 7 or rises above 7.8, death can occur. Many chemical reactions that take place in the body result in the formation of acid substances; for example, the formation of amino acids when proteins are digested. To avoid drastic changes in the blood pH when chemical reactions take place, the blood makes use of a buffer mechanism.

D. Applications in nursing

  1. Some pathogenic organisms thrive in an alkaline environment. To control infection by these organisms the physician may prescribe mild acidic medications; e.g., vinegar douches.

  2. Severe acidosis can occur in uncontrolled diabetes mellitus and starvation. Symptoms may be relieved by administration of alkalines such as sodium bicarbonate and sodium lactate.

  3. Excessive vomiting and too frequent irrigation of a gastric tube can cause alkalosis due to loss of digestive acids.

  4. The kidneys play an important role in acid-base regulation. If the kidneys are severely damaged, the patient will suffer from uremic acidosis. Urea deposits on the skin of a patient in uremia can be neutralized by mild sodium bicarbonate solution baths, thus relieving some discomfort from these deposits.

  5. Soap left in the bed linens of a patient with a severe dermatitis can be very irritating. Rinsing the linen in a vinegar solution will remove the alkaline soap deposits.

  6. Strong acids have a corrosive action on wood, cloth, and skin. Thus the skin must be protected from leakage of digestive juices when a patient has a gastrostomy or colostomy.

  7. Antacid drugs such as aluminum hydroxide gel act to neutralize the acidity of gastric juices in a patient with gastric ulcer.

  8. The antidote for poisoning or burns by a strong alkali is a dilute solution of an acid, such as acetic acid.

  9. The antidote for poisoning or burns by an acid is milk of magnesia or milk of lime.

10. Fatty acids are the end products of fat digestion and are used as body fuel.
E. Salts—compounds which have only one property in common, that is, the ability to carry an electric current.
   1. Salts may react with acids, bases, or with each other to form another salt.
   2. Salts are the most numerous and useful inorganic and organic compounds.
   3. Examples of salts used in medicine:
      a. Aluminum acetate (Burow's solution) used to treat skin diseases.
      b. Sodium chloride (table salt)—used in solution of 0.9 per cent strength as physiologic saline solution for intravenous therapy, wet compresses, etc.
      c. Calcium gluconate—used as source of calcium to replace that lost or to provide sufficient calcium when there is an imbalance in the body.
   4. Inorganic salts (sodium chloride, potassium chloride, calcium chloride, calcium phosphate, etc.) are essential to life and health.
      a. Build and repair tissues.
      b. Maintain normal contractility of muscles and irritability of nerves.
      c. Assist in holding substances in solution in the body fluids.
      d. Help maintain proper acid-base balance in the body.

VI. **Solutions**
   A. A solution is a homogeneous mixture of the molecules of two or more substances. The individual molecules are distributed so evenly that there is no visible distinction of substances.
   B. Components of a solution
      1. Solvent—the substance in which the molecules are dissolved.
         a. Solvents may be liquids, gases, or solids.
         b. Water is the universal solvent, but fats and oils will not dissolve in water.
         c. Ether, alcohol, and carbon tetrachloride dissolve fats and greases.
      2. Solute—the substance being dissolved.
         a. Amount of solute used in proportion to amount of solution affects the concentration of the solution. The more solvent used for a certain amount of solute, the weaker will be the concentration of the solution.
   C. Use of solutions
      1. Most substances enter into chemical reactions much more readily when in solution.
         a. Many drugs given in solution.
         b. Properties of acids and bases evident only when they are in solution.

   2. Examples of solutions used in medicine
      a. Glucose for intravenous therapy.
      b. Normal saline for irrigations, soaks, I.V. therapy.
      c. Ringer's solution—contains chlorides of potassium, calcium, and sodium, given to replace the salts essential to the body tissues.
   D. Properties of true solutions
      1. Diffusion—movement of molecules from an area of relatively high concentration to one of lower concentration.
         a. Examples—escape of molecules of alcohol or ether from the container to the air immediately after the cover is removed. We know this occurs because we can smell the alcohol or ether.
            Another example—absorption of glucose or drugs from intestinal tract into the bloodstream.
         b. Diffusion can lead to the spread of cancer cells when they enter a body cavity.
         c. Diffusion is the result of motion of molecules apparently in an effort to achieve even distribution.
      2. Osmosis—the selective flow of a solvent, usually water, through a membrane.
         a. Membrane is semipermeable; that is, will allow passage of a solvent but not passage of the solute.
         b. Molecules of the solvent will move from less concentrated solution to more concentrated. This is the opposite of diffusion but both have the effect of equalizing concentrations of the various solutions in a given area.
         c. Examples of osmosis
            1. Swelling of dried fruits or vegetables when soaked in water.
            2. Withdrawal of fluids from body tissues and their deposition in the intestinal tract when a "saline" cathartic is given. In this way watery stools are produced.
            3. Filtration—passage of water and its solutes through a membrane as a result of greater pressure on one side of the membrane. Example— formation of urine as a result of the filtering action of the nephron cells of the kidney.

VII. **Oxygen**
   A. Most abundant and probably most important of all the elements because it forms compounds with almost every other element.
   B. All forms of living matter need oxygen to carry on their activities.
   C. Properties of oxygen
      1. Transparent, colorless, odorless gas.

2. Slightly heavier than air.
3. Supports combustion (burning).

D. Some uses of oxygen
1. Used for slow combustion of foodstuffs in the body to produce heat and energy.
2. Oxidation (chemical change that takes place when oxygen unites with other substances) necessary for utilization of food elements.
3. Pure oxygen used to prevent asphyxiation in respiratory distress.
4. Used with certain other gases for anesthesia by inhalation.

VIII. Nitrogen—occurs in a vast number of organic and inorganic compounds.

A. Constitutes 78 per cent of the dry air of the atmosphere.
B. Is the key element of proteins which are among the most important constituents of protoplasm of cells.
C. Nitrogen is as essential to life as oxygen.

IX. Terms to be learned

A. Gravity—a force between two bodies. The gravitational pull of the earth upon an object is called *weight*. Water seeks its own level because of gravitational pull.
B. Specific gravity—a measurement of density. The weight of a substance divided by the weight of an equal volume of water is the specific gravity of the substance. If the specific gravity of a liquid is less than one, then it is lighter (less dense) than water. If the specific gravity of urine is 12, then the urine is 12 times heavier than water.
C. Pressure—the amount of force exerted in a given area.
1. Positive pressure—greater than the pressure of the atmosphere.
2. Negative pressure—less than atmospheric pressure.
D. Manometer—a device used to measure pressure. Example—sphygmomanometer, used to measure blood pressure.
E. Barometer—an instrument used to measure atmospheric pressure.
F. Viscosity—fluid friction. Blood has a higher viscosity than alcohol.

Questions

1. When we use the term *matter* in chemistry we are referring to:
   1. all visible forms of life
   2. anything which can be seen or felt
   3. anything which occupies space and possesses weight
   4. any substance that is not found in living organisms
2. In solid matter, the particles of which it is made are:
   1. loosely packed with no space between them
   2. tightly packed with no space between them
   3. loosely packed with very little space between them
   4. tightly packed with very little space between them
3. Gases differ from solids in that the gases:
   1. take the shape of their container and are always invisible
   2. have no shape or boundaries
   3. have a definite shape
   4. have definite shape and boundaries
4. The simplest forms of matter are substances that cannot be broken down by ordinary chemical change. We call these simple substances:
   1. molecules
   2. elements
   3. properties
   4. particles
5. Which of the following descriptions are chemical properties?
   1. lighter than air and yellow in color
   2. liquid, heavier than air
   3. colorless, soluble in water
   4. reacts with other elements to form oxides.
6. Which of the following is *not* a true statement?
   1. All atoms of the same element have the same properties.
   2. Atoms are changed when they are chemically combined with other atoms.
   3. Atoms of most elements can combine with atoms of other elements.
   4. All elements are composed of atoms.

7. Oxygen is an element and so is hydrogen. When two atoms of hydrogen unite with one atom of oxygen:
   1. three atoms of water are formed
   2. one atom of water is formed
   3. two molecules of water are formed
   4. one molecule of water is formed
8. Hydrochloric acid (HCl) is composed of hydrogen and chlorine. A molecule of HCl is formed:
   1. by the union of one atom of hydrogen and one of chlorine
   2. when hydrogen and chlorine are chemically changed into other elements
   3. by the union of water and salt
   4. by the union of molecules of hydrogen and oxygen
9. Sugars and starches are carbohydrates, and are composed of three elements. They are:
   1. carbon, oxygen, and sodium
   2. carbon, sodium, and hydrogen
   3. oxygen, hydrogen, and carbon
   4. hydrogen, oxygen, and chlorine
10. Proteins contain:
    1. carbohydrates and fat
    2. carbon, hydrogen, oxygen, and nitrogen
    3. carbon, oxygen, and fat
    4. carbon and nitrogen
11. Table salt (NaCl) is composed of the two elements:
    1. oxygen and chlorine
    2. hydrogen and chlorine
    3. sodium and chlorine
    4. carbon and chlorine
12. Energy is not created, it is simply changed from one form to another. Simple sugars provide our body with energy because the sugars contain:
    1. energy in motion
    2. the ingredients necessary to produce energy
    3. potential energy that is changed to energy in motion when the sugars are chemically changed
    4. the oxygen needed to "burn" the sugar
13. In the electron theory the structure of an atom is described as:
    1. a miniature solar system
    2. a wheel
    3. an evenly balanced scale
    4. a clock
14. Atoms that are stable contain:
    1. only five electrons and protons
    2. an equal number of electrons and protons
    3. more protons in the nucleus than electrons in orbit around the nucleus.
    4. fewer protons than electrons
15. If the atomic number of an element is fourteen, then we know there are:
    1. fourteen nuclei in each atom
    2. fourteen electrons and no protons
    3. fourteen protons in its nucleus and fourteen orbiting electrons in each atom
    4. seven protons in its nucleus and seven orbiting electrons.
16. Isotopes are used in diagnosis and treatment of various diseases; An isotope of chlorine is an atom of chlorine that:
    1. has a different atomic weight than another atom of chlorine.
    2. is chemically less potent than an atom of natural chlorine.
    3. has different chemical properties than an atom of chlorine in its natural state
    4. has a different atomic number than a more stable atom of chlorine.
17. Unstable elements are called radioactive because they:
    1. emit rays as their nuclei disintegrate
    2. absorb rays from the atmosphere
    3. can be used to penetrate normal tissue for diagnostic purposes
    4. always have an equal number of protons and electrons in each atom

18. The Celsius scale is also called the centigrade scale. The prefix *centi* means:
     1. one tenth
     2. one hundredth
     3. one thousandth
     4. one ten-thousandth

19. On a centigrade scale, the boiling point of water is:
     1. 10 degrees
     2. 32 degrees
     3. 80 degrees
     4. 100 degrees

20. A patient having a body temperature of 36.6 degrees C. would have:
     1. a subnormal body temperature
     2. a body temperature within normal range
     3. an abnormally high body temperature
     4. a slightly elevated boy temperature

21. A reading of 104 degrees F. is equivalent to:
     1. 34 degrees C.
     2. 36 degrees C.
     3. 38 degrees C.
     4. 40 degrees C.

22. The term calorie refers to a measurement of:
     1. temperature
     2. degrees of heat
     3. quantity of heat
     4. amount of heat loss

23. Which of the following statements best explains why perspiration helps maintain normal body temperature?
     1. An evaporating liquid absorbs heat from the surrounding area.
     2. Water is a better conductor of heat than is skin.
     3. Moisture reduces friction between two surfaces.
     4. Moisture holds heat and prevents its escape to the surrounding air.

24. If a substance is changed so that its composition is permanently altered and a new and different substance is formed, we refer to this as a(n):
     1. biological change
     2. physical change
     3. chemical change
     4. anatomical change

25. When the foods we eat are acted on by digestive juices they have been:
     1. changed into new and different substances
     2. broken down into smaller particles
     3. made more liquid so they can be absorbed from the intestinal tract
     4. changed physically but not chemically

26. Which of the following is *not* characteristic of a catalyst?
     1. speeds up a chemical reaction
     2. slows down a chemical reaction
     3. becomes changed during a chemical reaction
     4. chooses the particular substance to which it is attracted during a chemical reaction

27. There are enzymes acting as catalysts in:
     1. the digestion of foods
     2. the metabolic processes within a cell.
     3. both of the above
     4. neither of the above

28. Acids and bases are called chemical opposites because they:
     1. are compounds of completely different elements
     2. have no properties in common
     3. have different functions in the body
     4. react with and tend to neutralize one another

29. The mild acid that is in vinegar is called:
     1. boric acid
     2. acetic acid
     3. citric acid
     4. lactic acid

30. Milk of magnesia is an example of:
    1. an organic salt
    2. an acid
    3. an inorganic salt
    4. a base
31. The term pH expresses the:
    1. density of a solution
    2. proportion of solute to solvent
    3. degree of pressure exerted by the blood
    4. degree to which a solution is acidic or basic
32. Death can occur if the pH of blood:
    1. falls below 7
    2. rises above 7.8
    3. either of the above
    4. neither of the above
33. Saliva is nearly neutral. This means that it has a pH of:
    1. 7
    2. 4
    2. 4
    3. 9
    4. 12
34. Vinegar douches are often ordered for the purpose of:
    1. destroying certain bacteria that thrive in an acid environment
    2. inhibiting the growth of organisms that thrive in an alkaline environment
    3. providing a local disinfectant to the vaginal area
    4. eliminating odor produced by certain types of organisms
35. Acidosis is a condition in which the blood is:
    1. neutral
    2. highly alkaline
    3. highly acidic
36. Improper use of a gastric suction apparatus with continued removal of gastric juices can produce:
    1. acidosis
    2. alkalosis
    3. a neutral blood pH
37. Skin irritation resulting from urea deposits in a patient with uremia can be relieved by bathing the skin with a:
    1. mild soap solution
    2. dilute vinegar solution
    3. baking soda solution
38. Soap deposits in clothing and bed linens can be removed by rinsing these articles in:
    1. a vinegar solution
    2. lysol solution
    3. warm salt water
39. The main purpose of protecting the skin around the outer opening of a gastrostomy or colostomy is:
    1. preventing infection
    2. avoiding decubitus ulcers
    3. preventing corrosion by acidic digestive juices
40. Antacid drugs act to:
    1. neutralize gastric alkalies
    2. neutralize gastric acids
    3. both of the above
    4. neither of the above
41. Emergency treatment of a burn by a strong alkali such as lye would include irrigating the area with:
    1. dilute acetic acid
    2. milk of magnesia
    3. baking soda solution
42. A saline solution is made of:
    1. sodium chloride and oxygen

    2. table salt and water

    3. glucose and water

    4. baking soda and water

43. A deficiency of inorganic salts such as sodium chloride, calcium phosphate, etc. in the body may result in:

    a. an upset in the fluid balance   1. all but d

    b. an increase in nerve irritability   2. b and c

    c. disturbances in muscular contractions   3. all of these

    d. an upset in the acid-base balance in the   4. all but a
        body

44. An aqueous solution is one in which:

    1. alcohol is the solute

    2. alcohol is the solvent

    3. water is the solute

    4. water is the solvent

45. To remove grease or oil from a piece of cloth, the best solvent would be:

    1. ether or carbon tetrachloride

    2. water

    3. alcohol or saline

    4. a strong alkali

46. To determine the concentration of a solution we must know:

    1. how much solvent is used

    2. the amount of solute that can be completely dissolved in the solvent

    3. how much solute is used

    4. the amount of solute and the amount of solvent used to prepare the solution

47. Solvents may be in the form of:

    1. liquids

    2. solids

    3. gases

    4. all of these

48. When diffusion occurs the molecules of a substance move from an area of:

    1. relatively high concentration to one of lower concentration

    2. concentration equal to that of the area to which it is moving

    3. relatively low concentration to one of higher concentration

49. A semipermeable membrane is one which will allow passage of:

    1. the solute but not the solvent in a solution

    2. both solute and solvent

    3. the solvent but not the solute

50. When dried fruits or vegetables are soaked in water they become saturated with water. This is an example of:

    1. osmosis

    2. diffusion

    3. filtration

51. Both osmosis and diffusion:

    1. remove liquid from an area of dehydration

    2. equalize the concentration of various solutions in an area

    3. prevent the free flow of solutions from one area to another

52. The formation of urine in the nephron of the kidney is an example of:

    1. osmosis

    2. diffusion

    3. filtration

    4. dilution

53. When a strong "saline" cathartic such as Epsom salts is taken, watery stools result because:

    1. fluid is withdrawn from the tissues into the intestinal tract through the process of osmosis

    2. the salts act on the nervous system and increase peristalsis

    3. the salts irritate the intestinal tract and cause an increased secretion of mucus

    4. the salts are always given with large amounts of water

54. Oxygen is essential to all living matter because it is:

    1. an important constituent of blood

2. one of the most abundant of all the elements
3. necessary for proper "burning" of foodstuffs taken into the digestive system
4. capable of uniting with almost all the other elements and forming a large variety of substances

55. When we say that oxygen supports combustion we mean that it:
   1. assists the burning of substances
   2. is explosive
   3. is necessary for life
   4. unites readily with all other elements

56. Oyxgen has many uses. These include:
   a. treatment of asphyxiation
   b. in combination with anesthetics
   c. in fire extinguishers
   d. as a disinfectant (hydrogen peroxide)

   1. all of these
   2. all but c
   3. a and b
   4. a only

57. In the process of external and internal respiration two gases are exchanged. These gases are:
   1. hydrogen and oxygen
   2. oxygen and carbon dioxide
   3. hydrogen and nitrogen
   4. oxygen and nitrogen

58. The key element of proteins, and therefore one of the most vital constituents of protoplasm, is:
   1. oxygen
   2. carbon
   3. hydrogen
   4. nitrogen

59. If the specific gravity of a urine sample is reported as 13, this means that the urine is:
   1. as dense as water
   2. thirteen times more dense than water
   3. one thirteenth as dense as water

60. A device used to measure pressure is called a:
   1. manometer
   2. speedometer
   3. thermometer

61. Viscosity refers to:
   1. molecular density
   2. fluid friction
   3. fluid weight

62. A suction machine exerts:
   1. pressure equal to that of the atmosphere
   2. negative pressure
   3. positive pressure
   4. a force that is neither negative or positive

UNIT 2   MICROBIOLOGY AND PATHOLOGY

I. Microbiology

A. Definition—the study of organisms that can be seen only with the aid of a microscope. Important in learning the cause and control of many diseases.

B. Microorganisms—living plants or animals, may be one-celled or many-celled. Bacteria and viruses are the two most familiar types of microorganisms.

C. Classification of microbes—there are many ways to classify microbes; categories increase as new organisms are discovered.

  1. Pathogenic—capable of causing disease.

  2. Nonpathogenic—generally considered to be harmless and sometimes beneficial to man.

  3. Bacteria—one-celled plants. Often grouped according to their shape and the arrangement of their cells when viewed under a microscope.

    a. Cocci—round or spherical; seen in characteristic arrangements.

      1. Streptococci—grow in chains, often attack the throat.

      2. Diplococci—grow in pairs, cause gonorrhea and meningitis among other disorders.

      3. Staphylococci—grow in clusters or bunches; responsible for a wide variety of infections.

    b. Rod-shaped, elongated. Called bacilli, they include the tetanus bacillus and tubercle bacillus.

    c. Curved rods. One type, similar to a comma in shape, is called *vibrio*; example is the cholera vibrio. Another form, the spirillum, resembles a corkscrew. Spirochetes are very similar to spirillum and are capable of twisting motions. Syphilis is caused by a spirochete called *Treponema pallidum.*

    d. Some bacteria form spores, which are thick granules that can resist boiling, disinfectants, and other unfavorable conditions for long periods of time.

    e. Pyogenic bacteria are pus-forming; e.g., Staphylococcus aureus.

    f. *Pseudomonas aeruginosa* is a major cause of bacterial infections in surgical patients because it frequently infects already injured tissues. It produces a blue-green pus. The organism thrives in moist places such as sinks and drains.

  4. Viruses—can be seen only through an electron microscope. Require living tissue for laboratory growth and study. Very adaptable and can change their characteristics, thus making them difficult to classify and study.

    a. Classification often based on size, nucleic acid composition, and affinity for certain types of tissues in the human body.

    b. Diseases caused by viruses range from encephalitis to influenza to many childhood diseases.

  5. Fungi—simple plants, only a very few types are pathogenic. Prefer warm, moist places to thrive. Fungal infections, called mycoses or mycotic infections, include athlete's foot and ringworm. Lung abscesses and kidney damage may occur when there is a generalized mycotic infection. Many fungal infections are dangerous and difficult to cure.

  6. Rickettsiae—named for their discoverer, Howard T. Ricketts. Resemble viruses in some of their living habits but can be seen with an ordinary microscope. Rickettsial infections include Rocky Mountain spotted fever and typhus fever. The organisms are almost always transmitted through the bite of lice, fleas, or ticks.

  7. Protozoa—classified as animals, much larger than bacteria, and are found in almost any body of water, pond, mud puddle, or sea. The best known protozoal infection is malaria; amebic dysentery is also of this type of infection.

D. Laboratory identification of microbes

  1. Acid-fast organisms—those which do not lose their stain when an acid has been applied to a smear of the specimen. The stain, a reddish dye applied to the smear, usually disappears when the acid is applied. However, the organisms that

cause tuberculosis and leprosy remain colored; they are therefore called acid-fast organisms.

2. Gram stain: Certain organisms will retain a bluish dye when it is applied and thus they become color-fast. Alcohol or other solvents will not remove the dye and the organism is said to be gram-positive. Pathogenic staphylococci and streptococci, the bacilli that cause diphtheria and tetanus, are gram-positive organisms. If the coloring can be removed with a solvent, the organism is classified as gram-negative. Examples of this type of organism are gonococci, epidemic meningococci, and the typhoid bacilli.

3. Other laboratory techniques for studying organisms:
   a. Culturing, in which bacteria are grown in a nourishing media such as broth or agar.
   b. Studying the ability of bacteria to ferment sugars.
   c. Numerous serologic (blood) tests.

E. Destruction of microorganisms (Table 1)
   1. Disinfection—removal or destruction of pathogenic microorganisms.
      a. Disinfectant—usually a chemical such as bichloride of mercury or phenol.
         1. Usually applied to inanimate objects.
         2. Chemical disinfectants not always effective against spore-forming bacteria.
         3. Germicide—same as a disinfectant.
   2. Antisepsis—use of an agent to prevent or combat infection by inhibiting the growth of bacteria.
      a. Antiseptics used to remove surface bacteria from living tissue; do not always kill microorganisms.
      b. Used in medical asepsis to prevent the spread of infection.
   3. Sanitation—rendering an object clean and relatively free from pathogenic organisms.
   4. Asepsis—the absence of all organisms capable of causing disease.
      a. Medical asepsis—destruction of organisms *after they leave* the body. Necessary to prevent the spread of infection from one person to another.
         1. Based on the principles of cleanliness and sanitation, "No single article can compare with soap in respect to the amount of sickness and death prevented by its use." The most important factor in the prevention of the spread of disease organisms is the *proper washing of hands.*

      2. Carried out by isolation of patients with communicable or infectious diseases, and careful handling and cleaning of all equipment that has come in contact with the patient.
   b. Surgical asepsis—destruction of organisms *before they enter* the body. Used in caring for open wounds and in surgical procedures.
      1. All objects coming in contact with an open wound must be absolutely free from organisms.
      2. Accomplished through the conscientious observance of strict aseptic technique.

5. Sterilization—destruction or complete removal of *all* living organisms in or on an object.
   a. Three factors determine the method used
      1. Type of organisms.
      2. Degree of contamination.
      3. Cleanliness of objects being sterilized. (Only inanimate objects can be rendered sterile; living tissue must be treated with an antiseptic.)
   b. Methods of sterilization
      1. Chemicals—phenol, Lysol, alcohol, etc.
         a. Factors influencing effectiveness of the chemical—proper strength, allowing sufficient time for solution to act, cleaning objects by removing organic material such as blood, mucus, etc., before sterilizing.
         b. Most chemical agents are poisonous and should be handled with care.
         c. All solutions should be labeled clearly, giving name, strength, and the date solution was made.
      2. Dry heat—similar to a baking oven.
         a. Used for glassware, delicate surgical instruments, or materials that may be damaged by moisture.
         b. Less effective than moist heat, so higher temperature must be used (320° F.) for at least 1 hour.
      3. Boiling—one of the oldest methods used.
         a. Objects must be completely submerged in boiling water.
         b. Timing begins when water begins to boil.
         c. Spores NOT killed by boiling.
      4. Autoclaving—steam under pressure, similar to pressure cooker used for canning foods.
         a. Most dependable method used.

b. Articles must be correctly wrapped or placed in proper containers.

II. Etiology of Disease
A. Etiology defined as the study of causes of disease.
B. Causes may be specific or predisposing.
  1. Predisposing causes—person becomes ill because he is more susceptible or has a tendency toward the disease.
    a. Examples—age, heredity, sex, physical condition.
    b. Environment can present predisposing causes—temperature, humidity, etc.
  2. Specific causes—immediate or definite; that is, those specific things which interfere with the normal functioning of the body's cells.
    a. Oxygen deficiency—some cells are more sensitive (brain cells, for example) than others (heart muscle). All need oxygen to survive.
      1. Obstruction to blood flow.
      2. Anemia and other blood dyscrasias.
      3. Inadequate intake of oxygen, as in lung disorders.
    b. Trauma—injury.
      1. Physical—as in extremes of heat and cold, a violent blow to or penetration of the body, radiation, and electrical trauma.
      2. Chemical—poisons, abuse and misuse of drugs and other chemicals; for example, alcohol, detergents.
    c. Genetic disorders—inherited disease or tendency toward a disease; transmitted through the genes. Examples include blood disorders such as sickle cell disease and hemophilia, metabolic disorders, imbalance of genetic material (for example, Down's syndrome or mongolism).
    d. Congenital defects—abnormal development during fetal life; individual is born with the condition.
    e. Parasites—organisms which live off their hosts.
    f. Obstruction—closing off of a hollow organ.
    g. Deficiency diseases—result of inadequate intake or improper utilization of nutrients.
    h. Degenerative diseases—cells and tissues lose their ability to function properly. *Necrosis* is death of the cells; *sclerosis* is hardening of tissues.
    i. Neoplasms—new growth of cells.
    j. Infections—invasion by pathogenic organisms.

III. Pathology
A. Pathology defined as a study of the changes brought about in the tissues of the body as a result of disease or injury.
B. Changes produced by diseases classified as:
  1. Changes in structure of cells and tissues—example, neoplasm.
  2. Functional changes—example, congestive heart failure.
  3. Chemical changes—example, diabetes.
C. Body's defense against illness and injury
  1. Skin and mucous membranes—external defenses
  2. Internal defenses—inflammatory process and antigen-antibody reaction.
    a. Inflammatory process—initiated by foreign substances such as pathogenic organisms or chemical or mechanical injury.
    b. A process by which the body releases additional fluid and blood elements to combat the invader.
    c. External signs—redness, heat, swelling, pain, loss of motion.
  3. Internal changes
    a. Vascular changes—increased flow of blood to area (congestion).
    b. Leukocytosis—increase in white cell count. Leukocytes transported to local area.
    c. Exudation—removal of dead bacteria, damaged tissue cells, and blood cells.
    d. Repair—construction of new tissue on framework of granulation tissue.
    e. Antigen-antibody reaction—the events that take place in the body when antigens enter the body and stimulate the formation of specific proteins (antibodies) which act against the antigens.
  4. Immunity—a specific resistance to disease, made possible through the formation of antibodies.
    a. Types of immunity
      1. Natural—species, race, sex, cell and tissue resistance, and an individual ability to manufacture immune bodies.
      2. Active—accomplished by having an attack of the disease or by artificial means (vaccines—weakened or harmless living organisms; *bacterins*—dead organisms; *toxoids*—modified toxins).
      3. Passive—to fetus from mother, or by artificial means (immune serum containing ready-made antibodies; gamma globulin).
    b. Antitoxins—substances which neutralize the toxins produced by certain types of bacteria.

Table 1.   Destruction of Microorganisms*

CHEMICAL	ACTION	USES
Phenol (carbolic acid) 88 per cent	Antiseptic: destroys bacteria, but some spores and viruses may be resistant.	Disinfect excreta, sinks, toilets, etc.
Lysol 2 to 5 per cent	Antiseptic: more active than phenol.	Disinfect excreta, sinks, bedpans, etc. Not used on living tissue.
Alcohol 70 per cent	Inhibits growth of bacteria.	Cleanse the skin prior to injections; for rinsing hands or disinfecting thermometers.
Boric acid 2.5 per cent	Slows growth of bacteria.	Cleansing mucous membranes of nose and throat; as vaginal irrigation; eyewash.
Argyrol (silver compound) 10 to 25 per cent	Mild antiseptic.	Infections of mucous membranes of eyes, nose, throat, bladder.
Hydrogen peroxide 10 to 20 per cent	Antiseptic.	Clean infected wounds; irrigate mouth; gargle.
Bacitracin and neomycin	Antibiotics: inhibits the growth and multiplication of bacteria.	Applied locally to infected wounds, mucous membranes of eyes, throat.

*There is no ideal disinfectant that destroys all microorganisms on all types of animate and inanimate objects.

c. Antibacterials — substances which act against specific bacteria.
d. Allergy — an exaggerated reaction to substances which in similar amounts do not produce such severe symptoms in most persons.
   1. Symptoms — include redness, increased secretion of mucus, swelling of mucous membranes. Skin rash and itching also present in some allergies. Severe reaction may be fatal.

2. Allergens — substances capable of producing an allergic reaction. Certain drugs such as antibiotics, local anesthetics, and the immunizing agents are among the more common agents producing a severe allergic reaction.
3. Treatment — in a severe allergic reaction epinephrine (Adrenalin) is administered immediately. Other drugs that may be used to control allergy are antihistamines and cortical steroids.

Questions

1. A microorganism is best defined as:
   1. any living organism
   2. living organisms that cause disease in the body
   3. any living plant or animal that is so small it can be seen only with the aid of a microscope
   4. a tiny single-celled animal that can be seen only through a magnifying lens
2. Microbiology is an important part of medical science because:
   1. all diseases are caused by microorganisms
   2. the study of microorganisms has led to the discovery of the cause and cure of many diseases
   3. it is a study of the ways in which disease affects the tissues of the body
   4. infectious diseases are still the major cause of death in the U.S.
3. Pathogenic organisms are those that are:
   1. extremely small or invisible to the naked eye
   2. capable of producing disease
   3. harmless to the body tissues
   4. capable of producing an allergic reaction

4. Bacteria are classified as:
    1. plants
    2. animals
    3. yeasts
    4. molds
5. The shape of the streptococcus is best described as:
    1. spiral
    2. rod-shaped
    3. oval
    4. spherical
6. Diplococci are organisms that grow in:
    1. pairs
    2. chains
    3. clusters
    4. circles
7. Two diseases caused by diplococci are:
    1. cholera and syphilis
    2. whooping cough and measles
    3. meningitis and gonorrhea
    4. influenza and hepatitis
8. The staphylococcus is a type of bacteria that is:
    1. rod-shaped
    2. round and grows in clusters
    3. oval and grows in pairs
    4. round and grows in pairs
9. Bacilli are:
    1. spherical
    2. oval
    3. rod-shaped
    4. spiral
10. The causative organism of syphilis is a:
    1. spirochete called *Treponema pallidum*
    2. bacillus called the tubercle bacillus
    3. staphylococcus that grows in pairs
    4. comma-shaped organism classified as a vibrio
11. Spore-forming bacteria are:
    1. easily destroyed
    2. destroyed only by boiling
    3. resistant to many methods of sterilization
    4. much less dangerous than other types of bacteria
12. *Staphylococcus aureus* is the type of bacteria which causes boils and abscesses. It is called a pyogenic bacterium because it:
    1. is capable of rapid multiplication
    2. produces spores
    3. does not usually produce a fever in the patient
    4. is accompanied by the formation of pus
13. In the laboratory, viruses to be studied must be grown in:
    1. agar
    2. beef broth
    3. living tissue
    4. glucose solutions
14. Viruses may be classified according to:
    a. size
    b. composition of their nucleic acid
    c. shape and color
    d. affinity for specific tissues

    1. all of these
    2. a and d
    3. b, c and d
    4. all but c
15. Virus-caused diseases include:
    1. measles, chickenpox, and mumps
    2. influenza, encephalitis, polio
    3. all of the above
    4. none of the above

16. Fungal infections are called:
    1. mycoses
    2. mixed infections
    3. monilial
    4. melena
17. Fungal infections are most likely to occur:
    1. on the outer surfaces of the hands and feet
    2. in cool, dry areas
    3. in warm, moist places
    4. in warm, dry places
18. Rickettsial infections, such as Rocky Mountain spotted fever and typhus fever, are almost always transmitted by:
    1. direct contact with a person carrying the organism
    2. flies and mosquitoes
    3. contaminated water supply
    4. the bite of lice, fleas, or ticks
19. Protozoa are found in:
    1. desert areas
    2. almost any body of water
    3. mountainous regions
    4. the tropical regions only
20. The best known protozoal infection is:
    1. pneumonia
    2. cholera
    3. syphilis
    4. malaria
21. Examples of gram-negative organisms include:
    1. gonococci
    2. epidemic meningococci
    3. typhoid bacilli
    4. all of the above
22. The tubercle bacillus is identified as:
    1. gram-positive
    2. an acid-fast bacillus
    3. difficult to grow in a culture
23. One of the most common causes of hospital-acquired infections is *Pseudomonas aeruginosa* which:
    1. is easily destroyed bo soap and water
    2. is a type of virus
    3. cannot be destroyed by chemicals
    4. thrives in moist places
24. Medical asepsis is a technique used to:
    1. prevent the spread of infection during a surgical procedure
    2. eliminate all organisms from any objects coming in contact with a patient
    3. prevent the spread of disease from one person to another
    4. remove bacteria from all objects that come in contact with an open wound
25. Medical asepsis is carried out by:
    1. sterilizing all objects in the patient's environment
    2. administering antibiotics to the patient in an effort to prevent infection
    3. observing strict aseptic technique when giving any kind of nursing care
    4. observing the basic principles of cleanliness and sanitation
26. One very simple nursing procedure that is considered the most important in preventing the spread of infectious diseases is:
    1. isolation of all patients suspected of having an infection
    2. wearing rubber gloves when performing nursing procedures for surgical patients
    3. washing the hands thoroughly before and after each contact with a patient
    4. sterilizing the hands with a strong germicide at least once a day
27. Strong disinfectants such as phenol or carbolic acid are used to:
    1. sterilize the skin
    2. kill the bacteria on instruments, equipment, and other inanimate objects
    3. inhibit the growth of bacteria but not to destroy them
    4. remove all bacteria from open wounds or sores containing pathogenic organisms

28. Antiseptic solutions are generally used to:
    1. check the growth of bacteria on the skin or mucous membranes
    2. destroy bacteria on instruments or hospital equipment
    3. disinfect water supplies, sewage, etc.
    4. kill all bacteria in open wounds or sores
29. Which of the following may render a chemical ineffective in destroying micro-organisms?
    a. improper strength of solution
    b. a solution that has been left standing too long
    c. a solution that is too cold
    d. a solution that will not destroy spores or viruses

    1. all of these
    2. all but c
    3. a and b
    4. c and d
30. Surgical asepsis is based on the principle of:
    1. destroying bacteria as they leave the body
    2. destroying organisms before they enter the body
    3. isolating all patients who have an infectious disease
    4. basic cleanliness and sanitation
31. If an object has been rendered absolutely sterile this means that:
    1. it is free from most pathogenic organisms
    2. it has been thoroughly washed
    3. there are no living organisms in or on the object
    4. a disinfectant has been applied to the object
32. The most reliable method used for sterilizing hospital equipment so that it is free of spores and active bacteria is by:
    1. soaking in a strong chemical
    2. washing and drying it thoroughly after each use
    3. applying steam under pressure in an autoclave
    4. boiling the equipment
33. Delicate surgical instruments that must have sharp edges will last longer if they are sterilized by:
    1. applying dry heat
    2. soaking in chemicals
    3. boiling
    4. autoclaving
34. When an object is being sterilized by chemical means it is very important to:
    1. avoid soaking the object too long
    2. wash the article thoroughly to remove any blood, mucus, or other organic material before placing it in the chemical
    3. use a solution that will not damage living tissue
    4. rinse the article under running water before it is placed in the solution
35. In order for chemical sterilization to be effective, which of the following requirements must be met?
    a. the solution must be of proper strength
    b. the solution must be hot
    c. the object must be completely submerged in the solution
    d. sufficient time must be allowed for destruction of the bacteria

    1. all of these
    2. a and c
    3. b and d
    4. all but b
36. If a thermometer is being sterilized in the home, it would be best to:
    1. soak it in undiluted phenol
    2. hold it under a stream of running water and then wipe with an alcohol sponge
    3. wash it well with soap and water before placing it in alcohol or some other chemical disinfectant
    4. rinse it in alcohol before and after each use
37. To sterilize linens, gauze dressings, or other bandages in the home, it would be best to:
    1. boil them
    2. soak them in a mild disinfectant
    3. place them in an oven preheated to 350° F. and leave them there for at least 1 hour
    4. wash them in strong soap and very hot water

38. When boiling is used as a method of sterilization, the timing must:
    1. be started 5 minutes after the articles are placed in the water
    2. begin from the moment the article is placed in the water
    3. end at the exact moment boiling ceases
    4. begin only when the water has begun to boil
39. In order for an article to be considered completely sterilized by boiling, the nurse must be sure that:
    1. the article is completely covered by the boiling water
    2. she does not leave the article in boiling water too long
    3. distilled water is used
    4. a mild disinfectant has been added to the water
40. An article that has been boiled in water for 20 minutes should be considered free from:
    1. bacteria and their spores
    2. spores only
    3. all living organisms
    4. active bacteria but not their spores
41. The bones of an elderly person are more brittle than those of a younger person. If an elderly person falls and sustains a fracture we would say that his age is:
    1. a predisposing cause of the fracture
    2. an immediate cause of the fracture
    3. not relevant to the fracture
    4. a specific cause of the fracture
42. Serum hepatitis is caused by a particular type of virus. The virus is considered to be the:
    1. complicating factor in the disease
    2. predisposing cause of the disease
    3. specific cause of the disease
    4. result of the disease
43. Many of the symptoms of anemia and other blood disorders are a result of:
    1. inadequate oxygen supply to the cells of the body
    2. deficiency of minerals and vitamins essential to the production of blood cells
    3. lack of immune bodies necessary to combat disease
    4. chemical changes resulting from accumulation of toxins in the blood
44. In which of the following situations is there danger of chemical injury to the patient if the nurse is careless?
    1. application of hot water bottles or hot compresses
    2. preparation of solutions for enemas and douches
    3. application of bandages or dressings which might interfere with blood flow
    4. improper handling of radioactive substances
45. Genetic counseling should be included in the care of the patient with:
    1. infectious hepatitis
    2. chronic lung disease
    3. sickle cell disease
    4. iron deficiency anemia
46. When an individual develops an illness because of the entrance of microorganisms into the body it would be most accurate to say he has:
    1. an inflammation
    2. a neoplastic disease
    3. an allergy
    4. an infection
47. The word trauma refers to:
    1. bleeding
    2. infection
    3. injury
    4. new growth
48. The term necrosis means that:
    1. the tissues have become hardened and useless
    2. the cells of the tissue are dead and in a state of decay
    3. the tissues are inflamed
    4. there is a new growth of abnormal cells in the tissue

49. A defect which is present at birth is called:
 1. acquired
 2. an allergic reaction
 3. an inflammatory disease
 4. congenital

50. Down's syndrome (mongolism) is a genetic disorder. This means that the disorder is transmitted:
 1. by viral invasion of the placenta
 2. through the genes of one or both parents
 3. by bacterial infection immediately after birth
 4. by bacterial infection immediately before birth

51. If the tissues of the body have been irritated or injured, the body reacts by releasing additional fluid and blood elements into the affected area. When this reaction takes place we would say that the area is:
 1. inflamed
 2. infected
 3. necrotic
 4. cancerous

52. Arteriosclerosis is classified as:
 1. a traumatic disease
 2. an inflammatory disease
 3. a degenerative disease
 4. a neoplasm

53. The symptoms of an inflammation include:
 a. heat and redness in the area
 b. swelling of the area
 c. pain and hemorrhage
 d. formation of pus

 1. all of these
 2. all but b
 3. a and c
 4. a and b

54. The study of changes in the body brought about by illness or injury is called:
 1. etiology
 2. psychology
 3. microbiology
 4. pathology

55. The word pathogenic means:
 1. extremely small or invisible to the naked eye
 2. capable of producing disease
 3. harmless to the body tissues
 4. capable of producing an allergic reaction

56. When an inflammatory process begins there is an increased blood supply to the area. This is called:
 1. exudation
 2. leukocytosis
 3. suppuration
 4. congestion

57. An abscess results from the body's attempt to:
 1. localize an infection
 2. increase the blood supply to the affected area
 3. decrease the blood supply to the infected area
 4. provide drainage for bacteria

58. The body increases its number of white cells when an infection occurs because:
 1. white blood cells contain oxygen, which the tissues need to destroy bacteria
 2. white blood cells destroy and ingest bacteria
 3. the formation of pus from white cells is necessary for the proper healing of an inflammation
 4. white blood cells aid in the clotting of blood

59. When we say that immunity is a specific resistance to disease, we mean that:
 1. immunity to one disease guarantees immunity to all other diseases that are infectious in nature
 2. the formation of antibodies against one disease will not provide immunity to another disease
 3. some antibodies can provide immunity to many different diseases
 4. once the body is stimulated to produce antibodies, it can build an immunity to all kinds of diseases

60. When a person is vaccinated he receives a vaccine which contains:
    1. ready-made antibodies
    2. specially prepared antitoxins
    3. an immune serum containing antibodies and antitoxins
    4. weakened or harmless living organisms

61. Tetanus toxoid contains modified toxins which:
    1. stimulate the body to produce antitoxins
    2. provide a passive immunity
    3. help the body neutralize poisons already present in the blood
    4. provide a natural immunity

62. Giving a patient an immune serum against a specific disease will provide him with:
    1. an active immunity that is permanent
    2. a natural immunity that is only temporary
    3. a passive immunity that is permanent
    4. a passive immunity that is only temporary

63. Whenever an immunizing agent is being given the nurse should be aware that:
    1. all immunizing agents are harmless
    2. severe allergic reactions may develop in very sensitive individuals
    3. these agents will provide only temporary immunity against the disease
    4. only the agents which contain living organisms are capable of producing a reaction in the patient

64. Allergens are substances which:
    1. provide the body with antibodies
    2. help the body destroy bacteria
    3. are capable of producing an allergic reaction in some sensitive individuals
    4. prevent an allergic reaction to some substances in our environment

65. Some of the common symptoms of an allergy are similar to those produced by an inflammation and include:
    a. formation of pus
    b. redness of the area due to dilatation of the local blood vessels
    c. increased secretions from the mucous membranes affected
    d. high fever and delirium

    1. all of these
    2. a and c
    3. b and c
    4. b and d

66. Allergy and immunity are similar in that they both:
    1. are the result of an infection
    2. are unfavorable reactions to a foreign substance entering the body
    3. cause very mild symptoms
    4. result from the formation of antibodies

UNIT 3   BODY STRUCTURE AND FUNCTION

I. The General Plan
  A. Directional terms
1. Superior—near head, above; inferior—away from head, below.
2. Cranial—near head; caudal—near lower end of spinal column.
3. Ventral (also anterior)—near belly or front; dorsal (also posterior)—near back.
4. Medial—near midline; Lateral—to the side.
5. Proximal—nearest to point of origin; distal—away from point of origin.

  B. Body cavities—compartments that hold various organs (Fig. 1).
1. Cranial—space inside the skull; contains brain.
2. Spinal—space inside the spinal column; contains spinal cord.
3. Thoracic—chest cavity; contains lungs, heart, trachea, esophagus, and thymus gland. A moist, smooth membrane called the *pleura* lines this cavity (parietal pleura) and covers the surface of each lung (visceral pleura). The space between the parietal and visceral pleura is called the pleural sac. The diaphragm separates the thoracic cavity from the abdominopelvic cavity.
4. Abdominopelvic—upper portion is abdominal cavity; lower portion, pelvic cavity. They are not divided by any structure.
    a. Abdominal cavity contains stomach, intestines (upper), liver, gallbladder, pancreas, and spleen.
    b. Pelvic contains lower part of intestines, urinary bladder, ureters, and reproductive organs.

II. Structural Units
  A. Cells—the basic units or "building blocks" of all living matter.
1. Smallest unit of living matter which can live independently and reproduce itself (excluding virus).
2. Varying in sizes and shapes—approximately 1/2000th of an inch.
3. Basic structure and function of all cells are similar; in addition, each performs special functions.

4. Principal parts:
    a. Cell membrane—thin membrane surrounding cell. Acts as initial line of defense and determines the substances accepted or rejected by the cell. The membrane and nucleus control cell activity.
    b. Cytoplasm—the main substance of the cell body. It is the storage and working area of the cell.
    c. Nucleus—consists of a nuclear membrane, nucleoli, and chromosomes within a matrix. Its functions concern heredity and control of the cell's functions.
5. DNA and RNA—nucleic acids through which the nucleus affects heredity.
    a. DNA—deoxyribonucleic acid, the substance of which genes are made. Chromosomes, which house the genes, are composed mainly of protein and DNA.

      DNA carries the genetic code of every living entity and keeps a record of all its characteristics—size, shape, and orderly development from infancy to death. Each of these characteristics that can be passed on to succeeding generations is recorded by the arrangement of molecules in the DNA. It also governs production of enzymes and the synthesis of proteins, both of which are essential to the nutrition and growth of cells.
    b. RNA—ribonucleic acid; it is called the "messenger" because it carries from the DNA instructions needed to manufacture proteins from amino acids.
6. Functions of the cell—each cell carries on many functions that are the same as the functions of the whole body.
    a. Respiration (breathing)—exchange of oxygen and carbon dioxide.
    b. Eating and digestion—food elements pass through cell membrane and are used (metabolized) by the cell. Metabolism—the sum of all processes involving the release of energy from food (catabolism) and converting food into more complex compounds (ana-

35

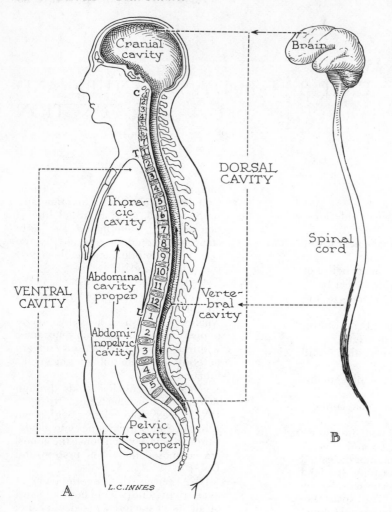

FIGURE 1. Body cavities as seen in a midsagittal section of head and trunk. *A*, Diagram of midsagittal section of head and trunk, showing vertebral column and body cavities. *B*, Organs of the dorsal cavity. (King, B. G., and Showers, M. J.: *Human Anatomy and Physiology,* 6th ed. Philadelphia, W. B. Saunders Co., 1969.)

bolism). The process involves many chemical reactions.

  c. Reproduction—primitive cells reproduce by a process of cell division called *mitosis*.

  d. Excretion—removal of waste products from the cell.

  e. Specialized functions—such as irritability and conductivity, which are characteristics of nerve cells, and elasticity, which is characteristic of muscle cells.

 7. Mechanisms by which substances enter and leave a cell include diffusion, osmosis, filtration, and active transport. The last requires an expenditure of energy on the part of the cell.

 8. Factors that influence the movement of substances through a cell membrane are:

  a. Size of molecule

  b. Electrical charge

  c. Solubility

B. Tissues—groups of cells that are similar in structure and function

1. Composition—made up of cells.
2. Types and functions

  a. Epithelial—forms glands, covers surfaces, and lines cavities.

  b. Connective—connects and supports various parts of the body.

  c. Nerve—conducts nerve impulses.

  d. Muscle—contracts to provide motion.

C. Organs—composed of two or more kinds of tissue

1. Composition and structure of organ will depend on its function; e.g., heart must act as pump, so it is composed chiefly of muscle tissue.
2. Organs perform more complex functions than tissues.

D. Systems—groups of organs

1. Body divided into systems for more organized study but no one system can function independently of other systems.
2. Body systems and general functions

  a. Integumentary (the skin)—protects the body against invasion of harmful agents.

b. Musculoskeletal system—support and motion.
c. Circulatory—transportation of nutrients and wastes, etc.
d. Digestive—intake of food; converting it into nutrients to be used by body cells.
e. Respiratory—exchange of oxygen and carbon dioxide.
f. Urinary—removal of certain wastes.
g. Reproductive—reproduction.

h. Endocrine—regulation of many body activities through chemical messengers called hormones.
i. Nervous—regulation and control of body activities.

III. Integumentary System (the Skin)
  A. Structure
    1. Composed of layers
      a. Epidermis
        1. Outer cells are flat, resembling

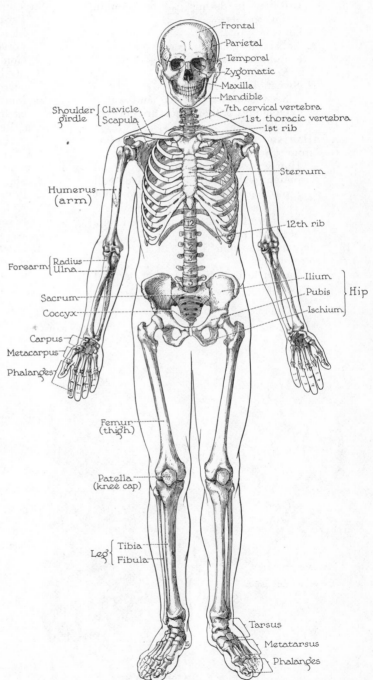

FIGURE 2. Anterior view of human skeleton. (King and Showers: *Human Anatomy and Physiology.* 6th ed.)

scales. Old ones continually flaking off and being replaced by new ones.
2. Deeper cells are more rounded.
3. Contains pigment (melanin) which gives skin its color.
b. Dermis (true skin)
1. Cells are scattered, with fibers between.
2. Contains blood vessels and nerves, roots of hairs, oil glands, and sweat glands.
3. Ridges in dermis can be seen in fingerprints.
2. Glands of skin
a. Sebaceous glands—secrete oil
1. Lubricate skin.
2. Keep hair and skin soft.
b. Sweat glands
1. Secrete waste products and water.
2. Openings of their ducts are pores of skin.
3. Hair and nails are structures that grow from skin
a. Hair grows from a cluster of cells at bottom of hair follicle. New hair will replace any that is cut or plucked out as long as these cells are alive. Nails are formed from hardened cells of the dermis.
B. Functions of the skin
1. Protection
a. Barrier to bacteria and other harmful agents.

b. Nerve endings in skin give warning of injurious agents in the environment.
2. Excretion
a. Urea and water are excreted through skin. Waste materials are excreted in very small amounts.
3. Regulation of body temperature
a. Insulation—keeps heat in.
b. Evaporation of perspiration cools skin.

IV. **The Skeletal System** (Figs. 2, 3, and 4).
A. Structure of the bones
1. Periosteum—outer covering; contains blood vessels, lymph vessels, and nerves.
2. Compact bone—makes up outside layer of bone; contains minerals, mainly calcium and phosphorus.
3. Marrow—spongy material that fills bone cavity.
a. Red marrow—manufactures red blood cells and some white blood cells.
b. Yellow marrow—soft, fatty tissue.
B. Functions of bones
1. Support and give shape to body.
2. Protect internal organs.
3. Help provide motion.
4. Form blood cells.
C. Types of bones
1. Long bones
a. Femur and tibia are examples.
b. Divisions (see Fig. 5)
1. Epiphysis contains red marrow.

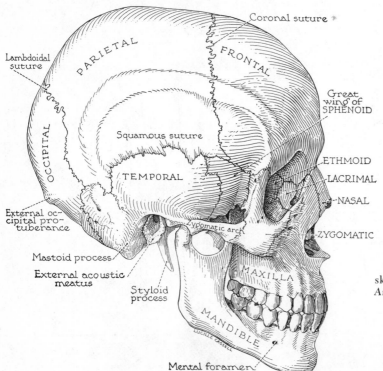

FIGURE 3. Lateral view of the skull. (King and Showers: *Human Anatomy and Physiology.* 6th ed.)

2. Diaphysis (shaft) contains yellow marrow.
2. Short bones
    a. Carpals and tarsals are examples.
    b. Used mainly for attachment of ligaments for motion.
3. Flat bones
    a. Cranium and sternum are examples.
    b. Used for protection and also formation of red blood cells.
4. Irregular bones
    a. Vertebrae are examples.
    b. Used for support and protection.
D. Processes—bony prominences or projections that serve as "landmarks" on the body and sometimes are areas of muscle attachment.
    1. Olecranon process—point of the elbow, upper part of the ulna.
    2. Iliac spine—upper pointed part of the front of the pelvic hip bone.
    3. Ischial spine—at the back of the pelvic outlet.
    4. Greater trochanter—rounded projec-

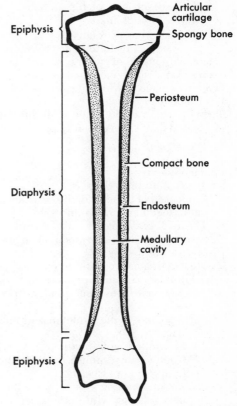

FIGURE 5.   Divisions of the long bone. (Anthony and Kolthoff: *Textbook of Anatomy and Physiology.* 9th ed., St. Louis, The C. V. Mosby Co., 1975.)

tions at the upper end and side portions of the femur.
E. Joints (also called articulations) are points of contact between two or more bones.
    1. Types
        a. Freely moveable joints are called *diarthroses.* Lined with synovial membrane and contain a fluid that acts as a lubricant to avoid friction during motion (Fig. 6). Examples include ball

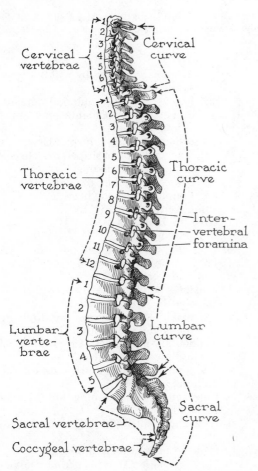

FIGURE 4.   Vertebral column from the left side. (King and Showers: *Human Anatomy and Physiology.* 6th ed.)

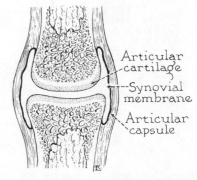

FIGURE 6.   Diagram of a synovial joint. (King and Showers: *Human Anatomy and Physiology.* 6th ed.)

and socket joint of hip and shoulder, hinge joint of ankle.

    b. Immoveable or relatively fixed joints — examples include bones of cranium.

F. Ligaments — made of strong white fibrous tissues that attach bones to other bones.

G. Tendons — made of white fibrous tissues that attach bones to muscles.

H. Bursa — a sac or cavity filled with fluid and so situated that it prevents friction in certain joints.

V. Muscular System

A. Structure of muscles (Fig. 7)
    1. Composed of bundles of fibers which are held together by connective tissue. These fibers contract and expand and therefore produce movement of an organ or a part of the body.
    2. Muscle tissues are of three main types:
        a. Voluntary (striated, or skeletal)
           1. Are made up of long, slender, striped cells.
           2. Attached to the skeleton and move its parts.
           3. Controlled by the will.
           4. Contract in response to stimulation by nerve impulses.
           5. Act in opposing groups, some members relaxing while others contract.
        b. Involuntary (nonstriated, smooth, visceral)
           1. Composed of spindle-shaped cells.

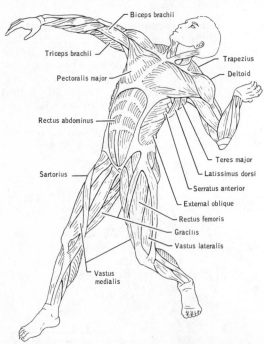

FIGURE 7.   Muscles of the anterior surface of the body. (Manner, H. W.: *Elements of Anatomy and Physiology*, Philadelphia, W. B. Saunders Co., 1962.)

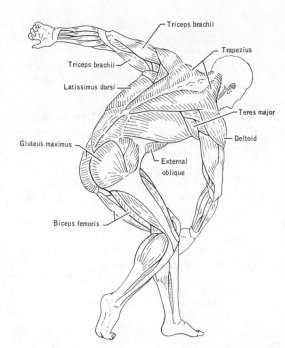

FIGURE 8.   Muscles of the posterior surface of the body. (Manner: *Elements of Anatomy and Physiology*.)

           2. Are not controlled by will but work automatically.
           3. Found in the internal organs, especially stomach, intestines, walls of blood vessels.
        c. Cardiac (branching, involuntary)
           1. A special type of striped muscle cell makes up this tissue.
           2. Not controlled by the will.
           3. Found only in the heart.

B. Functions of muscles (Fig. 8)
    1. Give the body shape.
    2. Provide motion.
    3. Give support to maintain posture.
    4. Produce heat and energy.

C. Muscular movements
    1. Flexion — bending the limb so that the angle at the joint is smaller.
    2. Extension — straightening the limb so that the angle at the joint is larger.
    3. Abduction — moving a part away from the midline of the body.
    4. Adduction — moving a part toward the midline.
    5. Contraction — a shortening and thickening of muscle fibers.
    6. Relaxation — a lengthening of the muscle fibers.

D. Terms used in relation to muscles
    1. Muscle tone — a state of partial contraction of a group of muscles; they remain poised, ready to go to work.
    2. Atrophy of the muscle — shrinkage of

```
┌─────────────────────────────────────────────────────────────┐
│                    PULMONARY CIRCULATION                      │
│                                                               │
│  Blood leaves right ventricle →right and left pulmonary       │
│  arteries ──→                                                 │
│  lung capillaries where carbon dioxide is released and oxgen  │
│  is picked up                                                 │
│  by blood cells →pulmonary veins →left atrium                 │
│                                                               │
│                                                               │
│                     GENERAL CIRCULATION                       │
│                                                               │
│  Oxygenated blood enters left atrium→left ventricle ──→       │
│                                                               │
│  aorta→arteries branching from aorta→capillaries in tissues   │
│                                                               │
│  of body→veins →superior and inferior venae cavae ──→         │
│                                                               │
│  right atrium→right ventricle.                                │
└─────────────────────────────────────────────────────────────┘
```

FIGURE 9.

muscle tissues, decrease in size due to disuse.
3. Muscle spasm—sudden involuntary contraction of a muscle.
4. Origin—the point at which the muscle is attached to a fixed part, e.g., bone.
5. Insertion—the end of the muscle that exerts power and movement.

VI. Circulatory System (Fig. 9)

A. Blood—red fluid within blood vessels; total volume averages 4 quarts in an adult male.
1. Functions
   a. Transportation of oxygen and carbon dioxide, etc. Also carries hormones.
   b. Nutrition—carries glucose, amino acids, fats, etc.
   c. Excretion—conveys waste products from tissues to kidneys and intestines for disposal.
   d. Regulation of body temperature.
   e. Helps maintain water balance of body tissues.
   f. Protection from disease by carrying immune bodies and other elements important in defense against pathogens.
2. Composition
   a. Cells
      1. Red blood cells (erythrocytes)
         a. Normal range 5 to 5.5 million per cu. mm.
         b. Manufactured in red bone marrow.
         c. Life span 3 to 4 months. Dead cells removed by spleen.
         d. Owe their color to a pigment called hemoglobin, which transports oxygen and carbon dioxide. Normal count for hemoglobin is 14 to 16 Gm. or 80 to 100 per cent.
      2. White blood cells (leukocytes)
         a. Normal range 5 to 9 thousand per cu. mm.
         b. Types of white cells—lymphocytes, neutrophils, eosinophils, monocytes, and basophils.
         c. Formed in red bone marrow and lymph tissues.
         d. Defend body against attacks of bacteria and other materials injurious to the body.
      3. Platelets (thrombocytes)
         a. Small, colorless cells about half the size of red cells.
         b. Average 500 thousand per cu. mm.
         c. Important in the clotting of blood.
   b. Plasma—straw-colored fluid part of the blood
      1. Contains antibodies, waste products, nutritive elements, hormones, and fibrinogen (which is manufactured by the liver).
      2. Serum is plasma with fibers removed.
   3. Blood types
      a. Four main groups—A, B, AB, and O.
      b. Rh negative and Rh positive refer to the absence or presence of a factor (a protein) that affects the clumping and destruction of red blood cells.

B. The heart and blood vessels
1. The heart—a hollow muscular organ lying a little to the left of the midline of of the chest.
   a. Function—acts as a pump to circulate blood through the blood vessels.
   b. Chambers
      1. Septum—a muscular wall dividing the heart into right and left halves.
      2. Each half is again divided into upper and lower quarters, with valves between them.
      3. Ventricles are lower chambers. Atria are upper chambers of the heart.
   c. Valves—one way type.
      1. Tricuspid—between right atrium and right ventricle.

2. Pulmonary—between right ventricle and pulmonary artery.
3. Mitral (also called bicuspid)—between left atrium and left ventricle.
4. Aortic—between left ventricle and aorta.

d. Heart composed of three walls or layers of tissue.
  1. Endocardium—inner lining.
  2. Myocardium—very thick muscular wall of heart.
  3. Pericardium—thin membranous sac surrounding the heart.

2. Arteries—large tubes which carry blood away from the heart.

  a. Have thick elastic walls which allow them to expand and contract.
  b. All arteries carry oxygenated blood (bright red) except the pulmonary arteries.
  c. Arterioles—extremely small arteries.

3. Veins—sometimes called the drainpipes of the circulatory system.
  a. Collect blood from capillaries and carry it back to the heart.
  b. Have thin walls; only slightly elastic, most have one-way valves to direct the flow of blood.

4. Capillaries—extremely small blood vessels that connect arteries and veins.

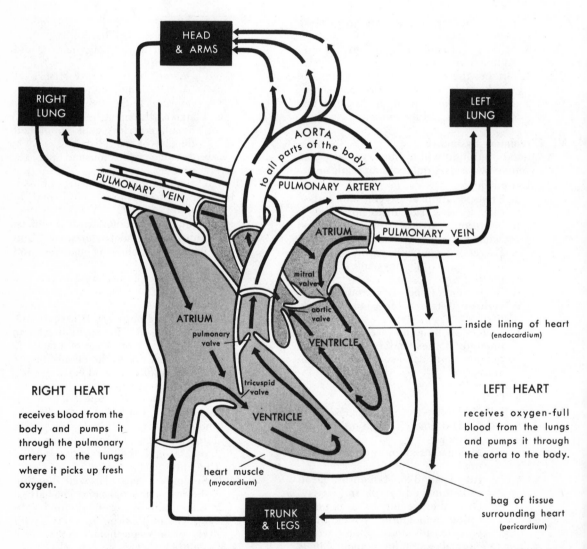

FIGURE 10.   The heart is really a double pump. One pump (the right heart) receives blood which has just come from the body after delivering nutrients and oxygen to the body tissues. It pumps this dark, bluish red blood to the lungs where the blood gets rid of a waste gas (carbon dioxide) and picks up a fresh supply of oxygen which turns it a bright red again. The second pump (the left heart) receives this "reconditioned" blood from the lungs and pumps it out through the great trunk-artery (aorta) to be distributed by smaller arteries to all parts of the body. (Courtesy of the American Heart Association.)

C. Circulation of blood (Fig. 10)
 1. Two phases of circulation
  a. General circulation—carries blood to all parts of the body except lungs.
  b. Pulmonary circulation—carries blood from heart to lung capillaries and back to the heart.
D. Lymphatics
 1. Lymph—a colorless fluid that is drained from the spaces around the cells of the body tissues.
 2. Lymph vessels—begin at periphery of body as close network of very small vessels.
 3. Lymph nodes—collections of lymphatic tissue that act as filters to assist the body in its defense against foreign agents.
 4. Functions of lymphoid tissue
  a. Removal of impurities such as dead blood cells, pathogenic organisms, malignant cells.
  b. Production of lymphocytes (a type of leukocyte).
  c. Production of antibodies.
 5. Tonsils—lymphoid tissue masses that filter pathogens from tissue fluid in the upper respiratory tract.
 6. Thymus—plays a key role in immunity and is essential to fetal growth. Most active during early years of life.
 7. Spleen—contains lymphoid tissue designed to filter blood.
  a. Located in the upper left quadrant of the abdomen.
  b. Functions:
   1. Destroys worn-out erythrocytes— iron and other products of decomposition returned for use in production of bile and new red blood cells.
   2. Serves as reservoir for blood that can be used in an emergency such as hemorrhage.
   3. Produces lymphocytes and monocytes and antibodies.

VII. Digestive System
 A. Structure—made up of organs of digestion in digestive tract and accessory organs of digestion.
  1. Organs of digestion (Fig. 11)—form the alimentary canal, which is a continuous passageway for food.
   a. Mouth—for receiving food and beginning the process of physical and chemical digestion.
    1. Teeth
     a. Incisors—for cutting food.
     b. Canines—for tearing food.
     c. Molars—for grinding food.
    2. Saliva—moistens food and contains secretions from three salivary glands.

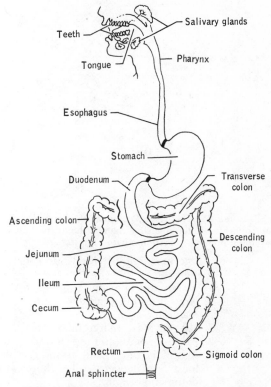

FIGURE 11.   Complete digestive system. (Manner: *Elements of Anatomy and Physiology.*)

   a. Ptyalin—an enzyme that changes some starches to sugar.
   b. Esophagus—long tube extending from pharynx (throat) to stomach.
    1. Propels food downward by wavelike contractions of its walls (peristalsis). This action moves food and wastes through entire digestive tract.
    2. Extends through thorax and diaphragm.
   c. Stomach—an elastic pouch that stores and churns food, changing it to semiliquid form (chyme).
    1. Glands in stomach secrete enzymes and HCl.
    2. Has two sphincter muscles—cardiac at upper end and pyloric at lower end.
   d. Small intestine—a hollow tube 20 to 22 ft. long. Divided into duodenum, jejunum, and ileum.
    1. All digestion completed in small intestine.
    2. Pancreatic duct and common bile duct empty into duodenum.
    3. Nutritive elements absorbed into bloodstream through villi in small intestine

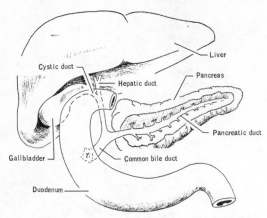

FIGURE 12. The liver, pancreas, and gallbladder are connected to the digestive tract by the ducts shown. (Manner: *Elements of Anatomy and Physiology*.)

e. Large intestine – divided into cecum, colon, and rectum.
　1. Absorption of water from waste in large intestine produces solid fecal material.
　2. No enzymes in large intestine.
　3. Anus – opening to the exterior.
　4. Appendix – a small blind tube located at ileocecal valve (between ileum and cecum).

2. Accessory organs of digestion (Fig. 12). Outside alimentary canal but provide digestive juices and enzymes essential to the digestion and absorption of food.
　a. Liver – the largest gland of the body
　　1. Produces bile, which passes through the hepatic duct into common bile duct.
　　2. Bile emulsifies (breaks down) fat globules.
　　3. Stores sugar as glycogen until needed for energy.
　　4. Removes toxins that have been absorbed from intestines.
　b. Gallbladder – small pouch under liver
　　1. Stores bile from the liver.
　　2. Releases bile when needed to aid in digestion of fats.
　c. Pancreas
　　1. Secretes pancreatic juices containing enzymes.
　　2. Pancreatic juices pass through pancreatic duct and empty into small intestine.
　　3. Islands of Langerhans – small microscopical clusters of cells in pancreas. Secrete insulin directly into blood to be used for proper utilization of glucose.

Table 2.　Digestion and Metabolism

NUTRIENT	DIGESTION		METABOLISM
CARBOHYDRATES	*Mouth* Some starches changed to maltose by ptyalin in saliva. *Stomach* No action. *Small Intestine* Lactose, Sucrose, Maltose } changed to glucose by enzymes { lactase, sucrase, maltase. Starch changed to glucose by amylopsin.		Glucose oxidized for heat and energy. Liver stores glucose as glycogen. Reconverted into glucose when needed for energy. Excess stored as body fat.
FATS	*Stomach* Fat-splitting enzyme lipase may act on fats, but considered of minor importance in digestion of fats in stomach. *Small Intestine* Bile emulsifies fats so that pancreatic enzyme lipase can digest them. Lipase breaks down fats into fatty acids and glycerol.		Fatty acids and glycerol changed into a new fat during absorption from intestine. Some new fat is oxidized for energy; excess is stored as adipose tissue (body fat).
PROTEINS	*Stomach* Pepsin, in presence of HCl, begins protein digestion. *Small Intestine* Erepsin and trypsin complete the breakdown of proteins. Proteins changed to proteoses, then to peptones, then to amino acids.		Amino acids used to build and repair body tissues. Liver uses amino acids to build proteins in blood plasma. Excess is converted into sugar and glycogen.

B. Functions (Table 2)
  1. Digestion—the physical and chemical breakdown of foods to prepare them for absorption into circulation.
  2. Absorption—passage of nutritive elements through villi in the walls of small intestine. These elements are amino acids, glucose, fatty acids, glycerol, etc. They are absorbed into circulation.
  3. Metabolism—takes place in the tissue cells. Is a series of chemical reactions that enable the body to use nutritive elements for building of cells and tissues and release of heat and energy.
    a. Anabolism—the chemical changes that allow cells to build and repair tissues.
    b. Catabolism—the chemical changes that break down nutritive elements for the formation of heat and energy.

VIII. **Respiratory System**
  A. Respiration
    1. Definition—the process of exchanging oxygen and carbon dioxide.
    2. Types
      a. External respiration (lung breathing)
        1. Takes place in alveoli of the lungs.
        2. Oxygen obtained from outside air passes through walls of alveoli into lung capillaries.
        3. Carbon dioxide leaves the blood in lung capillaries and passes through walls of alveoli to be exhaled into outside air.
      b. Internal respiration (cell breathing)
        1. Takes place in tissues of the body.
        2. Oxygen transported by blood cells in tissue capillaries passes into cells.
        3. Carbon dioxide leaving cells enters tissue capillaries and is transported in the blood back to the alveoli of lungs.
  B. Organs of respiration
    1. Nose
      a. Structure
        1. Nasal septum separates interior of nose into two cavities.
        2. Mucous membrane lines the nose. Contains cilia to trap foreign matter inhaled.
      b. Functions
        1. Warms, moistens, and filters air inhaled.
        2. Contains sense organ of smell.
    2. Pharynx—commonly called the throat
      a. Structure
        1. Two nasal cavities, mouth, esophagus, larynx, and eustachian tubes all have openings into pharynx.
        2. Tonsils and adenoids located in pharynx.
        3. Lined with mucous membrane.
      b. Functions
        1 Passageway for food.
        2. Passageway for air going to and from lungs.
    3. Larynx—the voice box
      1. Framework formed by cartilage rings.
        a. Epiglottis—acts as a lid to close off the larynx when food is swallowed.
        b. Thyroid cartilage (Adam's apple) largest and most prominent of cartilage rings.
      2. Vocal cords stretch across interior of larynx.
        1. Passageway for air to and from lungs.
        2. Produce sound.
    4. Trachea—windpipe
      a. Structure
        1. C-shaped rings of cartilage hold trachea open.
        2. Located in front of esophagus.
      b. Function
        1. Passageway for air to and from lungs.
    5. Bronchi, bronchioles, and alveoli
      a. Structure
        1. Trachea branches into right and left bronchi.
        2. Each bronchus branches into smaller and smaller tubes within each lung (bronchioles).
        3. Bronchioles end in grape-like clusters of microscopic sacs called alveoli.
      b. Functions
        1. Bronchi and bronchioles serve as passageways for air.
        2. Alveoli allow for exchange of gases between the air and the blood.
    6. Lungs
      a. Structure
        1. Three lobes in right lung, two lobes in left.
        2. Each lung has apex (narrow upper part) and base (broad lower part) that rests on diaphragm.
        3. Pleura—moist, smooth, slippery membrane that lines the chest cavity and covers the outer surface of the lungs. Prevents friction when lungs expand and contract.
        4. Pressure within pleural sac is less than that of atmosphere. If chest wall is punctured air will rush in and collapse lung.
      b. Function
        1. Respiration—exchange of oxygen and carbon dioxide.
  C. Muscles of respiration
    1. Diaphragm—large dome-shaped muscle.

When it contracts it flattens out and increases the size of the thoracic cavity.
2. External intercostals.
D. Control of respiration
1. May be controlled by will (muscles).
2. Nerves—respiratory center located in medulla oblongata of brain.
3. Chemical substances—carbon dioxide is respiratory stimulant.

IX. Urinary System (Fig. 13)
A. Kidneys—two bean-shaped organs, one on either side of the spine.
1. Structure
   a. Cortex—outer layer containing blood vessels and tubules.
   b. Medulla—inner part.
   c. Nephrons—microscopic functional units of the kidney (Fig. 14).
      1. Glomerulus—network of capillaries which filter water and chemical substances from the blood.
      2. Bowman's capsule—collects fluid filtered by glomerulus.
      3. Renal tubules—reabsorb water and chemical substances into the blood.
2. Function
   a. Secrete urine, normal daily output is 1200 to 1500 cu. cm.
B. Ureters—long narrow tubes, one from each

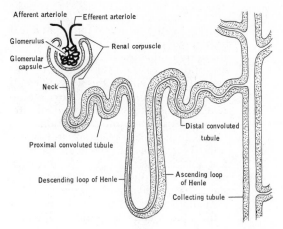

FIGURE 14.   Diagram of the renal unit, the nephron. Many renal units drain into the same collecting tubule. (Manner: *Elements of Anatomy and Physiology.*)

kidney. Drain urine from kidneys to urinary bladder.
C. Urinary bladder—elastic muscular organ capable of great expansion. Stores urine and aids in the process of voiding.
D. Urethra—the tube that extends from the bladder to the exterior of the body.
1. Lined with mucous membrane.
2. Length—1½ to 2 inches long in female; 6 to 8 inches long in the male.
3. Opening of urethra to outside is called urinary meatus. In the female the meatus is located between the clitoris and vagina. In the male it is located at end of penis.
4. Serves as passageway for urine from bladder to outside.

X. Female Reproductive System
A. Primary sex organs—two ovaries (female gonads).
B. Secondary sex organs—two fallopian tubes; uterus, vagina; vulva (external genitalia); breasts.
C. Ovaries—oval-shaped organs located on either side of uterus.
1. Contain graafian follicles, which, when stimulated by hormone from pituitary gland, rupture and release egg or ovum (called ovulation).
2. Functions
   a. Production of ova.
   b. Secretion of hormones (see Endocrine System).
D. Uterus—a hollow, muscular organ, approximately 3 inches long situated in abdominal cavity between bladder and rectum.
1. Composed of body, fundus, and cervix (neck of uterus).
2. Layers—endometrium, which is mucous

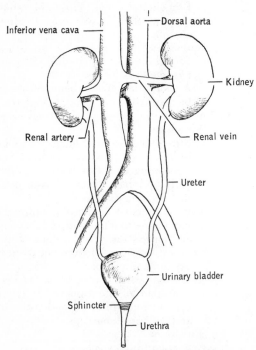

FIGURE 13.   The major organs and blood vessels of the excretory system. (Manner: *Elements of Anatomy and Physiology.*)

membrane lining that sloughs off during menstruation. Myometrium—network of smooth muscle fibers which form wall of uterus and give it great strength.
3. Eight ligaments anchor uterus in place. Normally, body of uterus lies over the bladder; cervix points downward and backward at right angles to vagina.
4. Functions
   a. Menstruation.
   b. Pregnancy.
   c. Labor.
E. Uterine tubes—extend from uterus. There is no direct connection from ovaries to tubes. Fimbriated (finger-like) end of each tube extends over ovary.
   1. Tubes lined with mucous membrane and cilia which propel the ova through tube.
   2. Function—serve as ducts for ovum from ovary to uterus. Fertilization of ovum takes place in tubes.
F. Vagina—birth canal
   1. Lies between rectum and urethra and urinary bladder.
   2. Functions
      a. Receives seminal fluid during copulation.
      b. Forms lower part of birth canal.
      c. Passageway for menstrual flow.
G. External genitalia (vulva)
   1. Mons pubis or pubic mound—lies over symphysis pubis, covered with hair after puberty.
   2. Labia majora and labia minora—large and small "lips." Contain numerous glands.
   3. Clitoris—located just behind labia majora.
   4. Vaginal orifice—located between rectum and urinary meatus.
   5. Perineum—a muscular structure covered with skin; forms the pelvic floor.
H. Breasts (mammary glands)
   1. Lie over pectoral muscles.
   2. Composed of glands in grape-like clusters.
   3. Nipples are bordered with a pigmented area called the areola.
   4. Function—lactation (secretion of milk).

XI. Male Reproductive System
A. Primary sex organs—two testes or testicles (male gonads).
B. Secondary sex organs—a series of ducts, accessory glands, and supporting structures (penis and scrotal sac).
C. Testes
   1. Structure
      a. Small oval glands.
      b. Located in the scrotal sac.

2. Functions
   a. Manufacture sperm (male sex cell).
   b. Secrete most of seminal fluid in which sperm are transported.
   c. Secrete the male hormone, testosterone.
D. Series of ducts—function as passageways for seminal fluid and sperm.
   1. Epididymis—thin tube which lies tightly coiled along the top and side of the testes.
   2. Seminal duct—an extension of epididymis.
   3. Ejaculatory duct—located inside prostate gland.
E. Prostate gland
   1. Lies just below the bladder and around the urethra.
   2. Adds a secretion to the seminal fluid making the sperm more active.
F. Supporting structures
   1. Scrotum—a skin-covered pouch suspended from the perineum. Serves as a container for testicles and ducts.
   2. Penis—composed of erectile tissue. Serves as supporting structure for urethra. Sperm are deposited in vagina by penis during copulation.

XII. Endocrine System
A. Endocrine glands
   1. Pour their secretions directly into the circulation.
   2. Hormones—chemical substances manufactured by the endocrine glands They regulate activities of various body organs.
   3. There are six organs definitely known to be endocrine glands.
      a. Pituitary gland
         1. Located in the cranial cavity at the center of the base of the brain.
         2. Divided into anterior and posterior lobes.
         3. Referred to as the "master gland" because it controls activities of other endocrine glands.
      b. Thyroid gland
         1. Located in the neck.
         2. Has two lateral lobes, one on either side of larynx.
      c. Parathyroid glands
         1. Usually four; adjacent to thyroid gland.
      d. Adrenal glands
         1. Located on top of kidneys.
         2. Divided into adrenal cortex (outer covering) and medulla (inner part).
      e. Islands of Langerhans
         1. Located in pancreas.
         2. Microscopic clusters of cells separate from pancreatic cells.

Table 3.   Functions of Endocrine Glands

GLAND	HORMONE	ACTION OF HORMONE
PITUITARY		
Anterior lobe	Thyrotropic hormone	Stimulates thyroid gland.
	Somatotropic hormone	Stimulates growth.
	Gonadotropic hormones (LH, FSH, LTH)	Affect growth, maturity, and functioning of primary and secondary sex organs.
	Adrenocorticotropic hormone (ACTH)	Stimulates cortex of adrenal glands.
Posterior lobe	Antidiuretic hormone	Decreases production of urine.
	Oxytocic principle	Stimulates uterine contractions.
THYROID	Thyroxin	Stimulates metabolism (catabolic phase).
PARATHYROID	Parathormone	Regulates blood calcium level.
ADRENAL		
Cortex	Hormones divided into three main groups:	
	Glucocorticoids	Tend to increase amount of sugar in blood.
	Mineralocorticoids	Tend to increase amount of blood sodium and decrease amount of potassium in blood.
	Androgens (male hormones)	Govern certain secondary sex characteristics. All corticoids important for defense against stress or injury to body tissues.
Medulla	Epinephrine (Adrenalin); "fight or flight" hormone	Elevates blood pressure. Converts glycogen to glucose when needed by muscles for energy. Increases heartbeat rate. Dilates bronchioles.
OVARIES	Estrone and progesterone	Stimulate development of secondary sex characteristics.
		Effect repair of endometrium after menstruation.
TESTES	Testosterone	Essential for normal functioning of male reproductive organs. Stimulates development of male secondary sex characteristics.
ISLANDS OF LANGERHANS, on pancreas	Insulin	Promotes metabolism of carbohydrates.

f. Ovaries (female sex glands)—located in abdominopelvic cavity.

g. Testes (male sex glands)—located in scrotal sac.

B. Functions of endocrine glands (Table 3)

XIII. Nervous System

A. Nerve cells (neurons)
  1. Structure—composed of cell body with extensions or processes called dendrites and axons. Unipolar neurons have only one extension, bipolar have two, and multipolar have three or more extensions. Number depends on function of neuron.
  2. Types of neurons
    a. Sensory (afferent)—conduct impulses to brain and spinal cord.
    b. Central (connecting)—conduct impulses from sensory neurons to motor neurons.
    c. Motor (efferent)—conduct impulses from central neurons to muscles or glands.
B. Divisions of nervous system
  1. Central nervous system—brain and spinal cord.
  2. Peripheral nervous system—spinal nerves and cranial nerves.
  3. Autonomic nervous system—ganglia on either side of spinal cord.
C. Organs of central nervous system—covered and protected by cranial bones, vertebrae, and meninges. Fluid between these coverings—spinal fluid.
  1. Brain—divided into cerebrum, cerebellum, and medulla oblongata.
    a. Cerebrum
      1. Largest part of brain.
      2. Controls mental processes such as memory, reasoning, intelligence, and will.
      3. Also controls voluntary movements.
    b. Cerebellum
      1. Smaller than cerebrum.
      2. Coordinates muscular movements.
    c. Medulla oblongata
      1. Called the midbrain.
      2. An enlarged extension of the spinal cord in cranial cavity.
      3. Center of many vital reflexes.
  2. Spinal cord—lies inside the spinal column.
    a. Reaches from occipital bone down to

Table 4.   Cranial Nerves

NUMBER	NAME	ORIGIN	DISTRIBUTION	FUNCTION
I	Olfactory	Nasal epithelium	Cerebrum	Sensory
II	Optic	Retina	Cerebrum	Sensory
III	Oculomotor	Midbrain	Eyeball muscles	Motor
IV	Trochlear	Midbrain	Eyeball muscles	Motor
V	Trigeminal	Pons	1. Ophthalmic branch – around the eye	Sensory
			2. Maxillary – upper portion of face	Sensory
			3. Mandibular – temple, ear, lower lip, teeth and gums of mandible, muscles of mastication	Mixed
VI	Abducens	Pons	Eyeball muscles	Motor
VII	Facial	Pons	Muscles of the face, taste buds, middle ear	Mixed
VIII	Auditory	Pons	1. Cochlear – cochlea of inner ear	Sensory
			2. Vestibular – semicircular canals	Sensory
IX	Glossopharyngeal	Medulla	Tongue and pharynx	Mixed
X	Vagus	Medulla	Abdominal viscera, heart	Mixed
XI	Spinal accessory	Medulla	Muscles of neck	Motor
XII	Hypoglossal	Medulla	Tongue and muscles activating hyoid	Motor

cartilage disc between first and second lumbar vertebrae.

   b. Conducts motor impulses from brain to muscles and glands of body, and conducts sensory impulses from sensory organs to brain.

   c. Serves as center for many reflexes.

D. Peripheral nervous system
   1. Cranial nerves (Table 4)
   2. Spinal nerves
      a. 31 pairs attached to spinal cord.
      b. Conduct impulses between spinal cord and parts of body not served by cranial nerves.

E. Autonomic (involuntary) nervous system
   1. Divided into sympathetic and parasympathetic
      a. Sympathetic controls involuntary functions in emergencies.
      b. Parasympathetic controls involuntary functions under ordinary circumstances.

XIV. Special Sense Organs

A. Eye (Fig. 15)
   1. Structure – wall of eyeball consists of three coats.
      a. Tough outer coating called *sclera*. Portion in front of eyeball is clear and is called the *cornea*.
      b. Choroid – middle layer, contains blood vessels. Hole in front of eyeball is the pupil. Circular band around pupil is pigmented and is the iris.
      c. Retina – third layer, contains rods and cones which are specialized cells that are sensitive to light.
   2. Function – bending or refracting light rays so that they focus on retina. Accomplished by
      a. Aqueous humor – watery fluid between cornea and lens.
      b. Lens – crystalline structure just behind iris.
      c. Vitreous humor – jelly-like substance filling space between lens and retina. Maintains spherical shape of eyeball.
   3. Conjunctiva – delicate membranous lining of eyelids. Covers front of eyeball.
   4. Lacrimal gland – located in upper, outer part of each eye socket. Produces tears,

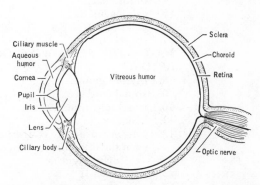

FIGURE 15.   Sagittal section of the eye, showing the major anatomical structures. (Manner: *Elements of Anatomy and Physiology.*)

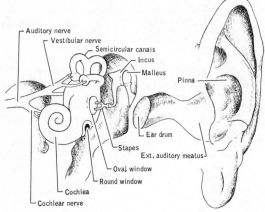

FIGURE 16.   The basic anatomy of the human ear.
(Manner: *Elements of Anatomy and Physiology.*)

which lubricate and cleanse surface of eyeball.

B. Ear (Fig. 16)
   1. Structure—has three main parts
      a. Outer ear composed of pinna (shell), auditory canal, and eardrum (tympanic membrane).
      b. Middle ear—actually a cavity in temporal bone. Connects with pharynx by means of eustachian tube. Three tiny bones in middle ear are hammer, anvil, and stirrups. These bones carry sound waves across middle ear from eardrum to inner ear.
      c. Inner ear—contains cochlea, which is spiral-shaped passageway for sound waves going to auditory nerve. Also contains semicircular canals, which are important for maintenance of proper body balance.
   2. Functions
      a. Transmission of sound waves to auditory nerve.
      b. Maintenance of equilibrium.

Questions

1. The term superior, when used as an anatomical direction, means:
    1. above normal
    2. near the lower end of the spine
    3. near the head
    4. above average in size
2. The ventral surface of the body is:
    1. the right side
    2. the left side
    3. the back
    4. the front or abdomen
3. The term dorsal means:
    1. posterior or toward the back
    2. anterior or toward the front
    3. posterior or toward the front
    4. anterior or toward the back

MATCH THE FOLLOWING ORGANS WITH THE CAVITIES IN WHICH THEY ARE LOCATED:

4. brain_____   1. abdominopelvic
5. esophagus_____   2. spinal
6. gallbladder_____   3. thoracic
7. spinal cord_____   4. cranial

MATCH THE FOLLOWING ORGANS WITH THE SYSTEMS TO WHICH THEY BELONG:

8. thyroid gland_____   1. circulatory system
9. spinal cord_____   2. digestive system
10. small intestine_____ 3. nervous system
11. heart_____   4. endocrine system
12. The organ that is concerned with respiration and separates the thoracic cavity from the abdominopelvic cavity is the:
    1. diaphragm
    2. trachea
    3. pleura
    4. sternum

13. The "building blocks" of all living matter are called:
     1. tissues
     2. ova (eggs)
     3. organs
     4. cells
14. The nucleus of a cell:
     1. allows for passage of substances into and out of the cell
     2. is the substance of which the cell is made
     3. governs many of the cell's activities, including reproduction
     4. rids the cell of its waste products
15. The substances DNA and RNA which affect heredity are called:
     1. genes because they are composed of genetic material
     2. nucleic acids because they are found in the cell nuclei
     3. amino acids because they are made of protein
16. The cell membrane is constructed so that:
     1. only harmless substances may enter the cell
     2. nutrients can enter the cell and waste products pass out of the cell
     3. oxygen and other gases are the only substances capable of penetrating it
     4. blood cells bringing oxygen and nutrients can pass through it
17. Factors that influence the movement of substances through a cell membrane include all of the following except:
     1. size of molecule
     2. electrical charge
     3. width of cell membrane
     4. solubility of substance
18. Which of the following is *not* a normal cell function?
     1. respiration
     2. reproduction
     3. excretion
     4. agglutination
19. The periosteum is the:
     1. spongy material that fills the bone cavity
     2. inner lining of the bone
     3. outer covering of the bone
     4. outside layer of bone that contains minerals
20. The part of the bone that manufactures red blood cells is called the:
     1. periosteum
     2. red marrow
     3. yellow marrow
     4. compact bone marrow
21. The cranium and sternum are examples of:
     1. long bones
     2. irregular bones
     3. flat bones
     4. short bones
22. The two minerals most important in the formation of bone are:
     1. iron and calcium
     2. phosphorus and calcium
     3. sodium and iron
     4. phosphorus and sodium
23. A trochanter roll is often used in the care of stroke patients. This is a device used to insure proper positioning of the:
     1. shoulder
     2. wrist
     3. cervical spine
     4. femur
24. Articulations are best defined as:
     1. bony prominences
     2. freely movable joints
     3. points of contact between two or more bones
     4. immovable joints

25. Movable joints are lined with a membrane and filled with a fluid that acts as:
    1. an adhesive to hold the bones of the joints in place
    2. a passageway for nutrients
    3. a barrier against infection
    4. a lubricant to prevent friction
26. Which of the following is *not* characteristic of the skeletal muscles?
    1. controlled by the will
    2. composed of smooth muscle tissue
    3. arranged in opposing groups so that when one set contracts the opposite set relaxes
    4. stimulated to move by nerve impulses
27. Which of the following does *not* apply to muscle tissues?
    1. give shape to the body
    2. provide motion
    3. manufacture red blood cells
    4. help maintain posture
28. Moving a limb away from the midline of the body is referred to as:
    1. flexion
    2. extension
    3. abduction
    4. adduction
29. When the hamstring muscles contract they:
    1. flex the lower leg, making the angle at the knee joint smaller
    2. extend the lower leg, making the angle at the knee joint larger
    3. flex the hip, making the angle at the knee joint larger
    4. extend the lower leg, making the angle at the hip joint smaller
30. When muscles have good tone they are:
    1. completely relaxed and flaccid
    2. always in a state of partial contraction
    3. smaller than normal
    4. permanently contracted
31. The muscle that abducts the upper arm at the shoulder joint is the:
    1. deltoid
    2. pectoralis major
    3. triceps
    4. biceps
32. Functions of the blood include all but:
    1. transportation of gases and nutrients
    2. transportation of waste products
    3. maintenance of water balance
    4. production of red blood cells
33. Red blood cells are also known as:
    1. leukocytes
    2. erythrocytes
    3. erythemacytes
    4. thrombocytes
34. Red blood cells owe their color to:
    1. bile
    2. iron
    3. fibrin
    4. hemoglobin
35. Another name for white blood cells is:
    1. leukocytes
    2. erythrocytes
    3. blastocytes
    4. leukoblasts
36. The normal range for a white cell count is:
    1. 3 to 5 thousand per cu. mm.
    2. 8 to 12 million per cu. mm.
    3. 3.5 to 5 million per cu. mm.
    4. 5 to 9 thousand per cu. mm.

37. Which of the following is *not* true of hemoglobin?
    1. an important constituent of all white blood cells and red blood cells
    2. a constituent of all red blood cells
    3. responsible for transporting oxygen to the body tissues
    4. responsible for transporting carbon dioxide
38. The straw-colored fluid part of the blood is called:
    1. lymph
    2. plasma
    3. tissue fluid
    4. serous fluid
39. The total volume of blood in the average man is:
    1. 3 pints
    2. 4 quarts
    3. 6 pints
    4. 2 quarts
40. The substance that is produced by the liver and is necessary for the clotting of blood is:
    1. fibrinogen
    2. thromboplastin
    3. prothrombin
    4. fibrin
41. The myocardium is the:
    1. sac surrounding the heart
    2. inner lining of the heart
    3. thick muscular wall of the heart
    4. major blood vessel serving the heart
42. The bicuspid valve is located between the:
    1. right and left ventricles
    2. right atrium and right ventricle
    3. left atrium and left ventricle
    4. left and right atria
43. A person suffering from mitral stenosis would have a defect of the:
    1. pulmonary valve
    2. bicuspid valve
    3. tricuspid valve
    4. ventricular valve
44. In a normal heart, the blood in the chambers of the right side of the heart would be:
    1. higher in oxygen content than that in the left side
    2. about equal in oxygen content with that of the left side
    3. equal in carbon dioxide content to that of the left side
    4. lower in oxygen content than that in the left side
45. The walls of the arteries are:
    1. very thin, allowing for expansion with each heartbeat
    2. thick, elastic walls which contract and expand
    3. composed of striated muscle tissue
    4. lined with a thick membrane which prevents their expansion
46. The flow of blood through the veins is directed by:
    1. rhythmic contractions of the vein walls
    2. gravity flow
    3. the force of the heart's contractions
    4. one-way valves within the veins
47. Blood flows from the heart through the aorta, and from there to:
    1. arteries to capillaries to veins
    2. arteries to veins to capillaries
    3. capillaries to arteries to veins
    4. veins to arteries to capillaries
48. The term lymph refers to the fluid that is:
    1. located within blood vessels
    2. drained from the spaces around the cells of the body tissues
    3. the liquid part of the blood
    4. obtained by removing fibrin from plasma

49. The lymph vessels are collections of lymphatic tissues that:
    1. destroy bacteria
    2. manufacture erythrocytes
    3. help the body by localizing infection and filtering foreign cells from the body tissues
    4. act as filters, thereby aiding in the clotting of blood
50. Other functions of lymphoid tissue include:
    1. production of lymphocytes and antibodies
    2. manufacture of pathogens
    3. maintenance of normal balance of liquid and solid in the blood
51. The spleen is located in the:
    1. posterior thoracic cavity
    2. upper left quadrant of the abdomen
    3. lower middle section of the abdomen
    4. upper middle section of the thorax
52. Which of the following is *not* a function of the spleen?
    1. destroys worn-out red blood cells
    2. produces lymphocytes, monocytes, and antibodies
    3. stores an emergency supply of blood
    4. manufactures red blood cells

MATCH THE FOLLOWING ORGANS WITH THEIR FUNCTIONS:

53. mouth_____
54. stomach_____
55. small intestine_____
56. large intestine_____

1. inner surface contains glands which secrete hydrochloric acid and enzymes
2. receives digestive juices from pancreas and liver
3. allows for absorption of water from wastes passing through
4. receives food and begins digestive process

57. The enzyme that changes cooked starches to sugar in the mouth is called:
    1. hydrochloric acid
    2. lactase
    3. maltase
    4. ptyalin
58. The complete process of digestion changes sugars and starches to:
    1. maltose
    2. glycogen
    3. glycerol
    4. glucose
59. Amino acids are used to build and repair body tissues. The amino acids are the end product of the digestion of:
    1. fats
    2. proteins
    3. carbohydrates
    4. vitamins
60. Of all the enzymes used in the process of digestion, the most important ones are those found in the:
    1. bile from the liver
    2. pancreatic juices poured into the small intestine
    3. gastric secretion
    4. secretions of large intestine
61. The sphincter muscle located at the lower end of the stomach is called the:
    1. cardiac muscle
    2. pyloric muscle
    3. duodenal muscle
    4. ileocecal muscle
62. Bile is important in digestion because it:
    1. dissolves meat fibers and makes them easier to digest
    2. digests simple fats
    3. breaks down fat globules so they can be more easily digested by enzymes
    4. changes complex sugars to glucose

63. The absorption of nutritive elements obtained from digested food takes place in the:
    1. stomach
    2. small intestine
    3. large intestine
    4. colon
64. The gallbladder:
    1. stores bile
    2. stores sugar as glycogen
    3. secretes bile
    4. contains glands which secrete digestive enzymes
65. All of the following are functions of the liver except:
    1. secretes bile
    2. stores bile
    3. stores sugar as glycogen
    4. removes toxins absorbed into the blood from the intestines
66. A substance secreted by the islands of Langerhans and important in the utilization of glucose is:
    1. epinephrine
    2. ptyalin
    3. pancreatic enzyme
    4. insulin
67. Metabolism is a series of chemical reactions that take place in the tissue cells. These reactions are necessary for:
    1. building tissue and storing fat
    2. building and repairing tissue and releasing heat and energy
    3. using nutritive elements to provide energy
    4. providing for elimination of waste products accumulated in the tissues
68. In general, the term respiration may refer to lung breathing or cell breathing, and simply means:
    1. the act of inhaling oxygen
    2. the process of exhaling carbon dioxide
    3. the combination of inhaling and exhaling
    4. an exchanging of oxygen and carbon dioxide
69. Which of the following is *not* a function of the nasal passages?
    1. warms and moistens inhaled air
    2. acts as a filter
    3. allows for absorption of oxygen through its mucous membranes
    4. serves as passageways for air
70. The organ commonly called the throat is the:
    1. larynx
    2. trachea
    3. esophagus
    4. pharynx
71. The epiglottis is:
    1. commonly called the "Adam's apple"
    2. the organ which acts as a lid to close off the larynx when food is swallowed
    3. the small covering over the pharynx which prevents aspiration of liquids into the lungs
    4. the structure containing the vocal cords
72. Hoarseness or inability to make voice sounds most likely would be a result of inflammation of, or injury to, the:
    1. trachea
    2. nasal cavities
    3. alveoli
    4. larynx
73. The exchange of oxygen and carbon dioxide between the outside air and lung capillaries takes place in the:
    1. bronchioles
    2. alveoli
    3. trachea
    4. pleura

74. Pressure within the pleural sac is:
    1. less than that surrounding the lungs
    2. less than atmospheric pressure
    3. more than atmospheric pressure
    4. the same as atmospheric pressure
75. Carbon dioxide acts as a:
    1. respiratory stimulant
    2. vasodilator
    3. respiratory depressant
    4. bronchodilator
76. The pleura is the:
    1. lower part of the lung
    2. main branch of the bronchial tree
    3. muscle most important in respiration
    4. smooth, moist membrane that lines the chest cavity and covers the outer surface of the lung
77. When the diaphragm contracts it:
    1. pushes upward against the lungs and causes them to deflate
    2. flattens out, allowing the lungs to expand and fill with air
    3. causes the intercostal muscles to relax and expand the chest wall
    4. pushes downward and inward, causing the lungs to deflate and expel air
78. Within the kidneys there are millions of microscopic units which carry out the function of producing urine. These functional units are called:
    1. neurons
    2. renal tubules
    3. nephrons
    4. renal cortex
79. In the process of producing urine, the kidneys must:
    1. dilute the chemicals and fluid absorbed from the blood
    2. concentrate the fluid withdrawn from the blood
    3. both filter and concentrate the urine before it reaches the kidney pelvis
    4. eliminate all waste products not removed by the intestines
80. The long narrow tubes that drain urine from the kidneys to the urinary bladder are the:
    1. renal tubules
    2. kidney pelvis
    3. urethras
    4. ureters
81. The length of the urethra is usually:
    1. 6 inches in the female, 2 inches in the male
    2. 2 inches in the female, 6 to 8 inches in the male
    3. 4 inches in the male and the female
    4. 8 inches in the male and the female
82. In the female the external urinary meatus is located between the:
    1. clitoris and vaginal orifice
    2. perineum and anus
    3. anus and bladder
    4. bladder and urethra
83. The functions of the ovaries include:
    1. production of ova (eggs) and secretion of hormones
    2. secretion of seminal fluid
    3. production of graafian follicles
    4. receptacle for fertilized ovum
84. The uterus lies in the abdominal cavity:
    1. just below the bladder
    2. above the bladder
    3. between the bladder and rectum
    4. directly below the vaginal orifice
85. The structures that serve as ducts for the ovum and are the site of fertilization of the ovum are called:
    1. ovaries
    2. vagina

    3. graafian follicles
    4. uterine tubes

86. The inner lining of the uterus is called the:
    1. perimetrium
    2. epimetrium
    3. myometrium
    4. endometrium

87. The lower part of the uterus narrows and forms a "neck" which is called the:
    1. fundus
    2. body
    3. cervix
    4. vagina

88. The muscular structure that forms the floor of the pelvis is called the:
    1. peritoneum
    2. parietal muscle
    3. mons pubis
    4. perineum

89. The mammary glands secrete:
    1. female hormones
    2. the menstrual flow
    3. milk
    4. a lubricating fluid

90. The organs of the male reproductive system that manufacture the male sex cells are called the:
    1. prostate gland
    2. testicles or testes
    3. epididymis
    4. Cowper's glands

91. The male hormone that is secreted by the primary sex organ of the male is called:
    1. estrogen
    2. estrone
    3. progesterone
    4. testosterone

92. The prostate gland is located:
    1. above the bladder in the abdominal cavity
    2. above the bladder around the ureters
    3. below the bladder around the urethra
    4. below the bladder in front of the urethra

93. Glands in the endocrine system are given this name because they:
    1. have ducts that lead to the circulation
    2. pour their secretions into the lymphatic system
    3. pour their secretions directly into the circulation
    4. always have more than one secretion

94. Hormones are:
    1. secreted by endocrine and exocrine glands
    2. chemical regulators secreted by endocrine glands
    3. primarily concerned with growth and normal functioning of the sex glands
    4. useful only in treating diseases of the reproductive systems

95. The endocrine gland located in the neck is called the:
    1. thymus
    2. pituitary
    3. thyroid
    4. adrenal

96. A deficiency in the hormone from the parathyroid gland will produce:
    1. gigantism
    2. dwarfism
    3. imbalance in the calcium level of the body
    4. decrease of potassium in the blood

97. A person having an increase in the production of thyroxin would be most likely to have:
    1. an increase in physical growth and a decrease in mental ability
    2. an increase in the level of blood sugar

    3.   a decrease in blood pressure
    4.   an increase in the metabolic rate

98. The hormone released by the medulla of the adrenal gland at times of emergency is called:
    1.   insulin
    2.   epinephrine or Adrenalin
    3.   medullin or Adrenalin
    4.   the pressor principle

99. The corticoids, which are hormones important for defense against stress or injury to the body, are secreted by:
    1.   the pituitary gland
    2.   the adrenal cortex
    3.   the adrenal medulla
    4.   the cortex of the thyroid gland

100. The two hormones secreted by the ovaries are important in the:
    1.   development of secondary sex characteristics and normal menstruation
    2.   maintenance of water balance in the body
    3.   regulation of the metabolic rate
    4.   transmission of sex-linked genetic traits

101. The central nervous system is composed of two organs. They are the:
    1.   cerebrum and cerebellum
    2.   spinal cord and cerebrum
    3.   brain and spinal cord
    4.   spinal nerves and cranial nerves

102. The meninges are:
    1.   membranous coverings of the brain
    2.   three layers of tissue that cover the brain and spinal cord
    3.   the bony layers of tissue covering the spinal cord
    4.   nerve cells on the outer surface of the brain and spinal cord

103. The part of the brain that controls the skeletal muscles is the:
    1.   cerebellum
    2.   cerebrum
    3.   medulla oblongata
    4.   pons

104. Muscular movements of the body are coordinated in the:
    1.   cerebellum
    2.   cerebrum
    3.   medulla oblongata
    4.   spinal cord

105. Many vital reflexes have their center in the:
    1.   cerebellum
    2.   cerebrum
    3.   pons
    4.   medulla oblongata

106. When a lumbar puncture is performed for the purpose of obtaining a specimen of spinal fluid, the needle is usually inserted between the third and fourth lumbar vertebrae because:
    1.   there is no spinal fluid below this point
    2.   the spinal cord can be penetrated most easily at this level
    3.   the spinal cord ends above the second lumbar vertebra
    4.   the vertebrae are smaller at this level

107. The spinal nerves conduct impulses between the:
    1.   brain and spinal cord
    2.   spinal cord and parts of the body not served by the cranial nerves
    3.   spinal cord and cranial nerves
    4.   brain and cranial nerves

108. An injury to the optic nerve will result in an impairment or loss of:
    1.   hearing
    2.   motion of the eyeballs
    3.   the ability to swallow
    4.   sight

109. A person having neural or nerve deafness would have some impairment in the function of the:
    1. olfactory nerve
    2. auditory nerve
    3. abducens nerve
    4. vagus nerve

110. The parasympathetic and sympathetic nervous systems are concerned with control of:
    1. voluntary movements
    2. the senses
    3. involuntary or automatic functions
    4. both voluntary and involuntary functions of the body

111. The eyeball is protected by a tough outer covering or coat called the:
    1. choroid
    2. sclera
    3. retina
    4. optic disc

112. When a corneal transplant is done the surgeon replaces the:
    1. middle layer of the eyeball
    2. circular band around the pupil
    3. normally clear portion of the sclera that lies in the front of the eyeball
    4. third layer of the eyeball that contains the nerve endings

113. The part of the eye containing the pigment that determines the color of the eye is called:
    1. iris
    2. pupil
    3. sclera
    4. retina

114. When light rays enter the eye they must be focused on the back wall of the eye to produce vision. The part of the eye that is sensitive to these light rays is called the:
    1. iris
    2. sclera
    3. retina
    4. lens

115. When we say that light rays are refracted by the eye we mean that they are:
    1. screened from the retina
    2. directed through the retina
    3. bent so they will focus on the retina
    4. lengthened so they will not damage the retina

116. The eyeball keeps its spherical shape chiefly because it is filled with a jelly-like substance called:
    1. lens
    2. vitreous humor
    3. aqueous humor
    4. lacrimations

117. An inflammation of the conjunctiva involves the:
    1. glands that produce tears
    2. delicate membrane lining the eyelids and covering the front part of the eyeball
    3. portion of the eye that contains the optic nerve
    4. circular band surrounding the pupil

118. Tears are produced by the:
    1. Cowper's glands
    2. orbital glands
    3. lacrimal glands
    4. optic glands

119. Tears flow across the eye to keep it moist and free from foreign particles. The tears are drained off by the tear duct, which is located in the:
    1. upper, outer corner of the eye
    2. lower, outer corner of the eye

      3. upper, inner corner of the eye

      4. lower, inner corner of the eye

120. The tympanic membrane of the ear is commonly called the:

      1. eardrum

      2. ear lobe

      3. middle ear

      4. mastoid

121. The eustachian tube leads from the:

      1. middle ear to the pharynx

      2. auditory canal to the eardrum

      3. malleus to the stapes

      4. middle ear to the inner ear

122. The auditory nerve receives sound waves from a shell-like structure called the:

      1. semicircular canal

      2. stapes

      3. cochlea

      4. pinna

123. The inner ear contains a group of structures important in the maintenance of body balance. These structures are known as the:

      1. cochleas

      2. tympanic membranes

      3. semicircular canals

      4. stapes

124. The middle ear contains the hammer, anvil, and stapes which are:

      1. shell-like bones that conduct sound waves

      2. membranes reaching from the inner ear to the outer ear

      3. three small sacs containing fluid

      4. very small bones that resemble the objects for which they are named

Part IV
NUTRITION

UNIT 1　NUTRITION IN HEALTH

I. **Nutrition—the Science of Man's Food Requirements**
   A. Requirements may vary according to age, activities, climate, etc.
   B. Balanced nutrition is essential to physical, mental, and emotional health.

II. **The Nutrients**
   A. Nutrients are chemical compounds found in foods, and are used to
      1. Provide heat and energy.
      2. Build and repair tissue.
      3. Regulate body processes.
   B. Foods are composed of six types of nutrients
      1. Carbohydrates
      2. Fats
      3. Proteins
      4. Vitamins
      5. Mineral elements
      6. Water
   C. Basic Seven food groups (daily requirements)
      1. Leafy green and yellow vegetables (1 or more servings).
      2. Citrus fruit, tomatoes, raw cabbage (1 or more servings).
      3. Potatoes and other vegetables and fruits (2 or more servings).
      4. Milk, cheese, ice cream (children—3 to 4 cups of milk; adults—2 or more cups).
      5. Meat, poultry, fish, eggs, dried beans, peas (1 to 2 servings).
      6. Bread, flour, whole grain or enriched cereals (every day).
      7. Butter and fortified margarine (some daily); fortified margarine has had vitamins A and D added.
   D. The four-group plan
      1. Milk group; some milk for everyone every day.
      2. Meat group; 2 or more servings. As alternates, dry beans, dry peas, nuts.
      3. Vegetable—fruit group; 4 or more servings.
      4. Bread-cereal group; 4 or more servings.
   E. A variety of foods in the diet is one of the best guarantees of an adequate diet.
   F. Some terms used in nutrition
      1. Calorie—a measurement of heat, just as a pound is a measurement of weight. One calorie is the amount of heat needed to raise the temperature of 1 kilogram of water 1 degree C.
      2. Cereals—the seeds of the grass family; e.g., corn, wheat, rye, oats, rice, barley.
      3. Enriched—restoring or replacing nutrients lost through refinement of cereals.
      4. Fortified—adding one or more nutrients not originally found in the food. Example, vitamin D in milk.
      5. Diet—simply, the daily intake of food.
      6. Cellulose—the fibers of a plant, practically indigestible in man, provide bulk in the diet.
      7. Glycogen—the form in which carbohydrates are stored in animal tissues.

III. **Carbohydrates**
   A. Starches and sugars are carbohydrates.
   B. The most economical and the quickest source of energy for the body.
   C. Make up about 50 per cent of the American diet.
   D. Kinds of carbohydrates
      1. Sucrose—cane, maple, and beet sugars.
      2. Fructose—found in honey and plants, especially fruits.
      3. Glucose—the form of carbohydrate that is in the blood. All other sugars must be converted into glucose before they can be used by the body tissues.
      4. Maltose—found in sprouting grains (malt sugar).
      5. Lactose—the carbohydrate found in milk.
   E. Carbohydrates produce 4 calories per gram.
   F. Excessive carbohydrates known to be a factor in causing tooth decay.

G. Extra carbohydrate taken into the body is stored as body fat.

H. Uses of carbohydrates in the body
 1. Provide heat and energy.
 2. Must be present for the normal oxidation of fats.
 3. Adequate carbohydrates in the diet minimize the oxidation of proteins for energy.

IV. Fats

A. Also composed of carbon, hydrogen, and oxygen but in different proportions.

B. Fats come from plants (invisible fats) and animals (visible fats).

C. One third of the calories in an American diet come from fats.

D. One gram of fat produces 9 calories.

E. Fats are found in many commonly used foods (egg yolk, meat, butter, nuts).

F. Uses of fats in the body
 1. Supply heat and energy.
 2. Carriers of the fat-soluble vitamins A, D, E, and K.
 3. Body fat serves as insulation for body heat, and pads some vital organs.
 4. Essential fatty acids needed for growth and for maintenance of body functions.

G. Food sources of fats
 1. Animal fats such as whole milk, cream, cheese, butter, meat, eggs, chocolate. (High in saturated fats.)
 2. Vegetable oils such as corn, nuts, olives, soybeans. (Unsaturated fats, liquid at room temperature.)

H. (Fats not easily digested, remain in the stomach longer than other nutrients, satisfy hunger longer.)

I. Mineral oil is not digested and prevents the absorption of vitamins A and D.

J. "Invisible fats" in chocolate, nuts, olives, corn, egg yolk.

V. Proteins

A. Complex organic compounds containing hydrogen, oxygen, nitrogen, and sometimes minerals.

B. Amino acids—the smallest units of proteins, essential to the building and repair of tissue.

C. (Kinds of proteins)
 1. Complete—contain all the essential amino acids. Animal proteins are complete proteins; e.g., meat, milk, fish, and eggs. Soybeans of plant origin but contain all essential amino acids.
 2. Incomplete—do not contain all the essential amino acids. Found in *plant life* with the exception of gelatin, which is an animal protein that does not contain all essential amino acids.

D. One gram of protein yields 4 calories.

E. Uses of proteins in the body
 1. Build and repair tissue.
 2. Provide heat and energy.
 3. Help maintain water balance.
 4. Needed for manufacture of chemicals, such as hormones, enzymes, antibodies, and other body proteins.

F. Protein foods are not stored in the body as such.

VI. Minerals

A. Calcium—99 per cent of the calcium in the body is found in the bones and teeth.
 1. Important in the formation of bone tissue and teeth.
 2. Other functions of calcium
  a. Helps muscles contract and regulates the heartbeat.
  b. Aids in the clotting of blood.
  c. Important for health and well-being at all stages of life.
 3. Rich sources of calcium
  a. Milk and milk products (it is difficult to meet the adult's daily requirements for calcium without including at least 2 cups of milk or its equivalent in milk products daily).
  b. Hard-shell fish such as oysters, shrimp, and clams.
  c. Leafy green vegetables are good sources.
  d. Oranges and figs are high in calcium.

B. Phosphorus—important element of every living cell.
 1. Ninety per cent of the body's phosphorus is found in the bones and teeth.
 2. Phosphorus helps maintain the normal acid-base balance of the blood.
 3. Sources of phosphorus
  a. Diets containing enough protein and calcium will be adequate in phosphorus.
  b. Milk and milk products, whole grain cereals, fish, nuts, poultry, and legumes.

C. Iron—very small amount in the body, but is of vital importance.
 1. Iron in the hemoglobin is responsible for carrying oxygen to the tissues.
 2. Used to manufacture new red blood cells.
 3. Vitamin C and calcium necessary for the proper absorption of iron from the intestinal tract.
 4. Need for iron increased
  a. During periods of growth.
  b. To replace losses in menstruation.
  c. During pregnancy and lactation.
 5. Sources of iron
  a. Liver or kidney.

Table 5.   Sources of Vitamins and Symptoms of Vitamin Deficiencies

VITAMIN	IMPORTANT SOURCES	DEFICIENCY SYMPTOMS
Fat-soluble A	Liver, fish liver oils, milk products, eggs, green leafy vegetables.	Night and glare blindness; inflammation and drying of the skin and mucous membranes.
D	Fortified milk, sunshine, fish liver oils.	Soft bones and teeth; bowed legs. Rickets is deficiency disease.
E	Green leafy vegetables, margarine, other vegetable oils.	Specific function in man unknown.
K	Green leafy vegetables, liver, cauliflower, cabbage.	Prolonged blood clotting time.
Water-soluble C	Citrus fruits (oranges, grapefruit, lemons, limes), strawberries, tomatoes, potatoes	Sore, bleeding gums; stiff joints; poor bone and cartilage formation, susceptibility to infections. Scurvy is deficiency disease.
B_1 (thiamine)	Pork, liver, other organ meats, whole grain cereals.	Anorexia; nervousness; fatigue.
B_2 (riboflavin)	Milk, liver, green leafy vegetables, eggs, whole grain cereals.	Retarded growth; scaly skin; lesions at corners of mouth.
Niacin	Liver, lean meats, dried beans and peas, whole grain cereals.	Skin lesions, fatigue, gastrointestinal disturbances.

      b. Enriched cereals.
      c. Green leafy vegetables.
      d. Dried beans and peas.
   6. Milk does not contain iron.
   7. Iron and copper needed for formation of hemoglobin.
   8. Iron lost if foods are cut into small pieces and cooked in too much water, or cooked too long.
D. Sodium and potassium—their functions closely related in the body.
   1. Functions
      a. Help maintain normal water balance.
      b. Regulate muscle irritability.
      c. Help maintain acid-base balance.
   2. Sources
      a. Both minerals are found in a wide variety of foods.
      b. Table salt contains sodium.
      c. Orange juice contains potassium.
   3. Excessive sweating may lead to deficiency of sodium.
   4. Diuretics sometimes deplete supply of sodium and potassium because these minerals are excreted by the kidneys.
   5. Iodine—essential to normal growth and development of thyroid gland.

VII. **Vitamins—Regulatory Substances Essential to Life and Growth**
A. Two groups: fat-soluble vitamins and water-soluble vitamins.

   1. Fat-soluble vitamins
      a. Are destroyed by rancidity.
      b. Are stored in the body.
      c. Are not destroyed by ordinary cooking methods.
   2. Water-soluble vitamins
      a. May be lost by improper cooking.
      b. Have little or no storage in the body.
      c. Can be lost by discarding the water in which the food was cooked or soaked.
B. Fat-soluble vitamins may be harmful if taken in excessive amounts.
C. Water-soluble vitamins excreted by kidneys.
D. Sources of vitamins and deficiency symptoms (Table 5).
E. Vitamin preparations do not take the place of well-balanced meals.

VIII. **Water—of Greater Importance than Any One Type of Food**
A. Functions
   1. As a solvent for all products of digestion.
   2. Helps carry nutrients to the cells and remove waste products.
   3. Aids in regulation of body temperature.
   4. Excretes waste products through the kidneys.
B. The daily intake of water should average 6 to 8 cups.
C. Vegetables and fruits are from 60 to 98 per cent water.
D. Milk is 87 per cent water.
E. Meat is 40 to 75 per cent water

UNIT 2   MENU PLANNING AND BUYING OF FOODS

I. **Planning Meals—Objectives Are to Include Foods Which Provide the Basic Nutrients and Are Appetizing As Well.**
  A. Factors to consider
    a. Use all the food groups in the Basic Four every day.
    b. Vary colors of foods on menu.
    c. Vary texture of foods; include some crisp and some soft.
    d. Choose foods that have compatible flavors.
    e. Vary type of foods used at one meal; i.e., include proteins, carbohydrates, and fats.

II. **Cost of Food**
  A. With proper planning an adequate diet need not be expensive.
  B. Planning menus in advance allows for more economical cooking because leftovers can be used to best advantage.
  C. Foods bought in season and in good supply are less expensive.
  D. Prepared foods cost more than those prepared at home (frozen foods, bakery products, etc.).
  E. Store foods properly to prevent waste and loss of nutrients.
  F. The following foods are very expensive in relation to the nutrients they contain: bacon, jams and jellies, carbonated drinks, potato chips, candy, pickles and relishes, bakery pies and cakes.
  G. "Empty calorie" foods supply only calories, no nutrients, e.g., candy, carbonated drinks.
  H. Foods containing a high concentration of sugar are irritating to the lining of the stomach.

III. **Food Handling**
  A. Wash the hands thoroughly before handling food and preparing meals.
  B. Cool leftovers before placing them in refrigerator.
  C. Any food that smells strangely or has a change of color or consistency should be discarded without being tasted.
  D. Be careful of foods that have been prepared in advance, especially those with cream, milk, or eggs in them, and place them in refrigerator until ready to be served. Bacteria grow rapidly in warm temperatures.

IV. **Food Fads and Facts**
  A. Misunderstandings about foods are often passed from one generation to another.
  B. Many people are influenced by faddists, who spread false information about foods.
  C. Some common fallacies and facts
    1. *Fallacy:* Acid fruits cause excessive acidity in the body.
       Fact: Acid fruits actually are made alkaline by the process of digestion. They do not cause acidity in the body.
    2. *Fallacy:* Fish is a brain food.
       Fact: No one food functions to build a special type of tissue. Although fish does contain phosphorus which is found in nerve tissue, this mineral also may be found in other foods.
    3. *Fallacy:* Certain foods will prolong life and preserve youth.
       Fact: The best assurance of a long and healthy life is a balanced diet containing a variety of nutritious foods. There are no "miracle" foods.
    4. *Fallacy:* Foods should not be left in their containers after they have been opened.
       Fact: Canned foods can be left in their original containers without danger. Acid foods may dissolve some iron from the can and change the taste slightly, but this is not harmful.
    5. *Fallacy:* Vitamin tablets or concentrates are necessary for guarantee of an adequate diet.
       Fact: Vitamins found in their natural state in foods are the best source. Unless there is a dietary deficiency or some disease present, concentrates are usually not necessary.

6. *Fallacy:* Certain foods such as fish and milk should not be eaten at the same meal.

  Fact: If the foods are unspoiled and are eaten in moderate amounts there is no combination of foods that will be harmful.

7. *Fallacy:* Toast is less fattening than plain bread.

  Fact: Toasting a slice of bread does not alter its caloric content, although it will make the starch more digestible.

8. *Fallacy:* Milk is a "complete" food.

  Fact: Although milk is a good source of complete protein, it does not contain vitamin C, iron, or cellulose.

9. *Fallacy:* Blackstrap molasses and raisins will prevent anemia.

  Fact: There is a very small amount of iron in these foods in comparison to other foods and more than 5 tablespoons of molasses are needed to meet the daily adult requirement of iron.

V. Food Cookery

A. Fruits and vegetables

  1. When dried foods are cooked they should be cooked in the water used to soak them.
  2. Discoloration of some fruits may occur after they have been peeled or cut. Juice from a citrus fruit can be used to prevent this discoloration.
  3. Frozen fruits should be served immediately after they have been thawed.
  4. Avoid soaking fruits or vegetables for long periods of time.
  5. Vegetables cooked whole or in large pieces and with the skins on retain their minerals and vitamins better.
  6. Place vegetables in boiling water for cooking, to preserve the nutrients.
  7. Cook vegetables only until tender. Overcooking destroys nutrients.
  8. Serve vegetables as soon as possible after cooking.

B. Protein foods such as meat, eggs, and milk products should be cooked at low temperatures. High temperatures toughen the protein and make the food less palatable.

C. Cooking fats at high temperatures forms products which are irritating to the intestinal tract. Fats which become liquid at body temperature are more easily digested than those which have a higher melting temperature.

D. Cooking foods obtained from plants softens the cellulose fibers and makes the food more digestible.

E. Cereals are cooked in order to soften the cellulose and make the starch easier to digest.

F. Bouillon and clear soups stimulate the appetite and the flow of gastric juices.

G. Pork and pork products must be cooked thoroughly to avoid the danger of *trichinosis*.

H. Shellfish from polluted streams may carry the organism that causes typhoid fever if not thoroughly cooked.

I. Terms used

  a. Bake—cook with dry heat.
  b. Simmer—cook just below boiling point.
  c. Broil—place under radiant heat.
  d. Sauté—cook quickly in a small amount of fat.

VI. Special Dietary Needs

A. Preschool children

  1. Metabolic rate high in this age group; nutrients essential for health and normal growth.
  2. Eating habits learned during this period. Children develop their eating habits by following the example of those around them.

    a. Mealtime should be relaxed; parents should appear casual about the child's acceptance of food.
    b. Food should not be used as a reward or bribe. Punishment should never consist of depriving the child of food.
    c. Give small servings and then give second helpings if child wishes them.
    d. Appetite may vary from one meal to another.

  3. Foods should be simple and separate; combinations such as in casseroles, etc., not as readily accepted at this age.
  4. Child prefers foods that can be handled with ease and without spilling. Finger foods such as raw fruits and vegetables, mashed potatoes that are fluffy and without lumps, and ground meats that are easy to chew are favorites of this age group.

B. Children from 6 to 12

  1. Nutritional needs of the child still must be met because he is continuing to grow.
  2. School may create some problems; increased activity, emotional upsets, change in routine.
  3. Between-meal snacks become a problem. High-calorie foods tend to dull the appetite and take the place of essential nutrients.

4. Breakfast must not be neglected; variety of foods can be increased at this age.

C. Adolescents from 12 to 20

1. A period of very rapid growth and intense physical activity and emotional adjustments. These factors increase the need for adequate nutrition.
2. Appeal to the importance of food to health, and its relationship to athletic ability and physical appearance. In this way the adolescent can be encouraged to develop good eating habits.
3. Boys at this age eat more than girls, have fewer fears of gaining weight and increasing their height. Need concentrated foods that will satisfy and contain essential nutrients.
4. Girls need foods rich in protein, iron, and other nutrients essential in the formation of red blood cells to replace those lost during menstruation.
5. Breakfast remains a problem; variety of foods and tendency to include foods not generally considered to be "breakfast" foods can help adolescent accept breakfast more readily.

D. The elderly

1. Lowered metabolism and decrease in activity may lessen the caloric requirements.
2. Poor appetite may be traced to lowered ability to digest and assimilate foods, poor teeth or ill-fitting dentures, emotional problems of loneliness and inadequacy, and chronic disease.
3. Small frequent feedings may be preferred to three large meals a day.
4. Older persons are likely to eat diets low in protein, vitamin C, and calcium.
5. Those who live alone may find cooking too exhausting and not worth the bother.
6. Many superstitions about food may be a factor in their refusal to eat a well-balanced diet.

E. Pregnancy and lactation

1. Diet of mother during pregnancy affects the physical health and development of the infant at birth.
2. Weight gain of no more than 22 pounds desirable.
3. Protein necessary because it is needed for formation of new cells and tissues.
4. Special effort must be made to substitute other foods for milk if mother is allergic to milk or refuses to drink it.
5. Iron and calcium important; also, iodine for proper functioning of thyroid gland.
6. High-calorie foods should be avoided.

Questions

1. A balanced diet can best be described as one that:
   1. includes foods that are high in mineral content
   2. eliminates foods that are high in caloric content
   3. meets the nutritional needs of each individual
   4. prevents severe nutritional deficiencies
2. One of the best guarantees of an adequate diet is:
   1. using a variety of foods in the diet
   2. avoiding fatty foods
   3. choosing foods of high caloric content
   4. eliminating carbohydrate foods from the diet
3. One guide for adequate nutrition is the four-group plan for daily intake. The types of foods included in this plan are:
   1. milk, meat, vegetable-fruit, and bread-cereal
   2. milk, meat, vegetables, and cereals
   3. milk, proteins, vegetables, and fruits
   4. milk, proteins, fruits, and bread-cereal
4. In the four-group plan it is recommended that the total daily intake include:
   1. 4 or more servings of meat
   2. 2 or more servings of bread or cereal
   3. at least 1 quart of milk for adults
   4. 4 or more servings of vegetables or fruits
5. As an *alternate* to serving of meat or fish the daily diet could include:
   1. whole grain cereals
   2. dried beans or dried peas
   3. green leafy vegetables
   4. potatoes

6. Fortified vitamin D milk has had vitamin D added to the milk because:
    1. milk does not naturally contain vitamin D
    2. milk contains vitamin C but no vitamin D
    3. the vitamin naturally found in milk is destroyed when the milk is pasteurized
    4. vitamin D is a water-soluble vitamin and is easily destroyed by heating
7. Cereals are foods which are:
    1. digestible only when cooked over a long period of time
    2. chiefly starchy foods
    3. obtained from seeds of plants belonging to the grass family
    4. obtained from wheat and oat plants
8. Starches belong to a group of nutrients called:
    1. fats
    2. carbohydrates
    3. proteins
    4. minerals
9. Which of the following foods would be considered the best source of "quick energy"?
    1. milk
    2. toast
    3. Karo syrup
    4. eggs
10. Nutrients which do not supply our bodies with energy include:
    1. carbohydrates
    2. proteins
    3. fats
    4. minerals
11. Cellulose is best defined as the:
    1. leaves of a plant
    2. most important constituent of cereal foods
    3. fibrous part or "skeleton" of a plant
    4. chief source of minerals in a plant
12. The main function of cellulose in the diet is to provide:
    1. bulk
    2. energy
    3. minerals
    4. vitamins
13. Carbohydrates are stored in animal tissues such as the liver in the form of:
    1. glucose
    2. glycogen
    3. galactose
    4. lactose
14. When cereals are refined many of their important nutrients are lost. The process of replacing these nutrients is called:
    1. fortification
    2. refinement
    3. supplementation
    4. enrichment
15. The body can use carbohydrates only after the sugars and starches in the diet have been converted to:
    1. glycogen
    2. sucrose
    3. glucose
    4. maltose
16. A food containing 20 grams of carbohydrates would have a caloric value of:
    1. 60
    2. 80
    3. 120
    4. 20

17. If fats were completely excluded from the diet the result would be a deficiency in:
    1. vitamins A, D, E, and K
    2. all the vitamins
    3. most of the minerals
    4. most of the essential amino acids

18. Fats are the most concentrated sources of energy because they provide more than twice the number of calories as carbohydrates. A food containing 15 grams of fat would have a caloric value of:
    1. 60
    2. 160
    3. 135
    4. 45

19. Fats are said to have a high satiety value. This means that fats:
    1. are high in caloric content
    2. delay hunger because they stay in the stomach longer
    3. are not digested in the body and serve only to fill the stomach
    4. stimulate the appetite

20. Fats are visible in some foods and the average person knows these foods to be fatty. Other foods contain invisible or "hidden" fats. These foods include:
    1. whole milk and cheese
    2. green leafy vegetables
    3. corn, chocolate, and egg yolk
    4. whole grain cereals

21. Fats are used by the body to provide:
    a. calories for heat and energy
    b. essential fatty acids for growth and maintenance of body functions
    c. essential amino acids for growth and repair of tissues
    d. calcium and iron

    1. all of these
    2. b and d
    3. c and d
    4. a and b

22. One cup of whole milk contains 12 grams of carbohydrate, 9 grams of fat, and 8.5 grams of protein. The total number of calories in one cup of whole milk is:
    1. 100
    2. 48.5
    3. 243.5
    4. 163

23. Fats are emulsified by bile in the digestive tract. This means that the fats are:
    1. converted into fatty acids and glycerol
    2. broken down into smaller particles so they can be digested
    3. converted into carbon dioxide and water
    4. acted on by the chemical enzymes in the stomach

24. Fats which come from plants are usually referred to as oils. These fats are:
    1. solid at room temperatures
    2. liquid at high temperatures only
    3. liquid at room temperatures
    4. solid at very high temperatures

25. Which of the following foods contain all the essential amino acids?
    1. gelatin
    2. nuts
    3. cereals
    4. eggs

26. Using mineral oil as a base for salad dressings or as a regular laxative is unwise chiefly because mineral oil:
    1. has no caloric value
    2. is a very strong laxative
    3. prevents the absorption of vitamins A and D
    4. prevents proper utilization of proteins in the body

27. Some protein foods should be included in every meal because proteins:
    1. are very quickly digested
    2. do not provide the body with energy
    3. are not stored in the body as such
    4. are usually the least expensive type of nutrient

28. Which of the following foods is richest in protein?
    1. cottage cheese
    2. dried beans and peas
    3. whole grain cereals
    4. beets and carrots
29. Proteins in the diet provide the body with amino acids and nitrogen. These substances are used by the body to:
    1. provide heat and energy
    2. produce body tissues, chemical secretions such as hormones and antibodies, and glandular secretions
    3. provide body fat for insulation
    4. manufacture red blood cells
30. A good source of protein for a person on a low calorie diet would be:
    1. pork
    2. cream cheese
    3. powdered skim milk
    4. black coffee
31. Nitrogen that is left after metabolism of proteins is changed to urea and excreted by the:
    1. lungs
    2. intestinal tract
    3. skin
    4. kidneys
32. High quality or complete proteins are those which:
    1. are most expensive to buy
    2. contain all the essential amino acids
    3. contain more nitrogen than other proteins
    4. are damaged by ordinary cooking methods
33. Generally speaking, the best source of complete proteins would be:
    1. animal products such as meat, fish, and eggs
    2. gelatin and cereals
    3. green leafy vegetables
    4. dried beans and peas
34. An example of a complete protein food that contains no fat is:
    1. hamburger
    2. egg white
    3. whole milk
    4. American cheese
35. A food that is plant in origin and contains all the essential amino acids is:
    1. corn
    2. nuts
    3. soybeans
    4. wheat
36. Calcium is an important mineral for adults as well as children because it:
    1. is necessary for the formation of sound teeth
    2. helps in the formation of strong bones
    3. helps muscles contract normally and regulates the heartbeat
    4. is necessary for the transmission of nerve impulses
37. In order to meet the *adult* daily requirement for calcium the diet should include:
    1. at least 2 servings of some citrus fruit
    2. at least 1 egg
    3. at least 2 cups of milk or milk products
    4. 1 serving of whole grain cereals
38. The two minerals most important in the formation of sound bones and teeth in the growing child are:
    1. iron and potassium
    2. iron and calcium
    3. potassium and phosphorus
    4. phosphorus and calcium
39. Iron is an important mineral in the body because it is used to:
    1. build new bone cells
    2. manufacture red blood cells

3. manufacture white blood cells
4. detoxify poisons in the liver

40. If you were planning meals that are rich in iron, which of the following foods should be included?

    a. liver at least once a week
    b. whole grain cereals
    c. dried beans and peas
    d. green leafy vegetables

    1. all of these
    2. a and d
    3. c and d
    4. b and c

41. Iron may be lost in the process of cooking if:

    a. an excessive amount of cooking water is used
    b. the food is cut into small pieces before cooking
    c. the food is not cooked long enough
    d. the food is overcooked

    1. all of these
    2. b and c
    3. a and d
    4. all but c

42. The mineral essential to the normal growth and activity of the thyroid gland is:
    1. iron
    2. iodine
    3. calcium
    4. phosphorus

43. Babies who are fed nothing but milk the first few months of their lives will develop anemia because:
    1. milk contains all the essential nutrients except vitamin C
    2. milk does not contain calcium
    3. there is little or no iron in milk
    4. evaporated milk is usually not fortified with vitamin D

44. The mineral that may be lost through excessive perspiration is:
    1. sodium
    2. calcium
    3. iron
    4. iodine

45. The mineral that is restricted from the diet when severe edema is present is:
    1. calcium
    2. potassium
    3. sodium
    4. iron

46. Fat-soluble vitamins are *not*:
    1. stored in the body
    2. destroyed by ordinary cooking methods
    3. found in animal fats
    4. destroyed when the fat becomes rancid

47. The best sources of vitamin C include:
    1. milk and milk products
    2. green leafy vegetables
    3. cereals
    4. citrus fruits

48. Fish liver oils are an important source of:
    1. calcium
    2. vitamin C
    3. vitamins A and D
    4. riboflavin

49. A deficiency of vitamin K results in:
    1. delay in the clotting of blood
    2. muscle spasms
    3. poor bone formation
    4. extreme irritability of the nerves

50. Fortified margarine has had which of the following vitamins added?
    1. A and B
    2. C and E
    3. A and C
    4. A and D

51. The vitamins in fortified margarine are most likely to be destroyed if the margarine is:
    1. used in cooking
    2. allowed to become rancid
    3. not kept in a warm, dark place
    4. melted by moderate temperatures
52. Which of the following foods can be considered most valuable as sources of thiamine, riboflavin, and niacin?
    1. whole grain cereals
    2. green leafy vegetables
    3. fortified milk
    4. potatoes and tomatoes
53. Scurvy is a deficiency disease resulting from an inadequate intake of:
    1. calcium
    2. phosphorus
    3. vitamin D
    4. vitamin C
54. Rickets is a disease affecting children who have a deficiency of:
    1. vitamin C, calcium, and sodium
    2. vitamin D and sodium
    3. vitamin D, calcium, and phosphorus
    4. vitamin A, vitamin D, and sodium
55. Which of the following statements is true regarding the intake of vitamin preparations?
    1. Only those who are ill need to take vitamin preparations.
    2. Taking an excessive amount of the fat-soluble vitamins is not harmful and probably will increase one's resistance to disease.
    3. Adults who do not drink milk should take extra vitamins to supplement their diet.
    4. Vitamin preparations do not take the place of well-balanced meals.
56. The citrus fruits include:
    1. apples and pears
    2. bananas and figs
    3. oranges, lemons, and limes
    4. grapes and plums
57. The water-soluble vitamins are excreted by the:
    1. intestines
    2. kidneys
    3. liver
    4. skin
58. The minerals used in the formation of hemoglobin are:
    1. iron and copper
    2. calcium and sodium
    3. iron and potassium
    4. calcium and copper
59. The one single item of greatest importance in the diet is:
    1. sugar
    2. sodium
    3. calcium
    4. water
60. Foods will be more appetizing if the meal is planned so that there is:
    1. a high proportion of carbohydrates
    2. a variety in color and texture of the foods
    3. an abundance of seasoning used
    4. a choice of at least three vegetables
61. If economy is a factor in the buying of food, which of the following practices would help decrease the cost of meals?
    a. buying foods that are in season
    b. preparing as much food at home as possible because specially prepared foods are more expensive

    1. all of these
    2. a and c
    3. all but d
    4. b and d

    c.   bearing in mind that expensive foods do
not always provide the most nutrients
for the amount of money spent

    d.   buying only the best grade of meats and
canned foods because these are less
expensive in the long run

62. "Empty calorie" foods are those which supply calories and nothing else. Examples of this type of food include:
1. peanuts and popcorn
2. carbonated beverages and candy
3. bakery products
4. dried fruits

63. Foods which contain a high concentration of sugar are:
1. irritating to the lining of the stomach
2. soothing to the lining of the stomach
3. not as quickly digested as fats
4. easily diluted by secretions from the stomach

64. Which of the following foods could be considered very expensive because of their cost in relation to the number of nutrients they contain?
1. bacon and eggs
2. jams and jellies
3. steak and potatoes
4. whole-grain cereals

65. Which of the following foods should be thoroughly cooked to avoid trichinosis?
1. roast beef
2. poultry products
3. shellfish
4. pork

66. If not properly cooked, shellfish taken from polluted water may be a source of:
1. trichinosis
2. typhoid fever
3. tapeworm
4. botulism

67. Custards and cream fillings should be eaten soon after preparation and refrigerated properly when stored because:
1. bacteria such as staphylococci multiply rapidly in these foods unless they are kept at low temperatures
2. the fat in these foods is poisonous if it becomes rancid
3. all minerals and vitamins are lost if these foods are cooked at temperatures high enough to destroy the bacteria in them
4. cooling these foods alters their taste and destroys the vitamins in them

68. If several persons became ill owing to food poisoning while on a picnic, which of the following foods would be most likely to be the cause?
1. potato salad
2. bananas
3. oatmeal cookies
4. iced tea

69. A mother of a small infant tells you that she does not give her baby orange juice because it causes the urine to be too acid and irritating. What is the best answer you could give her?
1. Acid fruits may cause an excess of acidity in the body and to counteract this she could give the baby a small amount of baking soda after the orange juice.
2. Acid fruits actually are rendered alkaline by the process of digestion. The irritation from the urine may be caused by improper rinsing of the baby's diapers.
3. Even though some people are allergic to orange juice she should give it to the infant because it is an important source of vitamin C.
4. Diluting the orange juice in water will dilute the acidity and make the urine less irritating.

70. A patient on a low-calorie diet asks you if she might have two slices of toast in

place of one slice of bread because toast is less fattening than bread. How should you reply?
1. Toasting bread does not change its caloric value.
2. Toast is less digestible than bread and she should use only those foods which are easily digestible while on a low calorie diet.
3. It would be better if she ate only one slice of toast and made up for the lost calories by substituting a fruit.
4. Toasting destroys the vitamins in bread and therefore toast is less nutritious than bread.

71. If you are told by a patient that she takes a little blackstrap molasses every day to prevent anemia and to guarantee a healthy old age, which of the following statements would be the best reply?
    1. Blackstrap molasses will prevent anemia but does not prolong life.
    2. Blackstrap molasses does not contain any iron but it has been proven to be an essential part of every diet.
    3. It would take a little over 5 tablespoons of blackstrap molasses to supply the daily iron requirement of an adult woman.
    4. There are no minerals or vitamins in blackstrap molasses.

72. A friend of yours is overweight and she has heard of a diet in which only lean meats are eaten and skim milk is taken as a beverage. She expects to lose 5 pounds a day on this diet. What advice should you give her?
    1. Too much protein can be harmful and she should supplement the diet with vitamin pills.
    2. The diet will probably work if she takes exercises while she is following the diet.
    3. It is not wise to follow any type of special diet without consulting a dietitian or physician for advice on its value.
    4. A diet of this kind does not provide many of the essential amino acids and the loss of 5 pounds a day is dangerous to one's health and well-being.

73. If an opened can of applesauce is left in the refrigerator overnight it would be correct to:
    1. discard the food because it is most likely to be poisonous
    2. realize that the taste of the food may be changed slightly, but this is not harmful
    3. heat the applesauce to destroy bacteria that have multiplied while the applesauce was cold
    4. realize that all nutrients in the food have been lost due to improper storage

74. Milk cannot be considered a "complete food" because it:
    1. does not contain any carbohydrates
    2. does not contain vitamin C, iron, or cellulose
    3. has no caloric content
    4. is rendered alkaline in the process of digestion

75. Which of the following methods of cooking would preserve the maximum number of nutrients in dried apricots?
    1. cooking them in the water in which they were soaked
    2. washing them thoroughly and then cutting into small pieces before soaking
    3. soaking them in orange juice and then discarding the juice before cooking
    4. lifting them out of the water in which they were soaking and immediately placing them in boiling water

76. When peeling vegetables prior to cooking them, minerals and vitamins are less likely to be lost if:
    1. the vegetables are not washed prior to peeling
    2. the vegetables are soaked in cold water overnight
    3. the skin is removed carefully so that only the thin outer layer is peeled
    4. the skin is scraped off and the vegetables are then soaked in warm water for several hours

77. The term *baking* means:
    1. cooking in a covered saucepan
    2. cooking by dry heat
    3. placing under radiant heat
    4. cooking at a very high temperature

78. Vegetables will retain practically all their mineral content and flavor if they are:
    1. cut into small pieces and boiled
    2. cooked over an open flame or hot coals
    3. baked in their skins
    4. cooked over a long period of time
79. Whenever possible, *raw* fruits and vegetables should be included in the menu because:
    1. cooking destroys the flavor
    2. excessive heat destroys minerals
    3. cooking removes the cellulose in plants
    4. cooking usually destroys some of the minerals and vitamins
80. The term *simmer* means:
    1. cooking in boiling water
    2. baking at a low temperature
    3. cooking just below the boiling point
    4. frying quickly in a small amount of fat
81. Clear soups are often used as a first course in meals because they:
    1. have no nutritive value but do help fill the stomach
    2. stimulate the appetite by increasing the flow of digestive juices in the stomach
    3. contain most of the nutrients and thereby guarantee a well-balanced meal
    4. inhibit the flow of digestive juices and slow down the process of digestion
82. Some fruits become discolored after they have been peeled or sliced. To avoid this discoloration it would be best to:
    1. heat the fruit before cutting
    2. soak the fruit in cold water after cutting
    3. add a small amount of juice from a citrus fruit
    4. rub the fruit with ice before cutting
83. Eggs are more digestible and retain their flavor best if they are cooked:
    1. at a very high temperature for a short period of time
    2. at a low temperature
    3. at a high temperature for a long period of time
    4. in combination with some other food that has a stronger flavor
84. Cooking cereals is done for the purpose of:
    1. removing the indigestible fibers they contain
    2. softening the cellulose and making the starch easier to digest
    3. preventing the loss of the vitamins they contain
    4. breaking down the sugars into glucose
85. When vegetables are cooked in water there will be a minimal loss of nutrients if the vegetables are:
    1. placed in boiling water and cooked only until tender
    2. placed in cold water and allowed to cook slowly over a period of time
    3. cooked until the cellulose has disintegrated
    4. cooked at temperatures just below the boiling point and allowed to simmer until all water has evaporated
86. If fats are subjected to extremely high temperature they soon reach the "smoking" point. When fats are heated in this manner they:
    1. are more easily digested
    2. will release their vitamins more readily
    3. are completely indigestible
    4. form products which are irritating to the digestive tract
87. The one meal most neglected by young people in America is:
    1. breakfast
    2. lunch
    3. dinner
    4. bedtime snack
88. A young mother of a 3-year-old child asks you what she can do to encourage her child to eat the meals he is served. Which of the following statements best describes the proper attitude toward feeding children?
    a. Never allow a child to eat his dessert until he has eaten all the food on his plate, and has thus deserved the "reward" of dessert.

    1. all of these
    2. all but b
    3. c and d
    4. b and d

    b. If you force a child to eat a little of everything and punish him when he refuses, he will eventually develop a liking for all foods.

    c. Children learn their eating habits from the adults around them.

    d. Try to develop a casual attitude toward eating and use a variety of foods to develop a variety of tastes for food.

89. Which of the following menus do you think would be most acceptable to a child 4 years old?
1. Tuna casserole, sliced tomatoes, baked potato, skim milk, and ice cream
2. Hamburger pattie, mashed potatoes, sticks of carrots and celery, milk, banana, and cookies
3. Tomato soup, fried fish, cole slaw, milk, and tapioca pudding
4. Creamed eggs, English peas, avocado and grapefruit salad, milk, and sherbet

90. If an adolescent in your family refuses to eat a nourishing breakfast, which of the following do you think would be the best solution to this problem?
1. Allow him to eat doughnuts with his cup of coffee but insist that he take his vitamin supplements.
2. Avoid discussing this with him if it seems to irritate him and encourage him to eat a good lunch at school.
3. Explain the value of a good breakfast and try varying the breakfast menu by using toasted cheese sandwiches, peanut butter and jelly, and other nourishing foods not generally considered to be breakfast foods.
4. Realize that he has almost reached the peak of his growth and probably does not need to eat as much as he did when he was much younger.

91. Adolescent girls need foods rich in protein, iron, and other minerals because:
1. they grow more rapidly than boys, at this age
2. girls usually need less energy because they are less active
3. these nutrients are needed for the formation of red blood cells lost during menstruation
4. the metabolic rate is higher in girls than in boys

92. A 14-year-old girl refuses to eat an adequate diet because she is afraid it will make her gain weight and grow taller. Which of the following statements would you choose as the best reply to her objections?
1. A well-balanced diet does not necessarily result in a gain in weight, and the nutrients in such a diet are needed if one is to look and feel his best.
2. Even though such a diet may result in a gain in weight, health is more important than one's physical appearance.
3. Young people usually do not appreciate the value of good eating habits, but they must learn to accept the advice of their elders.
4. Physical appearance may seem important to her now but she will learn as she grows older that good health is more important:

93. Since the physical activities of an elderly person are likely to be much less than those of children or middle-aged adults, the diet of a person over 70 years of age should be:
1. lower in protein content
2. higher in fat content
3. lower in caloric value
4. higher in carbohydrate content

94. The three nutrients most likely to be missing from the diet of an elderly person who prepares her own meals are:
1. carbohydrates, vitamins A and D
2. protein, iodine, and sodium
3. fats, iron, and calcium
4. proteins, calcium, and vitamin C

95. If Mrs. Jones, who is 74 years old, tells you that she does not prepare three meals a day when she is at home alone, it is most likely because:
1. she is not hungry and therefore is not lacking any essential nutrients in her diet

2. she is lazy and does not realize the importance of three regular meals a day
3. cooking exhausts her and mealtime has become a chore rather than a pleasure
4. she has decided that refusing to eat is a way of getting attention. If she gets hungry enough she will eat the food she needs

96. If an elderly relative in your home refuses to eat more than half the food prepared for him at each of the three meals, you might improve his intake of essential nutrients by:
    1. omitting one of the meals so he will be hungry and eat more at the other two meals
    2. giving him small frequent feedings in place of three large meals
    3. concentrating on carbohydrate foods that will provide him with energy, since he really does not need other foods at his age
    4. eliminating all fats from his diet and substituting foods that provide quick energy

97. When planning meals for elderly persons one should keep in mind that:
    1. their nutritional needs are much less than those of persons who are more active
    2. older persons instinctively know which foods are best for them
    3. diet has little effect on the health and well-being of elderly people
    4. older persons have a lowered ability to digest and assimilate foods

98. A young woman 20 years old tells you that she is pregnant and has heard that an adequate intake of milk is important during pregnancy. She asks you why milk is so important. What would be the best reply?
    1. Research has proven that milk is not as essential as many other foods and is of minor importance during pregnancy.
    2. Although milk is very important as a source of proteins and vitamins, a variety of foods should be included in the diet of the expectant mother.
    3. Milk is important in the diet during pregnancy only if the mother expects to breast-feed her infant.
    4. The proteins and minerals in milk are used by the body to build strong bones and teeth and healthy tissues; without these it is not possible for the fetus to develop properly.

99. A patient in the prenatal clinic tells you that she cannot tolerate the taste of milk and asks if it would be all right to omit milk from her diet. What would be the best reply to this question?
    1. Calcium tablets can take the place of milk in the diet.
    2. Taking cod liver oil will provide the vitamin D that is the most important nutrient in milk.
    3. It is difficult to replace all the nutrients in milk, and many of these nutrients are essential to the health and proper development of the fetus.
    4. If the mother does not drink enough milk during pregnancy she will not be able to breast-feed her baby.

100. In order to help this mother find a substitute for drinking whole milk you should tell her that:
    1. cheese, ice cream, and custards and soups made with nonfat dried milk will help supply the need for nutrients contained in whole milk
    2. there is not a substitute for drinking milk and she had best make up her mind to drink the milk if she is concerned with the health of her infant
    3. green leafy vegetables contain almost the same nutrients as whole milk
    4. eggs and lean meat are excellent substitutes for milk

101. The average weight gain considered to be desirable during pregnancy is:
    1. no more than one third the average weight
    2. calculated according to the size of infants born previously
    3. a minimum of 40 pounds
    4. 22 to 24 pounds

102. Which of the following foods do you consider to be most undesirable for a woman who is pregnant?
    1. eggs and cheese
    2. french fried potatoes, pastries, and nuts
    3. sherbets and canned fruit
    4. whole-grain cereals

Part V

BASIC NURSING

UNIT 1 PATIENT CARE

I. Introduction
A. Essentially, nursing care is doing for the patient those things which he cannot do for himself to assure physical and mental comfort and well-being.
1. Is an individual problem depending on each individual patient and his needs.
2. Ultimate goal is to restore the patient to his former state of health or help him adjust to his physical handicap.
B. Nursing care plan
1. A method of organizing the care so as to achieve best results.
2. Must be based on nursing problems of each patient and ways of solving these problems.
3. Two aspects
a. Medical care delegated by the physician.
b. Other responsibilities for patient comfort, personal hygiene, health education, etc.
4. Is a flexible plan so that it can be altered as the patient's needs and problems change, and as medical treatment changes.
5. Plan must take into consideration the patient's diagnosis, age, sex, social and cultural background, mental attitudes, and ability and willingness to help himself.
6. Needs of the patient may be met by a variety of individuals on the medical team, or those familiar with the patient's problems.
a. Physical needs—physician, professional and nonprofessional nursing service personnel, physical therapist, occupational therapist.
b. Emotional needs—physician, nursing

personnel, minister or rabbi, family and friends, clinical psychologist.
c. Spiritual needs—physician, nursing personnel, minister or rabbi, family and friends.
d. Financial needs—patient and his family, health insurance, voluntary and governmental agencies.
C. Effects of illness on patient
1. Physical handicap may be temporary or permanent. Rehabilitation of the patient is always kept in mind.
2. Emotional stress produced by illness. Reaction may be one of fear, anger, resentment, depression. Patient needs continued reassurance of nurse's interest in him *as a person.*
3. Illness may cause an individual to become more aware of his spiritual welfare and increase his need for spiritual guidance. Minister or rabbi is person most likely to be of assistance, but this does not relieve nurse of her responsibility to give patient moral support and recognize his spiritual needs.

II. Principles Governing Nursing Care
A. There are four general steps in every nursing measure: preparation, performance, aftercare, and recording and reporting.
1. Preparation
a. Nurse prepares herself by learning correct steps of the procedure.
b. Patient is prepared emotionally by having procedure explained, and physically by positioning and screening, draping, or other environmental changes as needed.
2. Carrying out procedure—nurse does this as taught and in a safe, comfortable, and efficient manner.

3. After-care of patient and equipment. Patient is made comfortable; used equipment is removed from room as necessary and is cleaned and returned to proper place.
4. The nursing measure and effects on patient are recorded and reported intelligently and accurately.

B. Nurses should establish good work habits.
1. Plan ahead so as to save steps and time. Assemble all needed equipment before starting procedure.
2. Work toward a "finished appearance," completing one assignment and replacing equipment before going on to next task.
3. Clean up any spills immediately and discard soiled linens as soon as possible.

C. Know your patient
1. Treat each patient as a person.
2. Develop an interest in his special needs.
3. Strive to learn all that you can about his particular illness, diagnostic tests, and medical treatment.

D. Good housekeeping and cleanliness are essential to the comfort and general welfare of the patient.

III. The Patient's Environment

A. Atmospheric conditions affect comfort and health.
1. Temperature—ideal is 65 to 72° F. (18 to 22° C.).
   a. Should be slightly higher during bed bath, may be lowered at night during sleep.
   b. Older persons and very small babies may require slightly higher temperatures.
2. Ventilation—needed to assure supply of fresh air and remove stale air.
   a. If windows are opened do not open windows or doors exactly opposite one another and create draft.
   b. Avoid drafts and sudden changes in temperature.
3. Humidity—amount of moisture in air in relation to temperature.
   a. Ideal is 30 to 50 per cent.
   b. High humidity with low temperature produces chilliness.
   c. High humidity with high temperature allows little or no evaporation of perspiration and causes discomfort.
   d. Low humidity dries out mucous membranes of nose and mouth and produces discomfort and irritation.

B. Physical conditions
1. Lighting—may be artificial or natural.
   a. Sunlight is more healing and cheerful, artificial light should be used only when necessary.
   b. Avoid glare on patient's eyes; overhead lights may be annoying to patient lying in bed.
   c. Floor lamps are placed so patient can adjust as desired.
2. Control of pests
   a. Screening of windows and doors essential.
   b. Cleanliness in utility rooms and kitchens of hospital.
   c. Avoid keeping meal trays on wards after patient has eaten; return to main kitchen.

C. Esthetic conditions
1. Term refers to conditions that are pleasing or displeasing to the senses.
2. Odors
   a. Bedpans, urinals, dressings, etc. removed from the patient's room immediately after use.
   b. Certain foods may be displeasing while they are being cooked.
   c. Nurses must avoid strong perfumes and colognes. Smoking leaves nurse's breath offensive.
   d. Illness may make a person more sensitive to odors.
3. Noises should be eliminated as much as possible.
   a. Noise stimulates the patient and may produce fatigue.
   b. Slamming doors, dropping equipment, etc. startles the patient and increases irritation and restlessness.
   c. Radios and televisions of other patients should be turned low.
4. Privacy
   a. The nurse has an obligation to respect and preserve the privacy and modesty of her patients.
   b. Screens, curtains, drapes are employed to provide physical privacy.
   c. Nurse must also consider personal privacy in spiritual and social matters.

D. Safety—the keynote of all care.
1. Utensils must not be chipped or cracked.
2. Electrical equipment must be in good working order, with no defects.
3. Floors clean and not slippery; mop up spilled liquids immediately. Keep floor clear of obstacles that may cause falls.
4. Place things within easy reach so patient will not fall out of bed trying to get them. Use side rails when patient is elderly, very young, disoriented or confused, or under sedation.
5. Be sure solutions for irrigation are at correct temperature.

6. Check temperature of hot water bottles and heating pads.
7. Correctly label all containers.
8. Restraints are used to restrict or limit the activity of a patient only when necessary and on written order of the physician. They must be removed at frequent intervals and the position of the patient changed. All restraints predispose a patient to pressure sores and stimulate resistance in an unconscious or conscious patient.

IV. The Patient's Unit
A. Unit refers to patient's room or the furnishings and equipment needed by each patient.
B. A disorderly room can create confusion and restlessness for the patient and indirectly affect his physical health and peace of mind. If a patient enjoys having his possessions around him and does not mind the clutter, his wishes may be respected as long as they do not serve as a source of infection.
C. Dirt and dust are carriers of disease.
D. General principles
 1. Hot water coagulates and hardens the albumin or protein wastes present in all excreta. Use cold water to remove excreta before washing utensil.
 2. Rubber goods—extreme heat ruins rubber; oil makes rubber soft and causes it to deteriorate; folding causes rubber to crack.
 3. Glassware—breaks and chips easily and is affected by sudden temperature change.
 4. Enamelware—chips easily; sudden temperature change causes cracking.
 5. Plastic—can never be boiled; thin plastic tears easily.
 6. Stainless steel—most expensive but very durable. Will dent if dropped.
 7. Type of cleanser or disinfectant depends on microorganisms present and degree of contamination.
 8. Damp cloth used for dusting.
 9. Equipment used must be cleaned and returned to its proper place immediately after use.
 10. Cleanliness is responsibility of all nursing service personnel, not just housekeeping department.
 11. Proper care of equipment prolongs its life and usefulness.
E. Care of flowers
 1. Change water in vases of cut flowers at least once a day.
 2. Discard dead flowers only with patient's consent.
 3. Water potted plants as needed.
 4. When preparing cut flowers, place in water and cut stems diagonally while under water.
 5. Water in flower vases can serve as a source of infection.

V. Bed Making
A. Purposes
 1. To make a comfortable and safe bed.
 2. To give the unit or ward a neat appearance.
B. General principles
 1. A bed made properly so that the bottom sheets are smooth and free of wrinkles provides comfort and prevents decubitus ulcers.
 2. In order to provide tight, smooth linen one must pull the linen tight rather than smooth and pat it into place.
 3. Linen should be kept close to the bed while it is being applied or removed from the bed. Fanning the linen stirs up dust and spreads bacteria.
 4. Linen is removed one piece at a time to check for articles left in the bed by the patient.
 5. Avoid touching your clothing with soiled linen.
 6. Complete one side of bed before going to other side.
 7. Use good body mechanics to avoid fatigue and muscle strain.
C. Types of beds
 1. Closed—top covers and spread pulled up to protect bottom linen. Made after patient is discharged.
 2. Open—top covers fan folded to foot of bed in preparation for patient.
 3. Occupied—one in which the patient is lying.
 4. Ether, anesthetic, or surgical bed—one prepared for return of patient who is in surgery. Top covers usually fan folded to side of bed, open side of bed facing door. They are sometimes folded to the foot.

VI. Personal Care of the Patient
A. Care of the skin—essential to health and a feeling of well-being.
 1. Purposes of the bath
  a. To refresh and relax the patient, thereby relieving fatigue.
  b. To cleanse the skin and protect it from breakdown.
  c. To increase elimination of wastes through the skin.
  d. To stimulate circulation.
 2. General principles of the bed bath
  a. Avoid chilling or exposing the patient.
  b. The temperature of the bath water should be 105 to 115° F. (41 to 46° C.) unless physician gives other orders.

c. Bath water should be changed at least once during the bath and more often if necessary.

d. Lengthy conversation during the bath may irritate or tire the patient. Use this time to *listen* to the patient if he apparently wants to talk.

e. Use long, smooth strokes when bathing the patient.

f. Bath cloth is folded into a mitt to prevent dripping water on linens.

g. Use soap sparingly and rinse well to avoid irritation of the skin.

h. Report any unusual redness, bruises, swelling, or cuts.

i. Oils and lotions help restore some of the natural oils of the skin. Alcohol has a drying effect.

j. If patient is paralyzed, each joint should be put through its full range of motion during the bed bath, unless contraindicated.

3. Tub baths

a. May be ordered to treat inflammation or infections of the pelvis.

b. Sometimes used to relieve pain and discomfort following rectal surgery, cystoscopy, or vaginal surgery.

c. Ambulatory patients allowed tub baths on order of physician.

d. The condition of the patient and his attitude determine the amount of supervision necessary.

e. If the patient becomes fatigued or dizzy he should be removed from the tub immediately. If help is needed to get patient out of tub, let water out of tub, wrap patient in a bath blanket and then go for help.

f. If patient is left in tub alone, nurse must remain within calling distance.

g. Cleanse tub thoroughly after patient has had bath.

4. Prevention and treatment of decubitus ulcers (bed sores):

a. Prevention of decubitus ulcers much easier than treatment and cure of them.

b. Prevention aimed at relieving constant pressure of the body's weight on any part of the body.

c. Decubitus ulcers occur most commonly over bony prominences and in obese or emaciated patients. However, they may occur in any patient unless care is taken to prevent pressure, friction, or irritation of the skin.

d. Nursing measures to prevent decubitus ulcers

1. Keep the skin clean and dry.

2. Keep bed dry and free of wrinkles.

3. Turn patient frequently and provide relief of pressure on any part of the body over a period of time.

4. Exercise care to prevent friction against the skin when turning patient or removing linen from the bed.

5. Use care when giving and removing bedpan.

6. Protect the skin from splints, casts, and restraints by padding them with cotton or foam rubber.

7. Bathe and gently massage pressure areas frequently.

e. Treatment of decubitus ulcers

1. Expose to air. Heat lamps and bed cradles may be used.

2. Apply medication as ordered.

3. Relieve pressure on area.

4. Other measures will depend on physician's orders.

B. Care of mouth and teeth

1. Purposes

a. To keep the mouth clean and moist.

b. To help prevent tooth decay and halitosis.

2. General principles

a. Correct toothbrush is one in which the bristles are set in tufts and evenly spaced along the working surface of the brush.

b. When brushing the teeth, hold brush at 45° angle and use a circular, scrubbing motion.

c. Choice of dentifrice up to the individual. Commercial dentifrices are basically the same, and serve only as an aid to cleansing. Most important factor is proper method of brushing.

d. Mouthwashes also are essentially the same. May reduce bacterial count in the mouth for a very short period of time, but tap water may be just as effective. It is the mechanical rinsing that is important. Mouthwash strong enough to destroy all microorganisms would be too harmful to tissues of the mouth. Most bacteria in the mouth will cause halitosis, but are not harmful to the body.

3. Special mouth care

a. If patient is unable to brush his own teeth, the nurse must do this for him.

b. Unconscious patient must have frequent mouth care.

1. Unconscious patients usually are mouth breathers and their mouths dry out quickly.

2. Teeth are cleansed with padded tongue blade and mouthwash.

3. Lips are lubricated with glycerin

and lemon juice mixture, cold cream, or small amount of mineral oil.

4. Care of removable dentures
   a. Cleanliness important; should be cleaned at least twice a day.
   b. Clean thoroughly with a brush under gentle stream of warm, never hot, running water. Be sure to pad lavatory bowl or place pan of water under teeth in case dentures are dropped.
   c. Dentures are removed by gripping firmly with tissues or gauze square and gently lifting.
   d. When dentures are not in use they should be kept in denture cup labeled with patient's name and room number.
5. Remember that dentures are expensive and valuable to the patient. Avoid chipping or breaking them when cleaning, and put them in proper place when not in use.

C. Care of the hair
   1. Daily brushing and periodic shampooing important to the health and appearance of scalp and hair; contribute to good grooming and sense of well-being.
   2. Special points to remember
      a. Tangles can be removed by wetting the hair with alcohol before combing.
      b. Long hair may be braided to prevent matting and tangling.
      c. Never cut a patient's hair without her permission, or the consent of the family.
      d. Do not neglect care of male patient's hair.
      e. Pediculi capitis (head lice) prevented by cleanliness. Treatment with medication done according to doctor's order. Nits (eggs) may be removed with vinegar and combing with fine tooth comb.

D. Care of the nails
   1. Purposes
      a. To improve the patient's general appearance.
      b. To avoid infection of the skin due to organisms lodging under the nails.
   2. General principles
      a. Soak hands well before cleaning nails. Avoid damaging the nails with sharp instruments when manicuring the nails.
      b. Push cuticle back with towel after soaking hands. Do not damage nail beds with sharp instruments.
      c. Shape fingernails with emery board. File or cut toenails straight across.
      d. Toenails should not be cut shorter than the tips of the toes.

E. Providing for elimination
   1. Elimination of wastes through kidneys and intestines of increased importance during illness.
   2. General principles
      a. Provide privacy for patient.
      b. Patient should be left alone unless contraindicated by weakness, delirium, etc.; be sure call light is within reach of patient being left alone.
      c. Bedpans and urinals are thoroughly washed and sterilized after each use.
   3. Use of bedpan
      a. Have patient flex knees and lift himself by pushing with soles of feet.
      b. Slide bedpan into position. If patient cannot lift himself, the nurse places her hand under the small of his back and lifts gently. If patient is completely helpless, turn him on side, place bedpan against buttocks and turn back onto bedpan.
      c. Elevate head of bed unless otherwise indicated.
      d. Place toilet paper and call light within reach.
      e. Remove bedpan promptly and cover immediately.
      f. Provide patient with materials for washing his hands.
      g. Observe contents of bedpan and record observations. Measure urine if output is being recorded. Save specimen if indicated.
   4. Giving and removing urinal
      a. Male orderly usually assists helpless male patients.
      b. If patient can help himself, place urinal under top linens so patient can grasp handle.
      c. Leave patient after placing call light within reach.
      d. After removing urinal, provide patient with materials to wash his hands.
      e. Observe contents, measure, or save specimen as indicated.
   5. The incontinent patient
      a. Incontinence—inability to control defecation or urination.
      b. Special problems—skin breaks down more readily, odor offensive and embarrassing to patient.
      c. Frequent and regular use of bedpan often prevents embarrassing accidents and soiling of linens.
      d. Large absorbent pads under patient facilitate frequent changing and help keep patient dry without changing bed linens.
   6. Nursing measures to induce voiding
      a. Sometimes necessary when patient

has urinary retention following vaginal or rectal surgery, or after delivery.
    b. Catheterization performed only on doctor's order and after other measures have failed.
    c. Have patient assume as nearly natural a position as possible.
    d. The sound of running water or pouring warm water over the vulva often stimulates voiding.
    e. Give bedpan as soon as requested.
    f. Provide privacy and relieve patient's anxiety or nervousness.
F. Nursing measures to induce sleep
    1. Quiet and darkness are desirable in inducing sleep.
    2. Reassure patient and help him relax.
    3. Provide adequate ventilation and sufficient warmth with lightweight blankets.
    4. A warm bath is soothing and relaxing. Cold baths and hot baths are both stimulating.
    5. Back rub promotes relaxation
        a. Use lotion or alcohol, unless contraindicated.
        b. The back is rubbed with long smooth strokes.
        c. Massage with both hands and work with a stronger upward than downward stroke.
        d. Give particular attention to pressure areas and bony prominences, the neck and shoulders, and lower back (sacrum).
    6. Always avoid indiscriminate use of drugs to induce sleep. Hypnotics are used after nursing measures fail.
    7. Help patient assume comfortable position and reassure him that the nurse is nearby should he need her.

VII. Body Mechanics
A. Posture—position or arrangement of the different parts of the body in relation to each other.
B. Good posture—the key to comfort, health, and appearance.
C. Posture affects efficiency.
    1. Good posture provides better mechanical use of the body.
    2. Good posture gives impression of grace, vigor, and good breeding.
D. Undesirable effects of poor posture
    1. Increases fatigue and strains muscles.
    2. Internal organs are displaced and cramped, leading to impairment of function; e.g., poor expansion of lungs, indigestion, constipation.
    3. Physical appearance undesirable.
E. Good standing position (Fig. 17)—head is held high and chin is in, abdomen flat

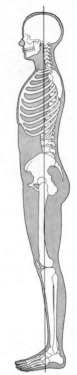

FIGURE 17.   Correct posture. (Turner, C. E.: *Personal and Community Health*, 12th ed., St. Louis, The C. V. Mosby Co., 1963.)

and back straight, shoulders back, knees slightly flexed, toes pointed straight ahead, and weight borne chiefly by ankles.
F. Good sitting position (Fig. 18)—"sit tall" without trying to hold certain parts of body

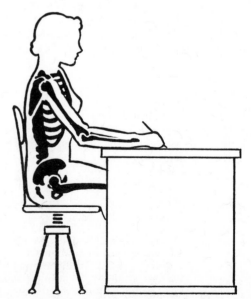

FIGURE 18.   Correct working posture for writing. (Courtesy Samuel Higby Camp Institute for Better Posture.)

in a prescribed position. Sit squarely on buttocks and thighs. Feet should be resting on the floor.

G. Lifting and moving
1. Body must be in correct alignment.
2. Feet placed far enough apart to provide a wide base.
3. Move an object toward rather than away.
4. Use muscles of legs, arms, shoulders, rather than of back and abdomen.
5. Flex the knees and place one foot slightly forward to maintain balance.

H. Moving patient from stretcher to bed
1. Place stretcher at right angles to bed. This requires three persons; one acts as captain and counts so that they all move in unison.
2. The three place their arms so that the patient's body and head are well supported.
3. If patient is conscious explain the procedure and enlist his cooperation.
4. Place patient on bed gently.

I. Turning patient onto his side
1. First, move patient over to side opposite that to which he is to be turned. Always move a patient TOWARD you.
2. Go to other side of bed and roll patient toward you. If patient's uppermost knee is flexed turning will be easier.
3. After turning patient onto his side support uppermost leg with pillow, and

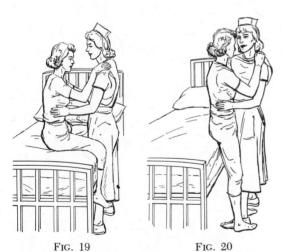

FIG. 19   FIG. 20

FIGURE 19. The nurse stands directly in front of the patient, with a wide base of support, pelvis stabilized, hands around the rib cage of the patient, and the upper arm of the nurse adducted to the body. One leg is placed between the patient's knees to break any possible fall of the patient. The patient leans forward with her arms on the shoulders of the nurse. FIGURE 20. The patient is then eased to a standing position on the floor and is ready to pivot to the chair with the nurse assisting. Note the body mechanics of the nurse. (Montag, M. L. and Swenson, R. S.: *Fundamentals in Nursing Care.* 3rd ed., Philadelphia, W. B. Saunders Co., 1959.)

support arm to prevent strain on shoulder and reduce the weight of his arm on chest.

J. Getting patient up into a chair (Figs. 19 and 20)
1. Be sure that chair is firmly anchored (if wheel chair, lock wheels so that it will not roll). Place chair beside bed.
2. Help patient to sitting position on side of bed.
3. Face the patient and ask him to place his hands on your shoulders. Place your hands under patient's armpits. Keep your feet far enough apart to give you a wide base.
4. Let patient slide gently to the floor.
5. Pivot and gently lower patient into chair. If using a wheel chair be sure that foot rests are folded up out of the way.
6. If patient is able to help himself and can use a foot stool, you may stand to the side of the patient to help him down. Place one arm around patient's back and the other under his axilla.

VIII. **Proper Positioning of Patient (Figs. 21, 22, and 23)**
A. Good posture in bed—position of the body should not vary from the standing position. Back straight and parts of the body adequately supported.
B. Promoting comfort through proper positioning
1. Pillows should be placed so that the body bends at the hips, not at the waist or neck.
2. Small pillows may be used to support the curves of the body.
3. Use of foot boards prevents foot drop because it keeps feet in normal position, and avoids strain on leg muscles.
4. Bed cradle supports the weight of the top covers and helps keep the feet in proper position (Fig. 24).
5. Keep top covers loose enough to allow movement of feet. Very tight covers may lead to foot drop.
6. Position of patient must be changed frequently to avoid fixation of joints and pressure areas on skin.
C. Therapeutic positions
1. Fowler's position—the head of the bed is raised or the patient is supported with pillows so that he is in a semisitting position. The knees are slightly flexed to prevent slipping down in bed.
2. Trendelenburg position—the head is lowered and the knees are slightly flexed to prevent slipping toward the head of the bed. Used for some types of surgery and in the treatment of shock.
3. Sims left lateral—patient is lying on left side with right knee and thigh flexed.

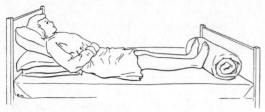

FIG. 21

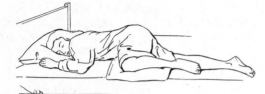

FIG. 22

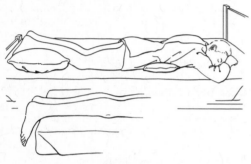

FIG. 23

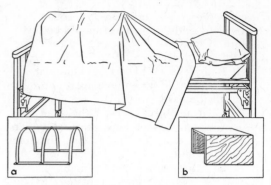

FIGURE 24. Cradle in position on bed. Inset *a* shows hospital-type cradle and inset *b* shows improvised cradle. (Montag and Swenson: *Fundamentals in Nursing Care.* 3rd ed.)

FIGURE 21. Patient lying on back. Blanket roll or footboard and pillows may be used to keep feet in correct position. Note support of patient's back with pillows. (Todd and Freeman: *Health Care of the Family.*) FIGURE 22. Patient lying on side. Pillow is placed under knee to maintain good alignment of back. (Todd and Freeman: *Health Care of the Family.*) FIGURE 23. Patient lying in prone position. Small pillow is placed under abdomen and under lower legs. Alternate position of feet may be used to maintain them in correct position. (Montag and Swenson: *Fundamentals in Nursing Care.* 3rd ed.)

    4. Orthopneic—back rest fully elevated, knees slightly flexed. Overbed table padded with pillows, patient's head rests on arms folded, supported by pillows. Used when patient cannot breathe lying down.

IX. **Exercises**
  A. Done to prevent atrophy of muscles, contractures and fixation of the joints.
  B. Types of exercise
    1. Active—those the patient can do himself.
    2. Passive—those that must be done for the patient.
  C. Special points to remember
    1. Be gentle and work slowly.

    2. Do not use force to move any part of the body.
    3. Do not fatigue the patient.

X. **Serving Foods and Fluids**
  A. Preparation of patient for meals
    1. Provide necessary articles so patient may wash his face and hands before eating.
    2. Position patient so that he will be comfortable and relaxed while eating.
    3. Place tray conveniently so that patient can reach all articles on it.
    4. Do not serve tray to helpless patient until someone is ready to feed him.
  B. General principles
    1. The manner in which the tray is arranged and served affects patient's appetite.
    2. Meals must be served so that hot foods are hot and cold foods cold when served.
    3. Mealtime should be a pleasant experience; avoid hurrying the patient.
    4. In some instances the physician is aided in his diagnosis and treatment of illness by the nurse's observation of a patient's eating habits.
    5. Meal trays of diabetic patients must be checked carefully after each meal to determine exact amount of food eaten.
    6. Special diets are a form of treatment and must be given as ordered by the physician.
    7. Most patients who do not need assistance prefer to be left alone while eating their meals.
  C. Feeding helpless patient
    1. Tray should be placed so patient can see the food being offered to him.
    2. Blind patients should be informed of various foods on tray.
    3. Food is offered in small amounts and in

Table 6.   Types of Hospital Diets

	CLEAR LIQUID DIET	FULL LIQUID DIET	SOFT DIET	REGULAR-HOUSE GENERAL-FULL
Characteristics	Temporary diet of clear liquids without residue. Nonstimulating, nongas-forming, nonirritating.	Foods liquid at room temperature or liquefying at body temperature.	Normal diet modified in consistency to have no roughage. Liquids and semisolid food; easily digested.	Practically all foods. Simple, easy-to-digest foods, simply prepared, palatably seasoned.
Adequacy	Inadequate: deficient in protein, minerals, vitamins, and calories.	Can be adequate with careful planning; adequacy depends on liquids used.	Entirely adequate liberal diet.	Adequate and well balanced.
Use	Acute illness and infections. Postoperatively. Temporary food intolerance. To relieve thirst. Reduce colonic fecal matter. 1 to 2 hour feeding intervals.	Transition between clear liquid and soft diets. Postoperatively. Acute gastritis and infections. Febrile conditions. Intolerance for solid food. 2 to 4 hour feeding intervals.	Between full liquid and light or regular diet. Between acute illness and convalescence. Acute infections. Chewing difficulties. Gastrointestinal disorders. 3 meals with or without between-meal feedings.	For uniformity and convenience in serving hospital patients. Ambulatory patients. Bed patients not requiring therapeutic diets.
Foods	Water, tea, coffee, coffee substitutes. Fat-free broth. Carbonated beverages. Synthetic fruit juices. Ginger ale. Plain gelatin. Sugar.	All liquids on clear liquid diet plus: All forms milk. Soups, strained. Fruit and vegetable juices. Eggnogs. Plain ice cream and sherbets. Junket and plain gelatin dishes. Soft custard. Cereal gruels.	All liquids. Fine and strained cereals. Cooked tender or pureed vegetables. Cooked fruits without skins and seeds. Ripe bananas. Ground or minced meat, fish, poultry. Eggs and mild cheeses. Plain cake and puddings. Moderately seasoned foods.	All basic foods.
Modification	Liberal clear liquid diet includes: fruit juices, egg white, whole egg, thin gruels.	Consistency for tube feedings: foods that will pass through tube easily.	Low residue – no fiber. Bland – no chemical, thermal, physical stimulants. Cold soft – tonsillectomy. Mechanical soft – requiring no mastication. Light diet – intermediate between soft and regular. Note: Because of trend toward more liberal interpretation of diets and foods, soft diet may be combined with light diet in some hospitals.	For a light or convalescent diet, fried foods, rich pastries, fat-rich foods, coarse vegetables, raw fruits may be omitted.

much the same way one would eat the food if feeding himself.

4. Alternate dishes.
5. Liquids should be given through a straw or drinking tube.
6. Allow patient to hold finger foods such as bread, fruit, or raw vegetables, and feed himself as much as possible.
7. Warn patient when hot or cold foods are being offered to him.
8. Do not make an issue over spilled foods or liquids when patient attempts to help himself.
9. Do not try to carry on continuous conversation while patient is being fed. Use a few well-chosen remarks to convey the idea that it is a pleasure to help him with his meal.

D. Gavage (tube feeding)
1. While patient is being fed he should be in upright position, at least 45-degree angle.
2. Specially prepared formula can be adequate to meet patient's nutritional needs.
3. Tube feeding usually given at rate of 250 cc. every 4 to 6 hours. It is warmed to room temperature
4. Diluting tube feeding and giving slowly prevents vomiting and diarrhea. Formula of 250 cc. usually diluted with 250 cc. water.
5. Mouth care one of most important aspects of nursing care while patient receiving tube feeding.

E. Types of hospital diets (Table 6)
F. Diet therapy
1. Definition—the use of special diets as a form of treatment for certain diseases.
2. Purposes of therapeutic diets
   a. To improve nutritional status or treat nutritional deficiencies.
   b. To maintain, increase, or decrease body weight.
   c. To rest certain organs of the body.
   d. To eliminate particular food constituents to which patient may be allergic.
   e. To adjust the composition of the diet to meet the ability of the body to digest, metabolize, and excrete certain nutrients or other substances.*

Questions

1. When planning the nursing care for a patient, the nurse should bear in mind that:
   1. all patients require constant attention
   2. the needs of the patient depend on his diagnosis more than his ability to help himself
   3. each patient is an individual with his own unique problems
   4. most patients are in the hospital because they are totally helpless and unable to care for themselves
2. The ultimate goal of nursing care is:
   1. complete recovery for every patient
   2. proper diagnosing and successful treatment of illness
   3. doing everything for the patient as long as he is entrusted to the nurse's care
   4. restoration of the patient to as near his former state of health as possible
3. One of the outstanding characteristics of a good nursing care plan is:
   1. flexibility to meet the changing needs of the patient
   2. adherence to hospital policies and rules
   3. consideration of the personnel available
   4. adequate organization of the work so it can be done quickly
4. Illness or injury may affect an individual:
   a. emotionally
   b. physically
   c. financially
   d. spiritually

   1. all of these
   2. b and d
   3. c and d
   4. a and c

5. Mr. Jones is admitted to the hospital for the first time in his life. He is convinced he has cancer and will not live much longer. This patient is very gruff and unpleasant during the admission procedure. Mr. Jones can probably be helped. most if the nurse:
   1. displays a sense of humor and encourages Mr. Jones to laugh his worries away
   2. ignores his bad humor and leaves his room as quickly as possible after admitting him
   3. is frank and tells him that things could be worse and there is no excuse for his bad manners
   4. realizes that fear is probably causing Mr. Jones to act this way and he needs assurance that she is interested in him

6. The person who is best qualified to meet the spiritual needs of a patient is most likely to be:
   1. the nurse who has cared for him the longest
   2. the doctor who knows his family history
   3. any member of the patient's family
   4. the patient's minister or rabbi

7. Whenever a minister or rabbi visits a patient the nurse should:
   1. stay with the patient in case he needs her
   2. notify the family immediately
   3. be sure a written order from the doctor has been obtained before allowing the visit
   4. provide the patient and his spiritual advisor with privacy and interrupt the visit only when necessary

8. If a patient asks you to pray with him you should:
   1. tell him it would be better if he waited until a minister visited him
   2. ask him if he is a member of your faith because you may not agree with his religious beliefs
   3. comply with his request, asking him if he has any special prayer he would like to say
   4. ignore his request, realizing that illness often causes a patient concern about his spiritual welfare

9. When carrying out a nursing procedure, the first thing the practical nurse should do is:
   1. report to the nurse in charge the effects of procedure on patient
   2. assemble the equipment and position the patient
   3. review the procedure in her mind to be sure she knows exactly how it is to be done
   4. explain the procedure to the patient so he will know the purpose and expected results of the procedure

10. A characteristic of good work habits is:
    1. being able to finish a task in a short period of time
    2. completing one assignment before going to another task, or working toward a "finished appearance "
    3. leaving equipment to be cleaned or replaced in one specific area until all assignments are completed and then attending to all equipment at one time
    4. planning tasks as you work so that interruptions will not interfere with getting the assignments completed

11. The ideal temperature for a sickroom is usually considered to be:
    1. 80 to 90° F. (27 to 32° C.)
    2. 60 to 80° F. (16 to 27° C.)
    3. 30 to 50° F. (−1 to 10° C.)
    4. 65 to 72° F. (18 to 22° C.)

12. Most modern hospitals have special ventilating systems to provide fresh air to patient's rooms. If there is no such system available the nurse must provide some means of cross ventilation in the rooms. In doing so she must be careful to avoid:
    1. allowing unfiltered air to enter the rooms
    2. creating drafts or sudden changes in room temperature

3. leaving windows open during the night
4. changing the humidity of the atmosphere

13. When there is only one window in a patient's room, adequate ventilation can be accomplished best by:
    1. opening the door and the window
    2. opening the window from the bottom
    3. using a window fan
    4. opening the window at the top and at the bottom

14. The ideal atmospheric humidity is considered to be:
    1. 70 to 90 per cent
    2. 60 to 70 per cent
    3. 50 to 60 per cent
    4. 30 to 50 per cent

15. The term *humidity* refers to:
    1. the percentage of fresh air in the atmosphere
    2. the amount of moisture in the air in relation to the temperature
    3. the amount of oxygen present in the atmosphere
    4. the barometric pressure of the atmosphere

16. When the temperature and relative humidity are both high, we become uncomfortable because:
    1. there is very little evaporation of perspiration
    2. we tend to perspire freely
    3. we become chilled easily
    4. there is an irritation of the respiratory tract

17. Which of the following atmospheric conditions is most likely to produce chilliness?
    1. low temperature and low humidity
    2. high temperature and low humidity
    3. high temperature and high humidity
    4. low temperature and high humidity

18. For a patient confined to bed the best type of lighting would be:
    1. an overhead light with wall switch near the door
    2. a bedside lamp placed so the patient can adjust the lighting
    3. direct sunlight through an unshaded window
    4. a table lamp with the shade removed

19. You have been taught that nurses must avoid strong perfumes and colognes while in uniform because:
    1. they are usually too expensive to buy
    2. one should never wear perfume to work
    3. the patients may not agree with the nurse's taste in perfumes
    4. most persons who are ill are very sensitive to odors and may be offended by strong perfumes

20. Loud talking and laughing in the hall, slamming of doors, or dropping equipment must be avoided because:
    1. noise produces stimulation and fatigue
    2. they are usually against hospital rules
    3. these may produce a gradual loss of hearing
    4. they may indicate a lack of interest in the patient and his welfare

21. Failure to use screens, curtains, and proper draping while performing a nursing procedure is considered to be:
    1. carelessness in following the steps of the procedure
    2. an invasion of the patient's privacy
    3. excusable if the nurse is in a hurry
    4. unimportant as long as the patient does not complain

22. If a nurse notices a puddle of water in the hospital hall she should:
    1. avoid stepping in it until someone cleans it up
    2. call the housekeeping department and ask that someone mop up the water
    3. mop up the water immediately to prevent an accident
    4. realize that keeping the hospital clean and safe is not her responsibility

23. Some hazards that may jeopardize the safety of patients in a hospital include:
    a. defective equipment   1. all of these
    b. careless labeling of containers   2. a and d

   c. failure to use side rails on all beds   3. b and c
   d. failure to check the temperature of solu-   4. all but c
      tions and hot water bottles

24. It is especially important that the sickroom be kept clean and orderly because:
   a. disorder creates mental confusion and   1. all of these
      indirectly affects the patient's peace of   2. a and c
      mind   3. all but b
   b. cleanliness is more important than   4. c only
      making the patient feel at home
   c. dirt and dust are carriers of disease
   d. most nurses need experience in house-
      keeping methods

25. The best method for removing mucus from an emesis basin is:
   1. submerging the emesis basin in hot water and then placing it in a small sterilizer
   2. rinsing in hot water and soaking in alcohol
   3. soaking for several hours in Lysol solution
   4. rinsing in cold water before washing in warm soapy water

26. When you are handling linen that has been removed from the bed, you should:
   1. avoid dropping it on the floor because it will get stained and will be difficult to launder
   2. hold linen away from your clothing so as to avoid spreading infection
   3. roll linen tightly and snugly against you to avoid spread of infection while taking it to the laundry chute
   4. wear gloves so as to avoid the necessity of washing your hands after the procedure is over

27. To remove dust from the furniture in a patient's unit it is best to use:
   1. an oily cloth
   2. a dry cloth
   3. a feather duster
   4. a damp cloth

28. Mrs. Wilson has received a bouquet of flowers and asks you to put them in a vase. When preparing the cut flowers you should:
   1. dry the stems thoroughly and cut them straight across
   2. place the flower stems in warm water for a few minutes and then plunge them into cold water in the vase
   3. place the stems in water and cut the stems diagonally while they remain submerged in the water
   4. break stems off and place in a container of warm water

29. Vases of fresh flowers should be handled with care in the patient's room because:
   1. they are expensive and difficult to replace
   2. they can serve as a source of bacterial contamination
   3. most patients prefer to keep their flowers as long as possible
   4. they are the property of the patient and his family

30. When Mr. Long is discharged his unit is prepared for the admission of another patient. If the bed is not to be occupied immediately what type of bed should be made?
   1. open bed
   2. unoccupied bed
   3. anesthetic bed
   4. closed bed

31. When making a bed a nurse can save steps and time if she will:
   a. assemble all needed linen before start-   1. all but c
      ing to make the bed   2. a and c
   b. tuck in bottom linen and top linen at foot   3. a and d
      of bed before going to head of bed   4. b and d
   c. complete one side of the bed before going to the other
   d. look for one of her co-workers and ask her to make one side of the bed while she makes the other

32. The bottom linen on the bed should be:
    1. pulled tight and tucked in well under the mattress
    2. smoothed out with the palm of the hand so there will be no wrinkling after the patient gets into bed
    3. applied loosely to prevent strain and tearing of the sheets
    4. smoothed out and tucked under the outer edges of the mattress
33. One of the best ways to judge whether or not a bed has been made properly is by:
    1. its appearance as soon as it has been made
    2. determining the comfort of the patient who has had to lie in it all day
    3. asking an experienced nurse
    4. determining the amount of linen used
34. In order to be sure that no personal belongings of the patient have been gathered up in the linen as it is removed from the bed, it is best to:
    1. remove the bottom linen first and shake it thoroughly
    2. loosen all the linen from under the mattress and then roll all top covers together
    3. remove the linen one piece at a time
    4. ask the patient to get out of bed so you can check for lost or misplaced articles
35. The main reason for using a cotton drawsheet over the bottom sheet is to:
    1. protect the bottom sheet in case the patient is incontinent or has drainage
    2. have some means for turning the helpless patient
    3. avoid daily changing of the bottom linen
    4. provide a means for tightening the bottom linen and keeping the sheet under the patient's body free of wrinkles
36. An open bed is one in which the top linens are:
    1. fan folded to the side
    2. removed from the bed
    3. fan folded to the foot of the bed
    4. pulled up over the bottom linens so that they are protected from dust and dirt
37. When making an ether bed in preparation for a patient's return from surgery it is important to:
    1. leave off the top linen until the patient is placed in the bed
    2. fan fold the top linens to the side so that the open end is toward the door
    3. fan fold the top linens to the foot of the bed and drape them over the foot board
    4. place the top linens so that the bottom linens are covered and protected from dirt and dust
38. You are assigned to give A.M. care to Mrs. White, a 56-year-old diabetic who has pneumonia. Before starting A.M. care you offer Mrs. White the bedpan. To avoid any unnecessary lifting of the patient, you should instruct Mrs. White to:
    1. turn on her side while you place the bedpan against her buttocks and then she can roll onto the bedpan
    2. push her feet against the foot of the bed and raise her up on her elbows
    3. lie flat in the bed and relax so she will be easier to lift
    4. flex her knees and push with the soles of her feet to raise her hips
39. While Mrs. White is using the bedpan it would be best if you:
    1. stayed with her and handed her the toilet tissue as she needed it
    2. stood outside the door until the patient calls for you
    3. left the room after placing the toilet tissue and the call light within easy reach
    4. took her temperature, pulse, and respirations to save time and get through with your work more quickly
40. After removing the bedpan, you should:
    a. cover it and place it on the foot stool
    b. cover the bedpan, take it to the utility room, and save a specimen of urine if one is needed

    1. a and d
    2. b and d
    3. a and c
    4. b and c

    c. provide Mrs. White with materials for washing her hands

    d. omit cleaning Mrs. White's hands because she will be getting a bath soon

41. While you are giving Mrs. White her morning care, she tells you that she is too tired to brush her teeth. While brushing Mrs. White's teeth for her, you should:
    a. use a circular, scrubbing motion
    b. use an upward stroke for the upper teeth and a downward stroke for the lower teeth
    c. brush the teeth crosswise
    d. hold brush at 45° angle

    1. a and d
    2. b and d
    3. c and d
    4. all but b

42. If you were asked the best type of toothbrush to use for cleaning the teeth, you would be correct in recommending a toothbrush with:
    1. bristles of uneven length within each tuft but an over-all surface that is flat
    2. an elevated tuft at the end of the brush and a flat surface for the remainder of the brush
    3. bristles of even length and a flat surface
    4. an uneven surface with tufts of uneven length

43. Many people feel that mouthwashes are important in removing all bacteria from the mouth. The practical nurse should know that:
    a. most mouthwashes are refreshing but will not destroy bacteria effectively
    b. most bacteria in the mouth may cause halitosis but are most often not harmful to the body
    c. bacteria in the mouth are easily destroyed by almost any kind of mouthwash
    d. mouthwashes are essential to good oral hygiene

    1. all but a
    2. b and d
    3. c and d
    4. a and b

44. Which of the following is true in regard to toothpastes?
    1. Toothpastes containing fluoride are best.
    2. Chlorophyll is the most important ingredient in toothpaste.
    3. There is little difference in toothpastes; the most important point in cleaning the teeth is proper brushing technique.
    4. Only toothpastes which contain an abrasive can effectively clean the teeth.

45. Mrs. Morgan is a 55-year-old patient who is on absolute bed rest for treatment of a heart condition. When you prepare the bath water for her bed bath, the temperature of the bath water should be:
    1. 70 to 80° F. (21 to 27° C.)
    2. 80 to 90° F. (27 to 32° C.)
    3. 105 to 115° F. (41 to 46° C.)
    4. 130 to 140° F. (54 to 60° C.)

46. To avoid dripping water on the bed linen and cooling the bath cloth during the bath, the cloth is:
    1. folded into a neat square
    2. rolled into a small roll
    3. only slightly dampened before soap is applied to the cloth
    4. folded into a mitt around the nurse's hand

47. It is recommended that bath water used for a bed bath be changed:
    1. at least once during the bath
    2. only if necessary
    3. only at the request of the patient
    4. at least once if it appears to be too soapy

48. The bath will be more relaxing and soothing to Mrs. Morgan if:
    1. long, smooth strokes are used to cleanse the skin
    2. circulation is increased by vigorous rubbing of the skin with the washcloth
    3. very hot water is used for the bath
    4. the linen is changed before the bath is given

49. To avoid irritation of the skin during the bath it is best to use:
    1. only medicated soap
    2. soap only if stains are to be removed from the skin
    3. soap sparingly and rinse well
    4. cold water for rinsing the skin

50. In choosing between body lotions and alcohol to massage the skin, it should be remembered that:
    1. alcohol is stimulating and increases circulation
    2. neither will be effective if it is not prewarmed to 130° F. (54° C.)
    3. they have about the same effect on the skin
    4. lotions tend to restore natural oils; alcohol has a drying effect on the skin

51. Mrs. Morgan has a tendency to develop decubitus ulcers because she is confined to bed. Factors which contribute to the formation of decubitus ulcers are:
    a. pressure caused by weight of the body on bony prominences
    b. wrinkles in the linen resulting from poor bedmaking technique
    c. obesity or emaciation
    d. maintenance of one position in bed without frequent turning to alternate site of pressure
    e. friction of the skin when the patient is turned or linen is removed from the bed

    1. all but e
    2. all of these
    3. a, c, and d
    4. all but c

52. While you are bathing Mrs. Morgan you notice a reddened area on her left shoulder just above the scapula. To prevent the formation of a bedsore it would be best to:
    1. place a rubber ring under her shoulders
    2. rub the area vigorously with the tips of your fingers
    3. gently massage the area and report your observation to the nurse in charge
    4. place a bed cradle on the upper part of the bed to remove the weight of the top covers from the patient's shoulders

53. During the bed bath the nurse may use this time to:
    a. observe the patient's skin for bruises, lacerations, swelling, etc.
    b. listen to the patient if he seems in the mood to talk
    c. cheer up the patient by engaging him in a lively conversation about the other patients in the ward
    d. question the patient to determine whether he has any hidden fears or problems he is reluctant to discuss

    1. all of these
    2. a and d
    3. b and c
    4. a and b

54. One of your patients is to receive a tub bath this A.M. You should plan your work so that:
    1. this patient is cared for first
    2. the tub bath is given at a time when you can stay with the patient or at least remain within calling distance
    3. the tub bath can be taken by the patient while you are feeding a helpless patient
    4. all other assignments are completed before starting this bath, since the patient will need your help

55. Proper cleaning of tub after a patient has had a tub bath is the responsibility of:
    1. the head nurse
    2. the patient
    3. the maid assigned to that unit
    4. the nurse assigned to the care of the patient taking the tub bath

56. Unconscious patients must be given mouth care frequently because they tend to breathe through their mouths, and this quickly dries the mouth and lips. In giving mouth care to these patients it is important to:
    a. help them rinse their mouths frequently with mouthwash

    1. all but d
    2. a and b

b. brush the teeth at least once a day using a dentifrice containing chlorophyll to prevent halitosis

c. clean the teeth with a padded tongue blade and mouthwash

d. lubricate the lips to prevent cracking

    3. b and d
    4. c and d

57. Lubricants that can be used for all patients who have dried and cracked lips include:
   1. castor oil or petroleum jelly
   2. mineral oil or petroleum jelly
   3. cold cream or glycerine with lemon juice
   4. olive oil or glycerine with sugar

58. The correct method for cleaning removable dentures is:
   1. brushing with an ordinary toothbrush in very hot water
   2. soaking in very cold water to remove mucus and food particles
   3. cleaning with soft cloth and baking soda to avoid scratching the surface of the dentures
   4. cleaning with a brush and dentifrice and rinsing under a gentle stream of running water

59. When dentures are not in use they should be:
   1. placed in the narcotic box under lock and key
   2. wrapped in tissues and placed in the patient's dresser drawer
   3. placed in a denture cup, labeled with patient's name and room number, and put in the drawer of the bedside table
   4. labeled correctly as a valuable and placed in the hospital vault

60. Nurses are instructed to keep a patient's hair clean and well groomed because:
   1. female patients are always more concerned about their appearance than male patients
   2. the patient usually cannot afford to pay for a professional hairdresser
   3. head lice are a constant danger to all bedridden patients
   4. cleanliness and daily brushing of the hair are important to the health of the scalp and the mental attitude of the patient

61. If a patient's hair becomes tangled it will be easier to comb if it is:
   1. cut short and then brushed, even though the patient does not wish to have her hair cut
   2. powdered with talcum to remove the oil
   3. dampened with alcohol before combing
   4. rinsed with vinegar solution before combing

62. The nits of pediculi capitis are the:
   1. outer covering of head lice
   2. eggs of body lice
   3. eggs of head lice
   4. female head lice

63. Nits closely resemble dandruff except that they cling to the hair. To facilitate removal of the nits from the hair it is best to:
   1. rub the hair with alcohol
   2. brush the hair with a nylon brush
   3. rinse the hair in vinegar and comb with a fine-toothed comb

64. The best time to clean the patient's fingernails is:
   1. during the bath after the hands have been soaked in warm water
   2. before the bed bath
   3. after breakfast
   4. before A.M. care is started

65. The safest method for shaping the fingernails is by using:
   1. a pair of nail clippers
   2. a pair of bandage scissors
   3. a razor blade
   4. an emery board

66. When caring for a patient's toenails the nurse should:
   a. cut the toenails along the side to prevent ingrown toenails

    1. all but b
    2. all but a

    b. cut the toenails straight across
    c. cut the cuticle with cuticle scissors
    d. cut the toenails so that they are even with
        the tips of the toes

    3. a and c
    4. b and d

67. If a patient is completely helpless and cannot lift her hips to get onto a bedpan the nurse can adjust the bedpan *most* easily by:
    1. elevating the head of the bed and the knee rest and sliding the pan under the hips
    2. placing her hand under the small of the back and lifting the entire torso while the bedpan is put in place
    3. elevating the foot of the bed and lifting the patient's buttocks
    4. rolling the patient onto her side, placing the bedpan against the buttocks, and rolling the patient onto the bedpan

68. If a male patient asks for a urinal a female nurse should:
    1. tell him to wait until an orderly is available to help him
    2. place the urinal under the top covers so the patient can grasp the handle, and then leave the room
    3. inform him that the urinal is in his bedside table for his convenience
    4. ask him to use a bedpan because female nurses cannot give urinals to male patients

69. Each time a patient uses the urinal the nurse is responsible for:
    1. saving a specimen
    2. providing him with toilet tissue
    3. providing him with materials for washing his hands
    4. measuring the output

70. The term urinary incontinence refers to:
    1. failure of the kidneys to excrete urine
    2. retention of the urine in the bladder
    3. incomplete emptying of the bladder
    4. inability to control urination

71. One of the best means by which the nurse can help establish a routine for incontinent patients and eliminate frequent changing of linens is:
    1. insertion of a Foley catheter
    2. frequent and regular administration of the bedpan
    3. catheterization every 8 hours
    4. use of waterproof materials to keep the linen dry

72. Inability to empty the bladder of urine is called:
    1. urinary suppression
    2. urinary incontinence
    3. residual urination
    4. urinary retention

73. Nursing measures that may be used to induce voiding include:
    a. catheterization with a very small catheter
    b. elevating the head of the bed and assisting the patient to a natural position for voiding
    c. providing privacy for the patient
    d. pouring warm water over the vulva while patient is on the bedpan
    e. restricting the intake of fluids

    1. all of these
    2. all but a
    3. a, c, and e
    4. b, c, and d

74. Miss Lowell has difficulty sleeping while in the hospital. Some nursing measures that could be taken to induce relaxation and encourage sleep for Miss Lowell are:
    a. bathing her face and hands and tightening the bottom sheets of her bed
    b. leaving the overhead light on in case Miss Lowell wishes to read before going to sleep
    c. providing adequate ventilation
    d. giving a back rub and providing an extra blanket for warmth

    1. all of these
    2. all but e
    3. a, c, and d
    4. d only

    e. giving the patient a sedative each night at bedtime so she will get into the habit of going to sleep at a certain time

75. A good back rub promotes relaxation and helps prevent pressure sores. A back rub is most relaxing if the back is:
1. rubbed with short brisk strokes
2. vigorously massaged with the fingertips
3. rubbed with a circular motion and kneaded with the thumbs
4. rubbed with long smooth strokes, exerting more pressure on the upward stroke than the downward stroke

76. While giving the back rub, the nurse should also increase circulation to the areas over bony prominences by gently massaging the:
1. lumbar region and buttocks
2. sacral region, neck, and shoulders
3. ribs and buttocks
4. lumbar vertebrae and ribs

77. Good posture has been called the key to comfort, health, and appearance. The term *posture* means:
1. the manner in which one holds different parts of the body in relation to each other
2. a pose or unnatural stance
3. the complete relaxation of all parts of the body
4. the complete rigidity of all muscles of the body

78. When one is standing in a position of good posture the weight is borne chiefly by the:
1. instep of each foot
2. toes of the forward foot
3. toes of both feet
4. ankles of both feet

79. When one is in a good sitting position the feet should be:
1. resting on the chair rung
2. kept at least 12 inches apart
3. resting on the floor
4. dangling so that only the toes touch the floor

80. To assure a good posture while sitting one should:
1. sit so that most of the weight is borne by one hip and then shifted to the other
2. sit squarely on the buttocks and thighs
3. flex knees at such an angle that the weight is borne by the buttocks only
4. sit so that most of the body weight is resting on the sacrum

81. The nurse can best avoid straining her back while lifting and moving patients in bed if she will:
1. keep her back straight and her knees flexed
2. bend her back and straighten her arms and legs
3. lean forward so that her back is bent slightly and the shoulders rounded for protection
4. relax her abdominal muscles and tighten her leg and arm muscles

82. It is easier to maintain one's balance while lifting and moving a patient if:
1. the feet are kept close together and in line with each other
2. the ankles are slightly flexed and the knees held rigid
3. the knees are flexed and the feet are held together
4. the feet are far enough apart to provide a wide base, and one foot is placed forward

83. Poor posture can result in:
a. displacement and cramping of internal organs
b. increased fatigue
c. muscle strain
d. fixation of the joints
e. a slovenly appearance

1. all of these
2. a, b and e
3. all but d
4. c, d, and e

84. If three persons are available for moving a patient from a stretcher to the bed, the stretcher is placed:
    1. outside the door of the patient's room
    2. against the wall, parallel to the bed
    3. at right angles to the head of the bed
    4. at right angles to the foot of the bed

85. When three persons move a patient from the stretcher to the bed:
    1. two persons stand on one side of the bed and the third stands by the stretcher
    2. they all lift at the count of "three" and carry the patient to the bed
    3. one person stands at the head of the stretcher and counts while the other two lift
    4. they lift the patient by grasping the edges of the sheet on the stretcher and pull him onto the bed

86. If you wished to turn a partially paralyzed patient onto his right side, you would *first*:
    1. stand on the right side of the bed and move the patient toward you
    2. stand on the left side of the bed and move the patient over to this side
    3. stand on the right side of the bed and move the patient away from you
    4. stand on the left side of the bed and move the patient to the right side of the bed

87. It is easier to turn a patient onto his side if:
    1. the patient's uppermost knee is kept straight
    2. both of the patient's knees are flexed
    3. the knee of the leg on which he will be lying is flexed
    4. the knee and thigh of the uppermost leg are flexed

88. Proper support of the patient's uppermost leg and arm while he is lying on his side will prevent:
    1. strain on his muscles and will support the weight of the arm and leg
    2. him from rolling onto his back
    3. foot drop
    4. contractures of the leg muscles

89. To avoid a serious accident when getting a patient up in a wheel chair, the nurse must be sure that:
    1. the back of the chair is cushioned with a pillow
    2. a foot stool is used
    3. the wheels are locked and the foot rests are folded up out of the way
    4. she has at least two other persons to help her

90. After helping a patient to a sitting position on the side of the bed, the nurse can best help him into a standing position by:
    1. firmly grasping one arm and lifting him off the bed
    2. asking him to place his hands on her shoulders while she steadies him with one hand on either side of his chest
    3. standing on the foot stool and gently easing the patient off the bed
    4. holding the patient's wrists and pulling him off the side of the bed

91. One of the best ways of determining whether a patient has good posture while lying in bed is to:
    1. check to see if he is breathing properly
    2. ask him if he is comfortable
    3. imagine him in a vertical or standing position with the same posture
    4. ask a member of his family if he is accustomed to lying in that position

92. When pillows are used to support a patient's back, they should be placed so that the body bends at the:
    1. neck
    2. shoulder
    3. waist
    4. hips

93. Footboards are used to:
    1. keep the mattress from sliding to the foot of the bed

   2. help keep the top linens neat in appearance
   3. support the toes
   4. hold the feet in their normal position and prevent foot drop

94. If the position of a patient in bed is not changed frequently, he is most likely to develop:
   1. a skin infection
   2. fixation of the joints and decubitus ulcers
   3. toughening of the skin and paralysis
   4. an infection of the bones

95. The position used for patients who cannot breathe without difficulty while lying down is called:
   1. dorsal recumbent
   2. Sims' left lateral
   3. orthopneic
   4. Trendelenburg

96. A bed cradle may be used in the hospital or home to:
   1. provide warmth for the lower extremities
   2. give support to the patient's back
   3. eliminate the need for an overbed table
   4. support the weight of the top covers

97. The position usually recommended for administration of an enema is with the patient lying on his side with the uppermost knee and thigh flexed. This position is called:
   1. Sims' left lateral
   2. prone position
   3. supine position
   4. right lateral

98. A patient in Trendelenburg position is lying on his back with:
   a. his knees slightly flexed   1. a and d
   b. his knees and thighs flexed   2. a and c
   c. his feet lower than his head   3. b and d
   d. his head lower than his feet   4. b and c

99. Fowler's position is one in which the:
   a. patient is lying on his abdomen   1. a and d
   b. knee rest is slightly elevated   2. a and b
   c. head rest is elevated   3. b and d
   d. legs are extended and flat on the bed   4. b and c

100. When a doctor orders passive exercises for a patient this means that:
   1. the patient may do them whenever he wishes
   2. the lower extremities are exercised
   3. the patient must do weight-lifting exercises
   4. the nurse exercises the muscles of the patient by moving the extremities in a prescribed manner

101. Special exercises are ordered primarily because:
   1. they keep the patient's mind off his troubles
   2. they prevent atrophy of the muscles and other crippling complications
   3. most hospitals have physical therapists to administer these exercises
   4. it is not the responsibility of the nurse to prevent complications resulting from lack of exercise

102. When helping a patient with his exercises it is *most* important to:
   1. exercise all muscles of the extremities
   2. avoid using force when joints are stiff or muscles tight
   3. work quickly so the patient will not tire before the exercises are completed
   4. vigorously massage each part before it is exercised

103. If the nurse is responsible for serving meal trays it is most important for her to:
   1. remind the patient that he must eat all the food on his tray
   2. see to it that the patient's coffee is hot
   3. serve the tray graciously and display interest in the patient's appetite
   4. plan the menu so that the meals are nutritious and inexpensive

104. When serving a meal tray to a patient the nurse must always be careful to:
    1. place the tray in a convenient place, and position the patient so that he is relaxed and comfortable
    2. get the patient up in a chair so he will be in a natural position for eating
    3. rearrange the articles on the tray in the order in which the patient will eat them
    4. provide privacy for the patient by screening his bed or closing the door

105. Patients on special therapeutic diets should receive *only* the foods sent to them from the diet kitchen chiefly because:
    1. their hospitalization insurance does not cover regular meals in the hospital
    2. the dietitian does not plan for additional food for these patients
    3. these special diets are a form of treatment in the same way that medications are
    4. the patient may not enjoy eating other foods

106. The best way in which the nurse may help the physician determine a patient's eating habits is by:
    1. asking the patient's family what foods he prefers
    2. asking the patient if he always eats everything served to him at the hospital
    3. serving the tray to the patient herself and asking him to eat everything prepared for him
    4. checking the tray after the patient has eaten and accurately recording the amount and type of food eaten

107. If a patient assigned to you must be fed because he is blind, his meal tray should be:
    1. taken to his room and left there until you can get back to feed him
    2. left on the food cart until a member of his family comes to feed him
    3. brought to his room and fed to him immediately after it is served
    4. placed in the kitchen until someone can be found to feed him

108. Eating will seem most natural to the patient being fed if the nurse will:
    a. offer the various foods in much the same way she would eat them herself
    b. ask the patient to be careful so that no foods are spilled on the bed linen
    c. tell the patient what is on the tray and engage him in conversation while he is eating
    d. allow the patient to hold finger foods and feed himself as much as possible

    1. all of these
    2. a and b
    3. c and d
    4. a and d

109. It has been said that the nurse must sometimes be the "eyes of the blind." If this be true, what must the nurse remember when feeding a blind patient?
    a. He will not know what he has on his tray if she does not tell him.
    b. All blind persons have difficulty understanding the spoken word.
    c. He must be warned when hot or cold liquids are being offered to him through a straw.
    d. He will not be able to feed himself any type of food unless she guides his hand to his mouth.

    1. all of these
    2. c and d
    3. a and c
    4. b and d

110. Another name for tube feeding is:
    1. lavage
    2. gavage
    3. gorging
    4. intravenous feeding

111. Tube feeding is usually done:
    1. once a day
    2. twice a day
    3. continuously
    4. every 4 to 6 hours

112. When preparing formula just before administering tube feeding, it is best to:

      1. warm the formula to room temperature
      2. place the formula in a basin of chipped ice to keep it cool and prevent spoilage.
      3. heat the formula to just below boiling so that bacteria can be destroyed.

113. The ideal position for a patient being tube fed is:
      1. lying on his back
      2. sitting upright
      3. lying on his right side
      4. lying on his left side

114. The formula prepared for feeding by tube:
      1. is always deficient in protein
      2. is never adequate in meeting all the nutritional needs of the patient
      3. can be prepared so that all nutritional needs are met
      4. is usually deficient in mineral content

115. To help prevent vomiting and diarrhea in a patient receiving tube feeding, the nurse should:
      1. chill the formula before it is given
      2. give the formula undiluted, followed with a small amount of water
      3. administer the formula with a syringe so it can be given quickly
      4. dilute the formula and give it very slowly

116. When a patient is fed by tube his salivary glands are not stimulated. Because this is true, one important aspect of his nursing care would be:
      1. frequent mouth care
      2. administration of hydrochloric acid once a day
      3. exercises to stimulate peristalsis
      4. measures to relieve constipation

117. Which of the following liquids would not be allowed on a clear liquid diet?
      1. orange juice
      2. ginger ale
      3. tea
      4. sweetened black coffee

118. The liquids allowed on a clear liquid diet have which of the following characteristics in common?
      a. leave a moderate amount of residue in the intestinal tract
      b. are nongas-forming
      c. stimulate the secretion of gastric juices
      d. will not irritate the intestinal mucosa

      1. all of these
      2. a and c
      3. b and d
      4. b and c

119. Which of the following foods are not allowed on a full liquid diet?
      1. milk
      2. cereal gruels
      3. ripe bananas
      4. strained soups

120. A full liquid diet:
      1. is deficient in protein
      2. lacks the necessary minerals
      3. can be adequate with careful planning
      4. must always be supplemented with vitamin preparations

121. Patients who have a fever over a period of time would most likely be given a:
      1. full liquid diet
      2. soft diet
      3. clear liquid diet
      4. soft diet with additional liquids

122. If fruits are included in a soft diet they should be:
      1. served raw after being soaked overnight
      2. peeled and cut into small pieces
      3. only those fruits belonging to the citrus group
      4. cooked with skins and seeds removed

123. A patient on a soft diet is allowed:
      1. no seasoning
      2. as much seasoning as he desires

     3. only a small amount of salt and no vinegar

     4. a moderate amount of seasoning

124. A low residue diet is one that restricts foods containing:

     1. natural salt or sodium

     2. fiber or cellulose

     3. animal fats or plant oils

     4. chemical stimulants

125. Patients with ill-fitting dentures or other difficulties in chewing are more likely to enjoy their meals if the diet is:

     1. composed of nothing but liquids

     2. served cold

     3. a soft diet

     4. mostly made up of baby foods

126. A light or convalescent diet is one in which there is a restriction of:

     1. meat and vegetables

     2. fat-rich foods and rich pastries

     3. salt and other seasonings

     4. cooked fruits and vegetables

UNIT 2   PATIENT ASSESSMENT AND NURSING SKILLS

I. Observation
A. Observation simply means taking notice.
B. Intelligent observation is one of the most important duties of the nurse.
C. Must be accompanied by good judgment, prompt and accurate reporting.
D. Some important observations
 1. General appearance: state of nutrition; color and appearance of skin; abnormalities in shape, size, or function of a part.
 2. Behavior of patient: fatigue; restlessness; posture in bed; sleeping habits; eating habits; emotional behavior.
 3. Excretions and drainage: color, amount, consistency, odor.
 4. Abnormal discharge: origin, type, and amount.
E. Symptoms—any indication of disease or change in the condition of patient.
 1. Objective symptoms—those apparent to the observer; rash, swelling, discoloration, etc.
 2. Subjective symptoms—those felt by the patient; e.g., pain, nausea, itching.
F. Cardinal symptoms, also called vital signs.
 1. Body temperature, normally maintained at a fairly constant level.
 a. Normal range—36 to 37.4° C., or 97 to 99° F. when taken orally. Rectal temperature one degree higher. Axillary temperature one degree lower.
 b. Contraindications for taking oral temperature
 1. When heat or cold is being applied to the face.
 2. When patient is unconscious, delirious, irrational, or mentally ill.
 3. Children under 5 years of age.
 4. When patient is receiving nasal oxygen.
 5. Within 10 minutes after a hot or cold drink has been taken by patient.
 6. When patient is a mouth breather.
 c. Special points to remember
 1. Always wipe thermometer before reading.

 2. Wipe away from fingers, toward bulb.
 3. Rectal thermometers must be held in place while temperature is being taken.
 4. Never use oral thermometer for taking rectal temperature.
 2. Pulse—wave of distention caused by expansion of the wall of the artery with each heartbeat. Pulse beat referred to as pulse wave.
 a. Pulse can be counted most easily where arteries are near surface and over a bone. Wrists and in front of ear are most common sites.
 b. Both rate and character of pulse must be observed.
 c. Normal pulse rate varies with age and sex.
 Infants—110 to 120 per minute.
 Children—80 to 120 per minute.
 Women—65 to 80 per minute.
 Men—60 to 70 per minute.
 d. Rhythm refers to the pattern by which the heart beats are spaced.
 e. An irregular pulse varies in the spacing of intervals between beats.
 f. Volume refers to the strength of the pulsebeat. A *bounding* pulse is one of unusually full force. A *thready* pulse is described as being weak, with indistinct waves.
 g. Apical-radial pulse—the simultaneous counting of radial pulse (at the wrist) and heartbeat at apex of heart. One nurse counts radial pulse for one full minute while second nurse uses stethoscope to count rate of heart beat. Each pulse rate is recorded; the difference between the two rates is called the pulse deficit.
 3. Respirations—inhalation and exhalation of air into and out of the lungs.
 a. Both rate and character of respirations are observed.
 b. Normal rate
 Adults—14 to 18 per minute.
 Children—20 to 40 per minute, de-

pending on child's age. The younger the child the faster the rate.

c. Respirations should be counted in such a way that the patient is not aware they are being counted because respirations are partially under voluntary control, and it is difficult to breathe normally when one is being observed.

d. Respirations may be described as *deep* or *shallow*.

e. Other terms used

✓ 1. Stertorous breathing—noisy, snoring type.

2. Dyspnea—difficult or labored breathing.

3. Apnea—cessation of breathing.

4. Cheyne-Stokes respirations — periods of dyspnea followed by periods of apnea.

5. Kussmaul's respirations—gasping type (air hunger)

4. Blood pressure—the amount of force exerted by the blood against the walls of the blood vessels.

a. Systolic pressure is a result of contraction of the left ventricle of the heart. When taking blood pressure the first of a series of beating sounds heard through the stethoscope is the systolic pressure.

b. Diastolic pressure is a result of relaxation of the left ventricle. The last beat heard as the cuff is deflated is recorded as the diastolic pressure. When a beat is heard all the way down the gauge, the diastolic pressure is recorded as the point at which a muffling of the beat is first heard.

c. Normal range—90 to 120 systolic, and 60 to 80 diastolic.

d. Blood pressure recorded as a ratio, e.g., 90/60.

e. High blood pressure—*hypertension*, a symptom of a variety of diseases.

f. Low blood pressure—*hypotension*, less frequently found but may be present in shock, hemorrhage, certain endocrine disturbances.

G. Reporting observations

1. Practical nurse reports important observations to nurse in charge, immediate supervisor, or physician in charge of the case.

2. Good judgment essential in deciding which observations are important and require prompt reporting.

3. All members of nursing team responsible for accurate reporting even though final decision for action may rest with physician.

H. Recording observations

1. Charts are legal documents and may or may not be used as evidence in court. They also provide data for research and information for insurance claims and vital statistics.

2. Only standard abbreviations should be used.

3. When recording observations on chart be careful to record accurately. Avoid giving interpretation to statements made by patient; simply record his exact words.

4. Use short, descriptive terms; write legibly; include only the facts which are important.

5. Indicate the hour each time a notation is made.

6. Charts are to be signed by person writing the notes.

7. Errors are not erased from the chart; a line is drawn through the error, and the correction made immediately following the erroneous statement.

II. Admissions, Transfers, Discharges

A. Admission of patient

1. First impression of hospital often a lasting one.

2. Nurse legally responsible for proper care of patient's clothing and any valuables brought to the hospital, e.g., money, jewelry, etc.

3. Admission procedure varies in each institution; however, basic principles of courtesy, interest in the patient as a person, and intelligent observation of patient must be followed always and everywhere.

4. Observations should be recorded briefly and accurately. Most institutions have a checklist to be used during admission of a new patient. The items include:

a. General condition of patient—apparent state of health, degree of orientation, mental alertness.

b. Any obvious symptoms such as dyspnea, bleeding, coughing.

c. Condition of skin, rashes, bruises, cuts.

d. Special problems with sight, hearing, mobility.

e. Prostheses (dentures, hearing aid, glass eye, artificial limb).

f. Known allergies to drugs, food, etc.

g. Complaints of pain, dizziness, etc.

B. Discharge

1. Written order needed for discharge from hospital.

2. Patients leaving without permission of physician must sign release themselves, or have release signed by member of

family or other person accepting responsibility for their care.

3. Patients on special diet should be instructed in this diet by nurse in charge or dietitian.

4. Other instructions regarding medications, treatments, or special exercises must be given before patient leaves.

III. Diagnostic Examinations and Tests

A. The physical examination

1. May be done for diagnosis and treatment or as a means of preserving and maintaining health through early detection of disease.

2. Patient's history an important part of the physical examination, nurse should provide privacy for physician and patient while history is being taken.

3. Methods of examination (Fig. 25)

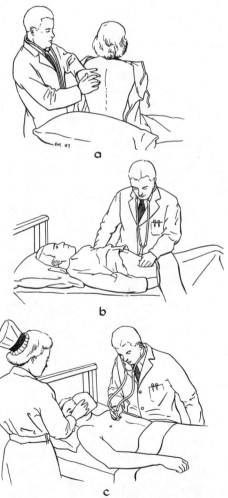

FIGURE 25. Methods of physical examination: *a*, percussion; *b*, palpation of the abdomen; *c*, auscultation. (Montag and Filson: *Nursing Arts*. 2nd ed.)

a. Inspection—requires adequate light and proper draping of the patient.

b. Palpation—feeling with the hands. Nurse responsible for helping patient relax and cooperate with the physician.

c. Percussion—tapping with the fingers to detect sounds and changes in sounds produced by various organs of the body.

d. Auscultation—listening to sounds within the body, usually with a stethoscope.

4. Nurse's responsibilities

a. Preparation of the patient mentally and physically.

b. Positioning of the patient (Fig. 26).

c. Assembling necessary equipment, which includes flashlight, tongue blades, percussion hammer, otoscope (for examination of the ear), ophthalmoscope (for examination of the eye), stethoscope. For vaginal examination rubber gloves, vaginal speculum, lubricant. For rectal examination rubber glove, lubricant.

d. Assisting patient onto bed or examination table and proper draping to avoid unnecessary exposure of the patient.

e. Room should be well lighted, privacy assured.

5. Positions used in physical examinations are shown in Figure 26.

B. Collection of specimens

1. General principles

a. All specimens must be correctly labeled and sent or taken to laboratory promptly.

b. Collect specimen at correct time.

c. Correct amount must be collected.

d. Laboratory slip should accompany specimen.

e. Avoid contaminating outside of container.

f. Never fill container completely. Use larger container if necessary.

g. Explanation is given to the patient and he is told exactly what is expected of him and how he can cooperate in the test.

2. Urine specimens

a. 60 to 100 ml. considered adequate for most tests.

b. For a routine urinalysis, the bedpan must be clean and the genitalia must be clean and free of discharge.

c. Clean-voided or "clean-catch" specimen requires thorough cleansing of external genitalia before specimen is obtained.

d. A midstream specimen is caught after

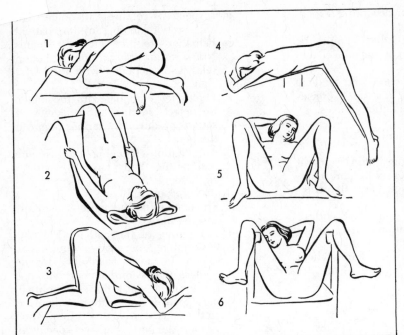

FIGURE 26. Positions used in physical examinations. *1*, Lateral or Sims's position (position may be right or left lateral). *2*, Trendelenburg position. *3*, Knee-chest or genupectoral position. *4*, Jackknife position. 5, Dorsal-recumbent position with knees flexed. *6*, Lithotomy, or dorsal-recumbent position with knees supported. (Harmer, B., and Henderson, V.: *Textbook of the Principles and Practice of Nursing*, 5th ed., New York, The Macmillan Co., 1955.)

the patient has voided a small amount and before the bladder is completely empty.

   e. A 24-hour specimen must include all urine voided within a 24-hour period. At beginning of test the patient voids and the specimen is discarded. Specimen is collected in special container which has a preservative in it.

   f. All other types of specimens, unless otherwise ordered, should be examined in the laboratory within 1 hour after collection; otherwise, the urine changes rapidly and laboratory readings will not be correct. If urine cannot be examined within the hour, the specimen must be refrigerated.

   g. Timed urine collections—specimens collected at specified times and placed in prelabeled containers.

   h. Containers sent from laboratory for special urine tests may contain a preservative which is highly caustic. If this liquid is spilled, the area should be rinsed thoroughly with running water to avoid burns.

   i. Tests for sugar and acetone.

1. Clinitest—for sugar in the urine. First specimen in the morning is discarded and a fresh specimen obtained shortly thereafter.
   a. Five drops of urine are needed.
   b. Clinitest tablets can cause severe burns to the mucous membranes.
   c. Color of urine may indicate negative, 1+, 2+, 3+, or 4+.

2. Tes-Tape—for sugar.
   a. End of tape is dipped into urine.
   b. Color of tape compared to color chart.
   c. Zero per cent (sugar-free) to 2 per cent or more.

3. Acetest tablets—for acetone.
   a. One drop of urine placed on tablet.
   b. Range from negative to slightly, moderately or strongly positive.

3. Sputum specimens
   a. Best to collect sputum specimen early in morning unless it is a 24-hour specimen.
   b. Use proper container.
   c. Instruct patient to cough and expectorate material brought up from lungs and bronchi.
   d. Outside of container should not be contaminated by sputum.

4. Stool specimens
   a. Fecal material collected in bedpan.
   b. Use extreme care to avoid contamination of hands or container.
   c. Material transferred from bedpan to waxed container with wooden spatula or tongue blade.
   d. All stool specimens should be sent to laboratory immediately because deterioration begins immediately.
   e. If stool is to be examined for ova and parasites it must be kept warm until examined.

C. Specimens for bacteriological studies
   1. Cultures are grown for bacteria present in body secretions, excreta, or exudate.
   2. Always remember that specimens col-

lected for culture are usually highly contaminated with living bacteria.
3. Use containers which are sterile and not cracked or broken.
4. Keep inside of container and stopper free from contamination from hands.
5. Avoid spilling specimen.
6. Do not fill container more than half way.
7. Use cork stopper and keep container in upright position once specimen has been obtained.

IV. Therapeutic Skills
A. Application of heat and cold
  1. General effects of heat applied to the body
    a. Prolonged application of heat produces muscular relaxation.
    b. Promotes suppuration (drainage from wounds or skin lesions).
    c. Helps localize an infection.
    d. Increases metabolic rate.
    e. Relieves congestion by increasing the flow of blood locally.
    f. Moist heat more penetrating than dry heat.
    g. Infants and elderly persons do not tolerate heat as well as others.
  2. Hot water bottle
    a. Applied by order of physician.
    b. Temperature of water—120 to 125° F. (48.8 to 51.6° C.).
    c. Fill bag one half with water, then expel air to prevent excess weight on part to which applied.
    d. Bottle should be covered to avoid burning patient.
    e. Refill bottle at least every 2 hours.
  3. Electric heating pad
    a. Check to see if pad is in good repair.
    b. Set thermostat on low at first. Never set thermostat on high.
    c. Cover pad well.
    d. Check skin often for redness.
  4. General effects of cold applied to the body
    a. Cold constricts blood vessels and reduces circulation of blood to a part.
    b. Helps control hemorrhage.
    c. Checks process of inflammation.
    d. Prevents suppuration.
  5. Ice caps, ice collars, and ice bags
    a. Test for leakage by filling with water, then remove water.
    b. Fill ice bags, etc. one half to two thirds with ice.
    c. Expel air within bag.
    d. Dry outer surface. Cover unless physician orders otherwise.
    e. Refill at least every 2 hours. Observe condition of skin each time refilled.

B. Irrigations
  1. General principles
    a. Use a steady, gentle stream to cleanse area being irrigated.
    b. Be sure of type of solution to be used, strength and temperature of solution.
    c. Amount of pressure used should be sufficient to reach desired area but not enough to force fluid beyond affected part.
    d. The greater the height of the container of solution the greater will be the pressure being exerted by the stream of solution.
    e. Aseptic technique must be observed if irrigation is ordered as sterile.
  2. Irrigation of the eye (conjunctival sac) (Fig. 27).
    a. Turn head to side so that affected eye is lower than other eye.
    b. Allow solution to run over eyelids to accustom patient to solution.
    c. Direct flow of solution from inner corner to outer corner of eye.
    d. Separate eyelids by exerting pressure on facial bones, NOT on eyeball.
  3. Irrigation of ear (external auditory canal)
    a. Keep stream flowing steadily but with very low pressure.
    b. Patient usually sitting for this procedure.
    c. Excessive pressure very painful and might spread infection to middle ear.
    d. Never obstruct the outward flow of the solution.
  4. Irrigation of throat (oral pharynx)
    a. Reaches more extensive area than by gargling.
    b. Temperature may be slightly higher than for other irrigations because mouth and throat are accustomed to hot liquids.
    c. Saline solution usually used.

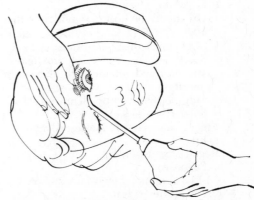

FIGURE 27.   Irrigation of the eye. (Sutton, A. L. *Bedside Nursing Techniques*. 2nd ed., Philadelphia, W. B. Saunders Co., 1969.)

d. Patient may be more comfortable sitting, with head bent forward slightly.

e. Instruct patient to hold his breath while solution is flowing.

5. Perineal irrigation (commonly referred to as perineal care)
  a. Type of solution may vary according to doctor's order but purpose is to cleanse the vulva.
  b. Teach patient to wipe area from front to back to eliminate contamination from anal region.
  c. Perineal pads are also removed from front to back.

6. Irrigation of vaginal canal (vaginal douche)
  a. Must be given under low pressure to prevent forcing solution through cervix and into uterus.
  b. Irrigation given with patient in dorsal recumbent position with knees flexed.
  c. Irrigating tip is gently rotated to cleanse folds in vaginal wall.

C. Treatments of colon
1. Cleansing enema
  a. Solution used usually tap water, saline solution, or soapsuds (1 quart is used). Soap irritating to the mucous membranes of intestine. Avoid soap bubbles which may produce excessive amount of gas in colon.
  b. Fluid container is held 18 to 24 inches above the patient's buttocks.
  c. Patient is placed in Sims's left lateral position.
  d. Insertion of tube into sphincter will cause an immediate spasm. If time is allowed for this spasm to pass, the tube can then be inserted easily and without discomfort.
  e. Return solution is carefully observed for color, content, and amount of feces.

2. Oil retention enema
  a. Given to soften feces.
  b. Oil should be heated to not more than 100° F. (37.7° C.) because it retains heat longer than water does.
  c. Small amount given (approximately 100 ml.) and retained for at least 30 minutes.
  d. May be followed by cleansing enema to evacuate bowel.

3. Fleet's enema—prepackaged retention enema.

4. Rectal suppositories
  a. Purposes
    1. To stimulate bowel movement.
    2. To relieve pain.
    3. As a means of administering medication.

  b. Inserted 3 to 4 inches into rectum, well past rectal sphincter.
  c. Base of suppositories melts at body temperature, thus should be handled as little as possible.

5. Rectal tube
  a. Inserted to relieve distention due to flatus in intestines.
  b. Rectal tube will achieve maximum results in 30 minutes; should be removed after this period of time and reinserted later.
  c. Be sure end of tube is wrapped or placed in container after insertion of tip in case of drainage from colon.

D. Treatments of urinary bladder
1. Catheterization—removal of urine via catheter
  a. Purposes
    1. To obtain sterile specimen.
    2. To relieve urinary retention.
    3. To prevent voiding, as in vaginal surgery, etc.
    4. To check residual urine left in bladder after voiding.
    5. To empty bladder before instilling medication or irrigating bladder.
  b. General principles
    1. Choose correct size catheter to avoid trauma to urethra and urinary meatus.
    2. Urinary system is considered to be sterile unless infection is present.
    3. Pause for a moment after inserting catheter to allow for passing of spasm of sphincter.

2. Irrigation of bladder
  a. Done to cleanse the bladder or for application of drugs to bladder lining. More effective if bladder is empty.
  b. Aseptic technique must be used.
  c. Amount and type of solution according to doctor's orders.
  d. Syringe and basin used for single irrigations; other apparatus may be used for continuous or intermittent irrigations.

3. Bladder instillation
  a. Antiseptic or bacteriostatic solutions may be instilled into bladder to treat infection.
  b. Technique similar to irrigation of bladder except that solution is left in bladder and is not siphoned back.

E. Bandages
1. Applied to hold dressings or splints in place, to apply pressure, or to support or immobilize a part.
  a. First, place part to be bandaged in a functional position. For example, ankle should be flexed, not extended.

    b. Apply bandage *from* extremity *toward* body.

    c. Change bandages frequently when a part is swollen.

    d. Place cotton or gauze between two body surfaces; for example, between toes, fingers.

    e. Pad all bony prominences and never place bulky knots over prominences.

    f. Apply even pressure when bandaging.

  2. Types of bandages

    a. Circular—to hold or anchor bandages and dressings. Each turn is placed so as to hold preceding turn firmly.

    b. Spiral—used on such parts as upper arms, trunk, and fingers. Overlap turns one-half or two-thirds.

    c. Figure-of-eight bandage—used to apply pressure, give support, or immobilize joints such as ankle or knee.

    d. Spica bandage—one that resembles the husks of an ear of corn. May be used to wrap thumb, shoulder, or foot.

    e. Recurrent bandage—consists of a series of turns passing back and forth over the part. May be used to retain dressings on the ends of fingers or the stump of an amputated limb.

    f. Triangular bandage—most commonly used as a sling for the arm. Apex of bandage is placed under elbow, ends are brought around neck and tied. Wrist is positioned slightly higher than elbow.

    g. Fundamental turns (see Fig. 28).

F. Binders

  1. Tailed binders used most often on abdomen.

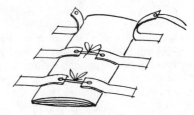

FIGURE 29. Montgomery straps. (Sutton: *Bedside Nursing Techniques*. 2nd ed.)

  2. Scultetus binder (many tailed). Ends overlap to secure binder, safety pin applied in vertical manner.

  3. T binder used to hold perineal dressings in place. Single T used for women, double T used for men.

G. Sterile technique (surgical asepsis)

  1. General principles

    a. Supplies must be considered contaminated and therefore no longer sterile if

      1. They become wet.

      2. A pin is inserted into a sterile package.

      3. They touch an unsterile object.

      4. They are handled by contaminated gloves or forceps.

      5. They are left uncovered.

    b. The covers of containers holding sterile supplies must be handled with care. If necessary to put cover down after it is removed, place upside down so that sterile side is up.

    c. The inside of containers must be kept sterile; the outside is contaminated

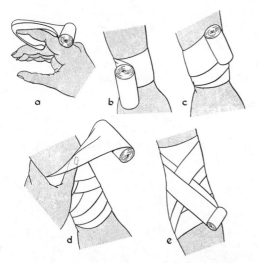

FIGURE 28. Fundamental turns in bandaging: *a*, Recurrent. *b*, Circular. *c*, Spiral. *d*, Spiral reverse. *e*, Figure-of-eight. Note position of roll of bandage in each instance. (Montag and Filson: *Nursing Arts*. 2nd ed.)

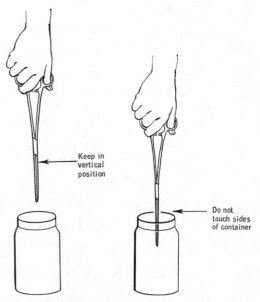

FIGURE 30. Handling pick-up forceps. (Sutton: *Bedside Nursing Techniques*. 2nd ed.)

and must not be touched with pickup forceps.

2. Handling sterile pickup forceps (Fig. 30).
   a. Pickup forceps are used to lift and handle *sterile articles*; must not touch sterile tray or equipment in process of placing articles on tray.
   b. ALWAYS hold tip end of forceps pointed downward and keep above waist level, *never* below.
   c. Remove and replace forceps so that they do not touch inside of holder.
3. Work to the side of sterile field. Do not bend over or breathe directly onto sterile field.

4. Assisting with sterile dressings
   a. Old dressings are wrapped in paper and discarded in utility room or incinerator, never in patient's room.
   b. Open sterile dressing tray before donning gloves if you will be wearing gloves.
   c. When preparing sterile field for doctor, place handles of instruments off edge of field so they can be picked up without contaminating tray.
   d. Anticipate doctor's needs. Inquire about special medications or applications needed before setting up tray.

Questions

1. Intelligent observation is one of the most important duties of the nurse. The term *observation* can be defined as:
   1. looking for symptoms of disease that will help you learn more about nursing
   2. taking notice of the patient and his environment
   3. watching the patient only when he is unaware that he is being observed
   4. obtaining information from the patient and his family by asking intelligent questions
2. A symptom is best defined as:
   1. any indication of disease
   2. a sign of improvement in the patient's condition
   3. an indication that a patient's illness is becoming more severe
   4. any indication of disease or change in the condition of a patient
3. Examples of subjective symptoms would include:
   1. nausea and vomiting
   2. rash and swelling
   3. itching and burning
   4. pain and discoloration of the skin
4. A normal range for body temperature when taken by mouth is:
   1. 99 to 100° F. (37.4 to 37.7° C.)
   2. 36 to 38° F. (2.2 to 3.3° C.)
   3. 97 to 99° F. (36.1 to 37.4° C.)
   4. 38 to 40° C. (100.4 to 104° F.)
5. A rectal temperature of 99.4° F. (37.4° C.) is considered to be:
   1. lower than normal
   2. higher than normal
   3. only three degrees above the normal range
   4. within the normal range
6. In which of the following situations would it be necessary to take a temperature rectally?
   1. after rectal surgery
   2. when the patient is unconscious
   3. when an axillary temperature cannot be taken
   4. when the patient is under 12 years of age
7. If a patient has just finished drinking a cup of hot coffee before his temperature is to be taken, the nurse should know that:
   1. a rectal temperature is contraindicated
   2. an oral temperature should not be taken for at least 10 minutes
   3. this will have no effect on an oral temperature
   4. the patient's temperature must be taken rectally

8. Before inserting a clinical thermometer, it is necessary to shake down the thermometer so that it registers:
   1. at least as low as room temperature
   2. below 96° F. (30.6° C.)
   3. lower than the patient's temperature at last reading
   4. all the way down to the tip at the end of the thermometer

9. When wiping a thermometer clean after removing it from the patient's mouth or rectum, the nurse must be sure to:
   1. wipe in the direction of the bulb, away from the fingers holding the thermometer
   2. wipe toward the fingers holding the thermometer
   3. rinse in cold water before wiping the thermometer
   4. wash with hot soapy water before wiping the thermometer

10. An axillary temperature is taken by placing the thermometer:
    1. under the forearm
    2. so that the bulb is in the armpit
    3. on the inner arm at the elbow and then bending the arm
    4. so that the thermometer is held lengthwise between the upper arm and chest

11. Before taking an axillary temperature it is most important to:
    1. rub the arm to increase circulation
    2. dry the armpit by patting the area with a towel
    3. help the patient to a sitting position
    4. turn the patient onto his back

12. When taking a rectal temperature it is most important for the nurse to:
    1. keep the patient on his left side
    2. insert the thermometer so that it is beyond the sphincter muscle
    3. use a lubricant with an oil base
    4. hold the thermometer in place while the temperature is being taken

13. The most common sites for taking a pulse are:
    1. the ankle and wrist
    2. over the jugular vein and at the wrist
    3. the wrist and temple
    4. the wrist and knee

14. A pulse of unusually full force is best described as:
    1. thready
    2. bounding
    3. irregular
    4. deep

15. When the spaces or intervals between pulse beats are uneven, the pulse is said to be:
    1. weak
    2. shallow
    3. irregular
    4. thready

16. A weak and rapid pulse which can be barely felt is called:
    1. shallow
    2. irregular
    3. bounding
    4. thready

17. In order to gain the most accurate count of an irregular pulse it is most important to:
    1. apply more pressure on the artery
    2. use the thumb to count the pulse
    3. use only one finger to feel the pulse
    4. count the pulse for one full minute

18. Which of the following is *not* true of an apical-radial pulse?
    1. a stethoscope is needed to count the apical pulse.
    2. One nurse can carry out this procedure if she is very careful to make a distinction between the two pulse rates.

    3. The difference between the apical pulse and the radial pulse is called the pulse deficit.

    4. Both pulses must be counted simultaneously for one full minute.

19. The normal rate of respiration varies with age. Which of the following statements best describes this variation in normal rates of respiration?

    1. An infant's rate of respiration is almost half the adult rate.

    2. The older a person, the faster is his rate of respiration.

    3. An infant's rate of respiration is normally much faster than an adult's.

    4. Elderly persons normally have a very high rate of respiration.

20. When counting a patient's respirations, it is most important for the nurse to:

    1. count the respirations in such a manner that the patient is not aware of her doing so

    2. ask the patient to lie down so she can get an accurate counting

    3. always count the respirations before the pulse is taken

    4. always count the respirations while a thermometer is in the patient's mouth

21. Stertorous breathing refers to:

    1. shallow respirations

    2. difficult breathing

    3. noisy or snoring type of breathing

    4. cessation of breathing

22. Cheyne-Stokes respirations are characterized by:

    1. periods of dyspnea followed by periods of apnea

    2. very shallow breathing

    3. periods of rapid breathing followed by periods of slow breathing

    4. noisy or snoring sounds during inspiration of air

23. Blood pressure is best defined as the:

    1. rate of the heartbeat

    2. amount of force exerted by the blood against the walls of the blood vessels

    3. amount of force exerted by the walls of the arteries as they constrict

    4. strength of the heartbeat

24. When taking blood pressure, the first in a series of sounds heard through the stethoscope is called the:

    1. diastolic pressure

    2. pulse pressure

    3. systolic pressure

    4. venous pressure

25. The diastolic blood pressure is determined by watching for the point at which:

    1. the first sharp sound is heard

    2. there is a cessation of sounds

    3. sounds change from muffled to sharp

    4. sounds increase in rate per minute

26. The normal range for blood pressure is generally considered to be:

    1. a person's age plus 100

    2. 90 to 120 over 60 to 80

    3. 120 to 150 over 100 to 120

    4. 140 to 180 over 120 to 140

27. Hypotension refers to:

    1. a narrow margin between the systolic pressure and the diastolic pressure

    2. abnormally high blood pressure

    3. any abnormality in blood pressure

    4. abnormally low blood pressure

28. In order to obtain an accurate blood pressure reading, it is most important that the:

    1. patient has received no stimulants such as coffee or tea within the past hour

    2. patient is lying down

    3. arm of the patient is well supported during the procedure

    4. cuff is kept inflated for at least 2 minutes before it is allowed to deflate gradually

29. When recording her observations of a patient, the nurse must remember that a patient's chart is:
    1. a legal document that may be used as evidence in court
    2. not a permanent record and is most important when the patient is in the hospital
    3. the property of the patient
    4. the property of the physician treating the patient

A nurse enters Mr. Brown's room to give him his medication and finds that Mr. and Mrs. Brown are involved in a heated argument about financial matters. When the medication is offered to Mr. Brown he refuses it, stating, "Those pills make me nauseated."

30. When charting the incident, the nurse should write:
    1. refused medication because they make him sick
    2. upset by argument with wife and therefore refused medication
    3. refused medication — stated the pills make him nauseated
    4. refused medication because of worry about cost of illness
31. The main reason for charting a patient's refusal of the medication is to:
    1. prove that the patient is difficult to get along with
    2. relieve the nurse of responsibility for giving medications to the patient
    3. inform the physician of the patient's reaction to the medication
    4. notify the nurses on duty that the patient will not cooperate with them
32. *Each time* a notation is made on a patient's chart, it is most important to include the:
    1. patient's name in the notation
    2. signature of the person making the notation
    3. time the notation was made
    4. name of the physician attending the patient
33. Correction of an error in charting should be made by:
    1. erasing the error with ink eradicator
    2. blacking out the error with a pencil or pen
    3. drawing several lines through the error
    4. drawing a single line through the error and writing the word "error" above it
34. If a whole page of notations has been made on the wrong chart the nurse should:
    1. draw a line through each notation
    2. draw an X through the page and write "error in charting" across the page
    3. erase the notations and start again
    4. remove the page from the patient's chart even though there may be correct notations on the other side

Mrs. Wilkins, age 48, is admitted to the hospital for surgery of the gallbladder. During the admission procedure she is very talkative and seems to be worried about having the surgery.

35. Which of the following terms best describes Mrs. Wilkins' emotional status?
    1. disoriented
    2. irrational
    3. uncooperative
    4. apprehensive
36. The nurse can help Mrs. Wilkins relax and feel more at home in the hospital if she will:
    1. take time to explain the hospital routine and show her where the bathroom, call light, etc. are located
    2. tell Mrs. Wilkins she has nothing to worry about because many people have had this same type of surgery
    3. tell the other patients in the ward how worried Mrs. Wilkins is so they can cheer her up
    4. ignore Mrs. Wilkins' worries because all patients having surgery are upset when admitted
37. If Mrs. Wilkins tells the nurse that a rash on her arms and legs is due to an allergy to a medication she has been taking, the nurse should:
    1. tell her not to worry about it because she probably won't receive that medication while she is in the hospital

2. record her observations of the rash and the patient's statement about its cause
3. realize that this is not an unusual situation since allergies are very common
4. conclude that Mrs. Wilkins' rash is probably the result of nervousness rather than an allergy

38. Even though the admission procedure varies in institutions, the one basic principle that never changes is:
   1. Time is not to be wasted and the procedure must be completed as quickly as possible.
   2. All patients are nervous when they are admitted to a hospital.
   3. The patient's first impression of the hospital is nearly always a bad one.
   4. Courtesy and interest in the patient are of primary importance during the admission procedure.

39. When patients bring valuables such as money or jewelry to the hospital with them, the person responsible for proper care of these valuables is the:
   1. nurse admitting the patient
   2. hospital administrator
   3. physician in charge of the patient
   4. patient himself

40. If a patient decides to leave the hospital against the advice of his physician, the nurse must:
   1. send a written report to the local police department
   2. ask the patient to sign a release, relieving the hospital and physician from responsibility
   3. restrain the patient by whatever means necessary
   4. warn the patient that he can never be readmitted to the hospital once he leaves

41. During a physical examination, the physician may detect sounds produced by various organs of the body by using the:
   1. otoscope
   2. stethoscope
   3. speculum
   4. percussion hammer

42. When a physician examines a part of the body by palpation it is the nurse's main responsibility to:
   1. provide adequate lighting
   2. have the necessary instruments on hand
   3. help the patient relax and cooperate with the physician
   4. distract the patient's attention from the procedure

43. While the physician is examining the chest by percussion the patient should be:
   1. lying on his back
   2. sitting upright
   3. lying on his left side with right knee flexed
   4. in lithotomy position

44. The instrument used to examine the eye is called the:
   1. ophthalmoscope
   2. otoscope
   3. stethoscope
   4. speculum

45. The position most often used for a pelvic examination is the:
   1. Trendelenburg
   2. prone
   3. knee-chest
   4. lithotomy

46. When assisting the physician with a vaginal examination, the nurse would need to assemble at least three articles. They include:
   1. sigmoidoscope, lubricant, and speculum
   2. tongue blade, otoscope, and rubber gloves
   3. stethoscope, tongue blade, and lubricant
   4. speculum, lubricant, and rubber gloves

47. While assisting a patient onto the examination table and draping the patient for examination, the nurse must be *especially* careful to:
    1. avoid chilling the patient
    2. provide adequate lighting   –
    3. assemble the instruments she will need
    4. avoid unnecessary exposure of the patient
48. Which of the following positions would NOT be used for a rectal examination?
    1. Trendelenburg
    2. Sims' position
    3. lithotomy
    4. knee-chest
49. The amount of urine considered adequate for most laboratory tests would be:
    1. 20 to 30 ml.
    2. 40 to 60 ml.
    3. 300 to 500 ml.
    4. 60 to 100 ml.
50. A sterile specimen of urine is obtained by:
    1. asking the patient to void in a sterile bedpan
    2. catheterizing the patient
    3. cleansing the external genitalia before the patient voids
    4. having the patient void directly into a specimen bottle
51. When collecting a clean-voided specimen for urinalysis the first thing the nurse should do is:
    1. give the patient a clean specimen cup and instruct her to void
    2. cleanse the external genitalia or instruct patient to do so
    3. explain the catheterization procedure to the patient
    4. give the patient a full glass of water to drink so the bladder will be full when the specimen is needed
52. If you were instructing a patient in the correct method for obtaining a midstream urine specimen, it would be best to tell him:
    1. "Please collect only the urine that is left after you have voided about one cup-full."
    2. "You should void a small amount first, to cleanse the urinary passage, and then void into the specimen cup."
    3. "Your bladder must be emptied completely, then you should drink a glass of water and save a specimen the next time you urinate."
    4. "When you feel a strong urge to urinate please void a small amount into the specimen cup."
53. A specimen of urine that includes all urine voided by the patient between 7:00 A.M. one day and 7:00 A.M. the following day is called a:
    1. clean-voided specimen
    2. specimen of the total output
    3. liquid tolerance test
    4. 24-hour specimen
54. When beginning to collect a specimen such as the one described in the previous question the nurse should ask the patient to:
    1. void and discard this specimen since the bladder should be empty when the test is begun.
    2. void directly into the large container used for collecting all specimens.
    3. drink one glass of water every hour so there will be sufficient urine to collect a specimen every hour.
    4. avoid drinking coffee or tea as this will cause an inaccurate testing of kidney function.
55. The best time for collecting a sputum specimen is:
    1. at bedtime
    2. in the midafternoon
    3. just before breakfast
    4. just after breakfast
56. A sputum specimen *must* contain:
    1. material coughed up from the lungs and bronchi
    2. nasal secretions

3. gastric contents
4. material produced by the salivary glands

57. A stool specimen consists of:
   1. urine
   2. sputum
   3. fecal material
   4. blood samples

58. Stool specimens usually should be sent to the laboratory immediately after they are collected, chiefly because:
   1. they are unsightly
   2. deterioration of the specimen begins almost immediately
   3. there is more danger of contamination than from any other type of specimen
   4. the specimen may dry out, and only liquid specimens can be examined

59. If a stool specimen is to be examined for ova and parasites, it is especially important for the specimen to be kept:
   1. refrigerated until examined
   2. warm until examined
   3. in an airtight container
   4. in a sterile container

60. A culture is done by:
   1. destroying all bacteria in a specimen
   2. examining the specimen for hidden blood
   3. growing bacteria under special laboratory conditions
   4. examining the specimen for ova (eggs) of bacteria

61. When assisting with the collection of a specimen for culture, the nurse must remember that the specimen is most likely to be:
   1. highly contaminated with living bacteria
   2. a stool specimen
   3. a large amount, usually 500 ml.
   4. collected by a laboratory technician or physician

62. The container for a specimen for culture must be:
   1. covered with a gauze square
   2. plugged with cotton
   3. filled completely
   4. examined carefully for cracks or chips before it is used

63. After a specimen for culture is obtained, it is especially important for the container to be:
   1. wrapped in tissue
   2. kept in an upright position
   3. refrigerated until it can be sent to the laboratory
   4. wrapped in a sterile wrapper

64. Which of the following is NOT a nursing responsibility in the collection of specimens?
   1. proper instruction of the patient
   2. determining the type of test to be done on the specimen
   3. accurate labeling of the specimen container
   4. choosing the type of laboratory procedure to be done

65. If you are collecting a 7:00 A.M. specimen to test for sugar and acetone, it is advisable to have the patient empty the bladder and then provide a fresh specimen 15 to 20 minutes later. The reason for this is:
   1. urine accumulated in the bladder during the night is more likely to contain bacteria and sediment
   2. the urine in the first specimen would be too concentrated to give an accurate reading
   3. the second specimen of urine is more likely to give an accurate indication of the amount of sugar in the blood stream
   4. the second specimen is more likely to give a higher reading of sugar because it would be more dilute

66. When collecting urine for a sugar and acetone test from a patient with an indwelling catheter, a more accurate reading will be obtained if the urine sample is taken from the:
   1. catheter

    2. drainage tubing

    3. drainage bottle

67. Clinitest tablets should be kept in the
    1. medicine cabinet with other oral drugs
    2. refrigerator to avoid decomposition
    3. narcotic cabinet to prevent their being misused
    4. workroom or other area where they are to be used

68. Heat may be applied to the body for ALL BUT ONE of the following reasons:
    1. to promote muscular relaxation
    2. to help localize an infection
    3. to promote drainage from wounds
    4. to help control hemorrhage

69. When moderate heat is applied to the body, the surface blood vessels:
    1. dilate
    2. constrict
    3. move closer to the surface of the body
    4. lose their elasticity

70. A hot water bottle is often used for the application of dry heat. The hot water bottle should be dried before it is covered and applied chiefly because:
    1. moist heat is less effective than dry heat
    2. water cools quickly and the hot water bottle will need to be changed almost immediately after it is applied
    3. the patient will not receive the benefit of the heat if the hot water bottle cover is wet
    4. moist heat is more penetrating than dry heat and the patient may be burned if the cover is wet

71. When applying any type of heat to a patient, the nurse must remember that:
    1. prolonged applications of heat will decrease circulation to the part
    2. heat cannot be tolerated by the body for more than 1 hour
    3. infants and elderly persons are usually more easily burned than other patients
    4. heat stimulates the growth of bacteria

72. The recommended temperature for water used to fill a hot water bottle is:
    1. 120 to 125° F. (49 to 51.6° C.)
    2. 90 to 100° F. (32 to 37.7° C.)
    3. 130 to 150° F. (54.4 to 65.5° C.)
    4. 65 to 75° F. (18 to 24° C.)

73. The main reason for filling a hot water bottle only half full of water is to:
    1. avoid having to change the water often
    2. prevent excess weight on the part to which it is applied
    3. prevent stretching of the rubber
    4. prevent cracking of the rubber

74. Before a heating pad is applied the nurse must:
    1. be sure it is in good repair, with no exposed wires
    2. check the cover to be sure it is not too thick
    3. remove the thermostat so the patient cannot adjust the temperature
    4. warn the patient that electric heating pads are very dangerous

75. The application of cold to the body has the effect of:
    1. increasing circulation to the part to which it is applied
    2. promoting muscular relaxation
    3. constricting blood vessels and reducing circulation to the part to which it is applied
    4. speeding up the process of inflammation

76. After an icebag or ice collar has been applied it usually must be refilled at least every:
    1. 15 minutes
    2. 3 hours
    3. 30 minutes
    4. 2 hours

77. To test an icebag or ice collar for leakage it is best to:
    1. fill it with ice and wait for an hour to see if it leaks
    2. fill it with air and squeeze to see if air escapes
    3. fill with water and check for leaks

      4.   cover it well and ask the patient to notify you if water seeps through the cover

78. To be sure that an irrigation procedure has the desired effect without harming body tissues, it is most important to:
1. use a steady, gentle stream to cleanse the area being irrigated
2. ask the patient to notify you when the irrigation becomes painful
3. allow the solution to trickle onto the area being irrigated
4. use only small gauge tubing for the irrigation

79. When administering an irrigation of any kind the nurse must remember that:
1. the higher the vessel containing the liquid, the greater is the pressure of the irrigating fluid
2. the higher the vessel containing the liquid, the less is the pressure of the irrigating fluid
3. the lower the vessel containing the liquid, the higher is the pressure of the irrigating fluid
4. it is the concentration of the liquid and not the level of the container that affects the pressure of the fluid

80. Since irrigations are often ordered for the purpose of cleansing an inflamed or infected part of the body, it is most important for the nurse to:
1. always use disinfectant solutions
2. use sterile solutions for all irrigations
3. allow enough pressure so that the irrigating fluid thoroughly washes all tissue surrounding the affected part
4. use only enough pressure to reach the affected area, but not enough to force fluid beyond that point

81. During an eye irrigation the head should be:
1. held upright
2. turned to the side so that the affected eye is uppermost
3. turned so that the affected eye is lower than the other eye
4. held so the irrigating fluid flows up over the upper lid

82. The flow of irrigating fluid is directed so that the solution runs:
1. from the inner corner of the eye to the outer corner
2. from the outer corner of the eye to the inner corner
3. from the top of the eye to the bottom
4. from the bottom lid toward the top

83. Whenever it is necessary to separate the eyelids in order to expose the eyeball, the finger and thumb are placed:
1. so that pressure is exerted on the eyeball
2. so that pressure is exerted on the facial bones
3. directly on the upper and lower eyelids
4. on the upper eyelid only

84. Excessive pressure must be avoided when an ear irrigation is being done chiefly because:
1. there is no way for the fluid to return during the irrigation
2. pressure will cause loss of consciousness
3. this may spread infection to the middle ear
4. the eardrum may be punctured

85. Gargling and irrigations of the throat are similar; however, the physician usually orders a throat irrigation when:
1. he wishes to have the irrigating fluid reach a more extensive area than can be done with gargling
2. the patient is semicomatose and unable to cooperate
3. the patient has had surgery of the trachea
4. the patient refuses to gargle

86. Solutions for gargling and irrigation of the throat may be slightly hotter than solutions for other types of irrigations because:
1. the throat is not lined with mucous membrane
2. there are more bacteria present in the mouth and throat
3. bacteria in the mouth and throat are easily killed by high temperatures
4. the mouth and throat are more accustomed to hot liquids

87. The most comfortable position for the patient during a throat irrigation is:
    1. lying on his back
    2. sitting up with head bent forward slightly
    3. sitting up with head held back as far as it will go
    4. lying face down on the bed
88. A perineal irrigation is done for the purpose of cleaning the:
    1. vaginal canal
    2. abdominal cavity
    3. vulva or external genitalia
    4. anal canal
89. To avoid contamination from the anal region while drying a patient after a perineal irrigation, it is necessary to:
    1. use sterile cotton balls
    2. wipe from front to back toward anal region
    3. wipe from back to front away from anal region
    4. cover the anal region with a sterile towel
90. If you were teaching a patient the best method for taking a douche at home, you should advise her to:
    1. lie down in the bathtub at home
    2. rent a bedpan and take the douche lying in bed
    3. sit on the commode and take the douche, since this is the most convenient way
    4. assume any position that is comfortable for her but be sure the tip is inserted at least 1 inch
91. The vaginal surface lies in folds. When instructing the patient you should tell her that the vagina will be cleaned more effectively if she will:
    1. elevate the container of liquid as high as possible so that the solution flows with a maximum force
    2. use a very strong Lysol solution
    3. use a solution that is at least 125° F. (51.6° C.)
    4. gently rotate the douche nozzle while the irrigating fluid is flowing
92. The amount of solution usually given in a cleansing enema is:
    1. ½ gallon
    2. 1 pint
    3. 1 quart
    4. ½ pint
93. It is recommended that the enema can should not be held higher than:
    1. 18 inches above the patient's buttocks
    2. 18 inches above the floor
    3. 6 inches above the patient's buttocks
    4. 36 inches above the patient's buttocks
94. The position recommended for administration of an enema is:
    1. lithotomy
    2. Sims' left lateral
    3. prone
    4. supine
95. When a soapsuds solution is given as an enema the soap has:
    1. a soothing effect on the mucous membranes of the intestine
    2. very little cleansing effect on the intestinal tract
    3. the effect of destroying all bacteria in the colon
    4. an irritating effect on the mucous membranes of the intestine
96. If the rectal tube is difficult to insert when administering an enema, it is best to:
    1. wait a few minutes until the lubricant has had effect
    2. tell the patient that she is uncooperative and must relax before you can give her the enema
    3. wait a while until the spasm of the sphincter muscle has passed and then continue to insert the tube
    4. report to the nurse in charge that the patient has refused the enema
97. When preparing a soapsuds enema you should:
    1. remove the suds and bubbles from the top of the solution before it is administered

    2.   stir the solution vigorously just before administering it

    3.   heat the solution to 125° F. (51.6° C.)

    4.   allow the solution to stand for at least 30 minutes to be sure all soap is dissolved

98.   Which of the following is the best example of charting the results of an enema?

    1.   good results

    2.   patient unable to tell if enema was effective

    3.   solution returned clear with small amount of constipated stool

    4.   patient stated she had good results

99.   An oil retention enema is given primarily for the purpose of:

    1.   stimulating peristalsis

    2.   softening fecal material

    3.   cleansing the bowel before diagnostic tests

    4.   relieving distention caused by flatus

100.   The oil for a retention enema should always be warmed before it is administered; however, it is important to remember that:

    1.   oil should not be heated to more than 100° F. (37.7° C.) because it retains heat longer than water

    2.   oil must be heated to 120° F. (48.8° C.); otherwise it will not flow freely through the rectal tube

    3.   oil will mix with water only after it has been heated

    4.   oil does not conduct heat as quickly as water and it must therefore be administered at a higher degree when given as an enema

101.   Before administering a retention enema it is most important to:

    1.   tell the patient that the enema must be expelled immediately after it is given

    2.   ask the patient to go to the bathroom to expel the enema

    3.   tell the patient the enema will be most effective if it is retained until the urge to evacuate is strong

    4.   warn the patient that the enema will not be effective unless it is retained for at least one hour

102.   The amount usually given for an oil retention enema is:

    1.   500 ml.

    2.   300 ml.

    3.   100 ml.

    4.   10 ml.

103.   While the nurse is inserting a rectal suppository the patient asks, "Will I have a bowel movement after this suppository?" To answer this question correctly the practical nurse must know that:

    1.   all rectal suppositories are given to relieve constipation

    2.   most rectal suppositories are given for relief of swollen hemorrhoids

    3.   rectal suppositories are given only when enemas are contraindicated

    4.   rectal suppositories are given for different reasons and the nurse should know the desired effect before inserting the suppository

104.   To decrease the patient's desire to expel the suppository, the nurse should insert it:

    1.   very quickly

    2.   at least 3 to 4 inches or well beyond the sphincter muscle

    3.   at least 1 inch into the rectum

    4.   after it has been heated to body temperature

105.   Rectal tubes are sometimes inserted to relieve distention caused by flatus. The word flatus refers to:

    1.   constipation

    2.   loose watery stools

    3.   gas in the intestinal tract

    4.   collapse of the intestinal tract

106.   A rectal tube achieves maximum results and should be removed after:

    1.   30 minutes

    2.   1 hour

    3.   2 hours

    4.   3 hours

107. Catheterization is performed as a sterile procedure because:
    1. there is danger of spreading the bacteria normally found in the urine
    2. the urinary system is considered to be sterile unless an infection is present
    3. most kidney infections are highly contagious
    4. most venereal diseases are spread by contaminated urine
108. Irrigation of the bladder is most effective if it is done:
    1. using a moderate amount of force
    2. when the bladder is full
    3. as a surgically sterile procedure
    4. when the bladder is empty
109. The specific solution to be used for irrigating the bladder should be:
    1. a very strong disinfectant solution
    2. prescribed by the physician
    3. clean, but need not be sterile
    4. determined by the nurse in charge
110. A bladder irrigation is similar to a bladder instillation except that in an instillation:
    1. the procedure is continuous and the flow of solution is not interrupted
    2. the solution used is always an antibiotic
    3. the solution used need not be sterile
    4. the solution is left in the bladder for a period of time and is not siphoned back immediately
111. The doctor has ordered a straight abdominal binder for an obese patient. It is the patient's second postoperative day following a cholecystectomy. The purpose of this binder would be to:
    a. hold the surgical dressings in place
    b. provide support for the abdomen and prevent strain on the sutures
    c. relieve abdominal distention
    d. eliminate frequent changing of the dressing

    1. a and d
    2. b and c
    3. a and b
    4. c and d
112. The type of bandage most commonly used as a sling for the arm is the:
    1. scultetus
    2. T binder
    3. square
    4. triangular
113. When applying a figure-of-eight bandage to an ankle, the first thing the nurse should do is:
    1. make at least three turns around the lower leg
    2. make two turns around the arch of the foot
    3. extend the ankle joint
    4. flex the ankle joint
114. When applying a bandage to the arm the nurse should:
    1. start at the end farthest from the body and wrap toward the body
    2. begin wrapping the area closest to the body and wrap away from the body
    3. start in the middle of the arm and wrap in either direction
    4. always begin at the elbow and wrap toward the wrist
115. If the nurse must bandage a foot, including the toes, which of the following would be most important?
    1. wrapping the foot more tightly than the toes
    2. placing padding under the ball of the foot
    3. placing gauze or cotton between the toes
    4. securing the bandage with a knot at the heel
116. Which of the following types of binders would be best for holding a rectal dressing in place?
    1. four-tailed binder
    2. straight binder
    3. T binder
    4. triangular
117. The scultetus binder most often is applied to the abdomen. Another name for the scultetus binder is:
    1. T binder
    2. straight binder

      3. many-tailed binder

      4. double T binder

118. When the arm is placed in a sling, the wrist should be:
    1. slightly higher than the elbow
    2. level with the elbow
    3. slightly lower than the elbow
    4. at least 6 inches lower than the elbow

119. In some cases when dressings must be changed quite frequently, the procedure will be less uncomfortable for the patient and easier for the nurse if the dressings are held in place with:
    1. wide strips of adhesive tape
    2. an abdominal binder
    3. a T binder
    4. Montgomery straps

120. If you prepared to catheterize a patient and found that the cotton wrapper around the tray was wet, you should consider the equipment to be:
    1 unsterile
    2. sterile
    3. unsterile but safe to use for this type of procedure
    4. safe to use as long as the wrapper is removed before the tray is set up

121 An object must be considered as contaminated if it is:
    1. handled with sterile pickup forceps
    2. handled with sterile gloves
    3. left uncovered for a period of time
    4. sterilized by any means other than submersion in a disinfectant

122. To properly place the cover of a container of sterile articles onto a table so that it is not contaminated, one must place the cover so that it is lying:
    1. sterile side up
    2. sterile side down
    3. on a clean paper towel
    4. on its side

123. To prevent contamination of the tips of pickup forceps, they must always be held:
    1. with the tips up
    2. with the tips down
    3. in a gloved hand
    4. in a horizontal position

124. Pickup forceps should be used to:
    1. remove contaminated dressings from a wound
    2. remove wrappers from sterile objects
    3. lift and handle sterile objects only
    4. lift and handle either sterile or unsterile objects

125. When using pickup forceps to remove sterile articles from a container, it is most important to:
    1. avoid touching the inside of the container with the forceps
    2. avoid touching the inside or outside of the container with the forceps
    3. hold the forceps so that the tips are higher than the object being lifted
    4. dry the tips of the forceps with a paper towel before picking up the articles with them

126. While working around a sterile field it is best to stand:
    1. to the side of the sterile field
    2. at least 3 feet from the sterile field
    3. directly over the sterile field to avoid dropping equipment on the floor
    4. with your back to the sterile field

127. If a physician requests additional sterile dressings to be placed on a sterile field, the nurse should:
    1. give him the container so he can reach in and get the dressings he needs
    2. remove the hemostat from the sterile field and use this to handle the sterile dressings
    3. use the pickup forceps to lift the dressings from the container and drop them onto the sterile field

      4. give the physician the pickup forceps so he can remove the dressings from the container

128. When soiled dressings are removed from a wound they should be:
 1. discarded in the patient's wastebasket
 2. placed at the foot of the patient's bed and discarded with the soiled linen
 3. autoclaved before they are discarded to prevent cross infection
 4. wrapped in paper and discarded in a closed trash can in the utility room or taken to the incinerator

129. If you were preparing to perform a sterile procedure such as catheterization, you would:
 1. don the rubber gloves before preparing the tray
 2. open the tray first and then don rubber gloves just before doing the procedure
 3. don rubber gloves before entering the patient's room
 4. use rubber gloves only if the patient has a contagious disease

Part VI

DRUGS AND THEIR ADMINISTRATION

UNIT 1   DRUGS

I. Sources of Drugs
A. Chemical compounds—agents that are prepared synthetically.
B. Plants—roots, bark, leaves, or other parts of the plant may be used.
C. Animal products—glandular secretions obtained from animals.
D. Certain food substances—vitamins and minerals.

II. Standardization of Drugs
A. Standards are necessary to guarantee purity and accurate strength of dosage.
B. Reference books used to describe the drugs, their use, and their action.
  1. United States Pharmacopeia (USP)
    a. Includes a list of approved drugs, their source, composition, use, dosage, and directions for compounding.
    b. Revised every 5 years so that new drugs are included, and old ones excluded if they are no longer used.
  2. National Formulary (NF)
    a. Published by the American Pharmaceutical Association.
    b. Contains the formulas of drugs.
  3. Physician's Desk Reference (PDR)
    a. Not an official listing of drugs; published by the manufacturers of drugs.
    b. Drugs are listed under trade names and generic names.

III. Forms of Drugs
A. Liquid preparations
  1. Solutions—contain a *solute* (the dissolved substance) and a *solvent* (usually a liquid, the substance in which the solute is dissolved).
  2. Elixirs—solutions containing alcohol, sugar, and water; e.g., elixir of Donnatal, terpin hydrate elixir.
  3. Tinctures—alcoholic or alcohol and water solutions; e.g., tincture of Merthiolate.
  4. Emulsions—suspension of fat globules and water.
  5. Lotions—soothing solutions, intended for soothing local application.
  6. Liniments—applied externally, produce a sensation of warmth to area applied.
B. Solid and semisolid preparations
  1. Capsules—drug is placed inside a gelatinous container which dissolves when swallowed. Capsules cannot be broken for smaller doses.
  2. Tablets—drug is compressed into a circular mold. Tablets may be scored so they can be broken into halves or fourths for smaller dosages.
  3. Pills—globe-shaped preparations, cannot be broken evenly for smaller doses. Some pills may be covered with a substance that is dissolved only by intestinal juices rather than gastric juices. These pills are *enteric-coated* and are not absorbed until they reach the small intestine.
  4. Suppositories—inserted into some body orifice. Have a base which will melt at body temperature.
  5. Ointments—mixtures with a fatty base; are applied externally.

IV. Actions of Drugs
A. Local effects—action of drug takes place

in area of skin or mucous membrane to which it has been applied.

B. Systemic effects—drug is absorbed into the blood and carried to the specific organ or tissues upon which it acts.

C. Side effects—usually undesirable effects which may result from administration of a drug. Side effects often limit the use of a drug.

V. Local Anti-infectives

A. General types—a single agent may have more than one type of action.
1. Antiseptic—inhibits growth of micro-organisms.
2. Bacteriostatic, antibacterial — inhibits growth of bacteria.
3. Bactericidal—kills bacteria.
4. Disinfectant, germicide—used on in-animate objects to destroy microorganisms.

B. Examples
1. Alcohol—70% ethyl alcohol is ideal per-centage for optimum antisepsis. Iso-propyl alcohol is twice as germicidal as ethyl alcohol and is more toxic.
2. Benzalkonium chloride (Zephiran). Safe to use on skin and mucous mem-branes in concentrations from 1:10,000 1:2000. *Caution*—inactivated by soap or detergent.
3. Methylrosaniline chloride (gentian violet). Used in strengths of 1:1000 to 1:100. Especially useful in fungus infec-tions.
4. Povidone-iodine (Betadine)—used in 1% to 1.5% solutions.
3. Staphene—has wide range of effects on many types of organisms.
6. Potassium permanganate—used in 1% solution as antiseptic but in 1:5000 solu-tion for vaginal irrigations and topical application.

VI. Vitamin Preparations

A. Characteristics
1. Required in small amounts.
2. Sensitive to light, heat, and oxidation—must be stored in a cool dark place in dark bottles.
3. Fat-soluble vitamins
a. Vitamin A—preparations include Stubil A, Aquasol A.
b. Vitamin D (Drisol, Dical-D)—enables body to deposit calcium and phos-phorus in the bones. Overdose leads to low calcium blood level, tetany, and eventual death.
c. Vitamin K (Synkayvite, Hykinone, Mephyton)—needed for formation of prothrombin.
4. Water-soluble

a. Folic acid—sold as Folvite.
b. Vitamin B_{12} (Coplex, Rubramin)—used in treatment of pernicious anemia
c. Vitamin C—ascorbic acid, cevitamic acid.

VII. Drugs Affecting the Body Systems

A. Musculoskeletal system
1. Analgesics—used to relieve pain
a. Aspirin—used to relieve pain of arthritis. Other salicylates such as sodium salicylate also used.
b. Phenacetin—relieves mild aches and pains.
2. Muscle relaxants—diminish muscular spasms.
a. Local applications of liniments such as oil of wintergreen.
b. Systemic relaxants—produce relaxa-tion and may also have tranquilizing affect.

B. Circulatory system
1. Heart stimulants—quicken the action of the heart. Example, epinephrine.
2. Heart tonics—slow and strengthen the heartbeat. Example, digitalis prepara-tions.
3. Heart depressants—slow the heart-beat. Example, quinidine.
4. Vasoconstrictors—produce narrowing of the blood vessels, raise the blood pressure. Example, Levophed.
5. Vasodilators—produce an increase in the size of the blood vessels. Example, nitroglycerin.
6. Coagulants—speed up the process of coagulation. Example, vitamin K preparations.
7. Anticoagulants—inhibit the formation of blood clots. Example, Dicumarol.
8. Hematinics—tonics that improve the production of hemoglobin and red blood cells. Example, iron preparations.

C. Respiratory system
1. Respiratory stimulants—increase the rate and depth of respiration. Example, carbon dioxide.
2. Respiratory depressants—slow down and deepen the respirations. Example, morphine.
3. Bronchodilators—relax and dilate the bronchi. Example, aminophylline.
4. Cough mixtures
a. Sedative cough mixtures—reduce irri-tation and lessen the desire to cough. Example, Cheracol.
b. Expectorants—induce expectoration by increasing secretion of mucus in the respiratory tract. Example, potas-sium iodide.
5. Specifics for pulmonary tuberculosis—

effective in destroying tubercle bacilli. Examples, streptomycin, para-aminosalicylic acid (PAS), and isoniazid hydrochloride (INH).

D. Digestive system
1. Antacids—counteract gastric acidity. Examples, milk of magnesia, Amphojel.
2. Digestants—used to aid the process of digestion; usually replace substances normally found in digestive juices. Example, hydrochloric acid.
3. Emetics—induce vomiting. Example, apomorphine.
4. Antiemetics—relieve nausea and vomiting. Example, Dramamine.
5. Cathartics—act to empty the colon. Example, cascara sagrada.
6. Antidiarrheics—soothe the intestinal tract and quiet an overactive bowel. Example, Kaopectate.

E. Urinary tract
1. Diuretics—increase the flow of urine. Example, Mercuhydrin.
2. Urinary antiseptics—used to treat minor infections of the urinary tract. Example, Urotropin.

F. Reproductive system
1. Uterine stimulants (ecbolic)—increase contractions of the uterine muscle. Example, ergotamine tartrate (Gynergen).
2. Uterine sedatives—decrease uterine contractions; used as antiabortives. Example, Lutrexin.
3. Emmenagogues—induce or increase menstruation. Example, progesterone.

G. Central nervous system
1. CNS stimulants—increase the activity of the brain, medulla, and spinal cord. Example, caffeine sodium benzoate.
2. CNS depressants—reduce activities and reflexes controlled by the brain and spinal cord. Example, opium.
3. Hypnotics—produce sleep. Example, barbiturates.
4. Anticonvulsants—reduce involuntary convulsive movements. Example, Dilantin.
5. Anesthetics—produce a loss of sensitivity to pain. Example, ether.

H. The endocrine glands
1. Secretions from the endocrine glands are called *hormones*. They are chemical substances which are carried by the blood to various organs of the body and directly affect certain activities of these organs.
2. Pituitary gland—divided into two lobes.
   a. Anterior lobe secretes several regulating hormones called the tropic hormones; e.g., thyrotropic hormone affects the thyroid gland, adrenocorticotropic hormone (ACTH) affects the cortex of the adrenal gland.
   b. Posterior lobe secretes hormone pituitrin, which stimulates uterine contractions; sometimes used to induce labor in obstetrical patients.
3. Thyroid gland secretes thyroxin. Thyroid extract given to relieve symptoms produced by underactivity of the thyroid gland.
4. Adrenal gland—divided into cortex and medulla.
   a. Cortex secretes a number of hormones essential to life; e.g., cortisone and hydrocortisone, used as anti-inflammatory agents.
   b. Medulla secretes epinephrine (Adrenalin).
5. Pancreas—islands of Langerhans are small clusters of cells located on the surface of the pancreas; they secrete the hormone insulin.
   a. Insulin activity (see Table 7)
      1. All types of insulin must be given by injection only.
   b. Strengths of insulin:
      1. May come as U40, U80, or U100.
      2. U40 indicates that there are 40 units of insulin per ml. of solution.
   c. Orinase and Diabinase
      1. Lower the blood sugar.
      2. Are *NOT* examples of oral insulin.

I. The eye
1. Eye washes—used to cleanse the eye and aid in removing foreign bodies. Examples, boric acid solution and normal saline.
2. Anesthetics—used to desensitize the eye during treatments. Examples, cocaine and Pontocaine.
3. Mydriatics—drugs which dilate the pupil. Example, atropine.
4. Myotics—drugs which constrict the pupil. Example, pilocarpine.

VIII. **Antihistamines—counteract the effects of histamine, thereby relieving the symptoms of simple allergic reactions and the common cold.**
A. Most dangerous side-effect is drowsiness. Patient should be cautioned against driving and working around heavy machinery when taking an antihistamine.
B. Examples include Benadryl, Chlor-Trimeton, Dramamine, Phenergan, Dimetane, Bonine.

Table 7.   Insulin Activity*

Name	Time and Route of Administration	Onset	Peak	Duration of Action	Most Likely Time for Insulin Reaction	Most Likely Time for Sugar in the Urine
Fast action						
Regular	15–20 minutes before meals, S.C. (I.V. in emergency)	Rapid, within 1 hour	2–4 hr.	5–8 hr.	10 A.M. to lunch	During night
Crystalline	Same	Same	Same	Same	Same	Same
Semilente	½–¾ hr. before breakfast, deep S.C. (never I.V.)	Same	6–10 hr.	12–16 hr.	Before lunch	Same
Intermediate action						
Globin	½–1 hr. before breakfast. S.C.	Within 2–4 hr. (rapidity increases with dose)	6–10 hr.	18–24 hr.	3 P.M. to dinner	Before breakfast and lunch
NPH	1 hr. before breakfast. S.C.	Within 2–4 hr.	8–12 hr.	28–30 hr.	Same	Before lunch
Lente	Same	Same	Same	Same	Same	Same
Slow action						
Protamine Zinc (PZI)	Same	Within 4–6 hr.	16–24 hr.	24–36 hr.	2 A.M. to breakfast	Before lunch and bedtime
Ultralente	1 hr. before breakfast, deep S.C. (never I.V.)	Very slow–8 hr.	Same	36 hr. plus	During night and early morning	

*Adapted from Bergersen and Krug, *Pharmac.* p. 627.

IX. Antibiotics (antimicrobials) — substances that kill or inhibit the growth of microorganisms. They are produced mainly by molds but some may be produced by bacteria and yeasts.
  A. Broad-spectrum antibiotics effective against many types of microorganisms.
  B. Penicillin — effective against gram-positive organisms.
  C. Streptomycin and dihydrostreptomycin — effective against gram-negative microorganisms, particularly the tubercle bacillus.
  D. Tetracyclines — have broad-spectrum activity. Prolonged use can lead to development of fungal infections in intestinal tract.
  E. Erythromycin — similar to narrow-spectrum activity of penicillin.
  F. Kantrex — most useful in treatment of urinary tract, respiratory tract, and soft tissue infections.
  G. Antifungal drugs — specifically used for treatment of fungal infections. Examples — amphotericin B, nystatin, griseofulvin.

X. Sulfonamides — inhibit the growth of bacteria and other microorganisms.
  A. Most often used in treatment of uncomplicated urinary tract infections.
  B. Examples — Gantrisin, Sulfathalidine, Thiosulfil, Madribon.
  C. Fluids should be forced while patient is taking a sulfonamide, and intake and output must be recorded. Usual toxic symptoms are nausea, vomiting, and other gastrointestinal disturbances.

XI. Tranquilizers and Antidepressants
  A. Tranquilizers — serve to calm the emotions without depressing the central nervous system.
    1. Used in certain types of mental illnesses.
    2. Examples, Equanil, Librium.
  B. Antidepressants — help overcome severe depression due to emotional disturbances.
    1. Some may relieve depression without stimulating the central nervous system.
    2. Examples, Ritalin, Tofranil.

UNIT 2   ADMINISTRATION OF MEDICATIONS

I. **Introduction**
   A. Administration of medications one of the most demanding of nurses' duties. Requires absolute accuracy; there is no "margin for error."
   B. To assure accuracy the nurse must be sure that
      1. The correct dose is measured.
      2. The correct medicine is poured.
      3. The correct patient is given the medication.
      4. The medicine is given at the correct time.
      5. The medicine is administered by the correct method or channel.
   C. To be sure that the correct medicine is given, the nurse must read the label *three* times
      1. When the container is taken from the shelf or cabinet.
      2. Before pouring the drug.
      3. When the container is being replaced in the cabinet or discarded in the wastebasket.

II. **Other General Rules for the Administration of Medications**
   A. Use a medicine card to accompany the medicine, thus eliminating error in administering the medication to the wrong patient.
   B. Wash hands before preparing the medication, but avoid handling any medication.
   C. Never take medicines from an unmarked container, or one that has a soiled label that is difficult to read. Have the pharmacist replace the label with one that is easily read.
   D. Medications are usually given by mouth except when otherwise ordered by the physician. For example, nitroglycerine tablets.
   E. Do not leave medications in a patient's room unless the medicine is cough syrup, or there is a specific order from the physician to leave the medicine at the bedside.
   F. Do not mix medications in the same container unless directed to do so. A chemical change may occur and a precipitate will form.

   G. Remain with the patient until the medicine is swallowed.
   H. A drug should not be administered if there is any change in its color, consistency, or odor.
   I. Always identify the patient by checking his hospital identification bracelet.
   J. If, for any reason, a medication cannot be given, a note must be made on the patient's chart stating the name of the drug, its dosage, and the reason it was omitted.

III. **Routes of Administration**
   A. Oral (P.O.) – by mouth
   B. By injection
      1. Subcutaneous (S.C.) – under the skin, also called hypodermic.
      2. Intradermal – into the layers of the skin.
      3. Intramuscular (I.M.) – into the muscle tissue.
      4. Intravenous (I.V.) – directly into a vein.
   C. Local – directly onto the skin or mucous membranes.
   D. Rectal – by way of the rectum.
   E. Inhalation – inhaling into the respiratory tract.
   F. Sublingual – placed under the tongue and held until dissolved.

IV. **Pouring Liquid Medicines for Oral Administration**
   A. May be measured in ounces, drams, minims, cc., drops, and sometimes in teaspoons (Table 8).
   B. Hold container with label side toward palm of hand so that label is not soiled by medicine.
   C. Hold medicine glass at eye level. Place thumbnail at point to which medicine is to be poured.
   D. Never open more than one bottle at a time. This will help eliminate pouring wrong medication.
   E. Wipe the lip of the bottle after pouring and before replacing cap.
   F. When medicine is ordered in drops, use dropper provided with medication. Droppers vary in size and accurate dosage may not be given if correct dropper is not used.

128

Table 8. Comparison of Measuring Systems

METRIC	APOTHECARY	HOUSEHOLD
	Volume-Liquid	
	1 minim (m.)	1 drop
1 cubic centimeter (cc.)	15 m.	15 drops
4 cc.	60 m. or 1 fluid dram (fl. dm.)	60 drops or 1 teaspoonful (tsp.)
30 cc.	1 fluid ounce (fl. oz.)	2 tablespoonfuls (tbsps.) or 8 tsps.
250 cc.	8 fl. oz.	1 measuring cupful
500 cc.	1 pint (16 fl. oz.)	1 pint (2 measuring cupfuls)
1000 cc.	1 quart (32 fl. oz.)	1 quart (4 measuring cupfuls)
	Weight-Dry	
60.0 milligrams	1 grain (gr.)	
1 gram (Gm.)	15 gr.	¼ tsp.
4 Gm.	1 dram (dr.)	1 tsp.
28.3 Gm.	1 ounce (oz.)	2 tbsps.

G. If dosage is ordered in minims for oral administration, use minim glass to obtain accurate dosage.

V. Preparing Solid Medicines for Oral Administration

A. Tablets may be broken in half ONLY if they are *scored* (indented in the middle).
B. Pills and capsules may NOT be broken in half for administration of smaller doses.
C. Powders may be dissolved in water and given in solution, or they may be poured into a spoon and placed on the back of the tongue, then followed by a drink of water.

VI. Injections

A. Special points to remember
 1. When preparing a medication for injection, the following parts of the syringe must not be contaminated: tip, plunger, and inside of the barrel. The shaft of the needle must be kept free from contamination.
 2. Always cleanse the site of injection with some type of disinfectant before giving the injection.
 3. Be very careful to choose the correct *site* for the type of injection being given.
 4. After the needle is inserted, the plunger is drawn back. If blood returns, the needle is in a vein and must be withdrawn and another site chosen for the injection.
B. Subcutaneous injections
 1. May be given wherever there is subcutaneous tissue. Usually is given in upper outer arm, or in the thigh.
 2. A 2-ml. syringe with a ¾-inch (19-mm.), 25-gauge needle is usually used.
 3. Amount that can be safely given by subcutaneous injection should not exceed 2 ml.

4. Drug is deposited subcutaneously if needle is held at a 45-degree angle to skin and skin is pinched between thumb and index finger.
 5. Certain drugs, such as those put in oil, or the mercurial drugs, should not be given as subcutaneous injections.
C. Intradermal injections
 1. Given in an area where the skin and hair are scant, such as the inner part of the forearm.
 2. A ⅜- or ½-inch (10- or 13-mm.) long, 25-gauge needle is used. Dosage usually very small.
 3. Needle is inserted at a 10- to 15-degree angle to the skin.
 4. This type of injection most often used for diagnostic tests or for administering certain types of vaccines.
D. Intramuscular injections
 1. Area selected for injection usually either buttock, in the upper, outer quadrant (drug is deposited into the gluteus maximus); thigh and deltoid muscle also used. NOTE: When injection is given into the buttock it is very important to choose the correct site, otherwise, SERIOUS INJURY MAY BE DONE TO THE SCIATIC NERVE, OR A LARGE BLOOD VESSEL MAY BE ENTERED.
 2. Needle should be at least 1½ inches (38 mm.) long, or longer if muscle is large; 20- or 22-gauge needle usually used. Size of syringe depends on amount of medication to be given; as a rule the amount should not exceed 5 ml. for an intramuscular injection.
 3. Needle is inserted at a 90-degree angle to the skin. The skin is stretched to insure deep deposit of drug.
 4. Whenever possible the patient is placed in prone position and asked to turn

his toes in during an injection into the gluteus maximus. This position relaxes this muscle and makes the injection less painful.

VII. Administration of Medication to the Eye
A. Special points to remember
1. O.D. refers to the right eye; O.S. to left eye; O.U. to both eyes.
2. Use sterile dropper, cotton balls. If infection is present in the eye use a separate dropper for each eye.
3. Patient should be lying down or with head tilted back.
B. Instilling eye drops
1. Remove secretions that may be present in eye or on eyelid.
2. Instruct patient to look up, then instill drop into lower lid. Do not touch eyeball with tip of dropper.
3. After instillation, instruct patient to rotate eyeball to spread medication evenly.

VIII. Administration of Ear Drops
A. Special points to remember
1. Medications for the ear should be warmed to prevent discomfort. DO NOT OVERHEAT.
2. Do not force air into the canal when giving ear drops.
3. Instruct patient to turn head so that it is tilted away from the affected side.
4. After drops are instilled the head is kept tilted for a few minutes to prevent leakage of drops from the ear.
B. Instilling ear drops
1. Remove secretions from external ear, using cotton-tipped applicator.
2. Straighten ear canal by gently pulling ear lobe upward and backward for adults; downward and backward for infants and small children.

IX. Special Precautions in Administration of Certain Drugs (see Tables 9 and 10)

X. Calculation of Drug Dosage – Metric System
A. Primary units are gram (Gm.) for solid measure and liter (l.) for liquid measure.
B. Secondary units are identified by prefixes.
1. *milli:* one-thousandth
   a. milligram (mg.) = 0.001 Gm. (1/1000 Gm.)
   b. milliliter (ml.) = 0.001 liter (1/1000 liter)
2. *kilo:* one thousand
   a. kilogram = 1000 grams
C. Fractional amounts in the metric system are expressed as decimal fractions. Examples:
1. One-tenth gram is written 0.1 Gm.
2. Five-tenths ($1/2$) gram is written 0.5 Gm.
D. Use ratio and proportion to determine fractional doses.
1. Ratios are expressions of the relationship between two quantities or two numbers.
   a. Example – 50 mg. per ml., as written on the label of a drug container, can be written as the ratio 50 mg.:1 ml.
   b. Example – 30 mg. per tablet can be written as 30 mg.:1 tablet.
   c. NOTE: When writing a ratio to express quantities of drugs, it is necessary to write *both* the number *and* the unit of measure – that is 30 *and* mg., or 30 mg.
E. A proportion shows equality between two ratios and can be thought of as a comparison.
1. A proportion is a kind of shorthand for writing the statement "30 mg. in one tablet equals, or is the same as, 60 mg. in two tablets."
2. Another way of saying this is, "If there are 30 mg. in one tablet, then there are 60 mg. in two tablets."

Table 9.   Special Precautions in Drug Administration

Drug	*Special Precautions*
Reserpine and hydralazine hydrochloride	Take blood pressure before giving; report if below normal range.
Cathartics and laxatives	Contraindicated in undiagnosed abdominal pain.
Cough mixtures	Should not be followed with water.
Digitalis preparations	Count pulse before giving; withhold and report to physician or nurse in charge if pulse is below 60/minute.
Hydrochloric acid	Given diluted and taken through a straw to prevent damage to the teeth.
Iron preparations	Given after meals to avoid gastric irritation.
Morphine sulfate	Count respirations; withhold and report if rate is below 12/minute.
Nitroglycerin	Usually given sublingually.
Potassium iodide	Discolors the teeth; should be given diluted in water and taken through a straw.
Streptomycin	Given deep into muscle tissue; sites of injection must be rotated.

Table 10. Drug Administration in Relation to Meals *

Take on an empty stomach (2–3 hours a.c.):
benzathine penicillin G
cloxacillin (Tegopen)
erythromycin
lincomycin (Lincocin)
methacycline (Rondomycin)
phenoxymethyl penicillin (penicillin V)
tetracyclines, except demethylchlortetracycline
   (Declomycin), which can easily upset the stomach

Take ½ hour before meals:
belladonna and its alkaloids, chlordiazepoxide
   hydrochloride (Librax)
hyoscyamine sulfate (Donnatal)
methylphenidate (Ritalin)
phenmetrazine hydrochloride (Preludin)
phenazopyridine (Pyridium)
propantheline bromide (Pro-banthine)

Take with meals or food:
aminophylline
antidiabetics
APC (acetylsalicylic acid, phenacetin, caffeine)
chlorothiazide, (Diuril) (Hydrodiuril)
diphenylhydantoin (Dilantin)
mefenamic acid (Ponstel)
metronidazole (Flagyl)
nitrofurantoin (Furadantin) (Macrodantin)
prednisolone
prednisone
rauwolfia and its alkaloids

reserpine (Serpasil)
triamterene (Dyrenium)
trihexyphenidyl hydrochloride (Artane)
trimeprazine tartrate (Temaril)

Do not take with milk:
bisacodyl (Dulcolax)
potassium chloride
potassium iodide
tetracyclines except doxycycline (Vibramycin)

Do not take with fruit juices:
ampicillin
benzathine penicillin G
cloxacillin (Tegopen)
erythromycin

Do not drink alcohol while taking:
acetohexamide (Dymelor)
antihistamines
chlorpropamide (Diabinese)
chlordiazepoxide (Librium)
chloral hydrate
diphenoxylate hydrochloride (Lomotil)
MAO inhibitors
meclizine hydrochloride (Antivert)
methaqualone (Quaalude)
metronidazole (Flagyl)
narcotics
phenformin hydrochloride (DBI)
tolbutamide (Orinase)

*© March, 1975, The American Journal of Nursing Co. Reprinted from *American Journal of Nursing,* Vol. 75, No. 3, p. 405.

3. The proportion contains two ratios and is written 30 mg.:1 tab. = 60 mg.:2 tab.
4. Each of the four parts of a proportion is called a term. The terms at the beginning and at the end of the proportion are called the *extremes.* The two middle terms are called the *means.*
   a. In a true proportion the product (result of multiplication) of the extremes must always equal the product of the means.
      1. Example: In the proportion 30 mg.: 1 tab. = 60 mg.:2 tab., 30 times 2 = 60, and 1 times 60 = 60. This is a true proportion.
F. Setting up a proportion.
   1. Read the dosage on the label of the drug to be given and write the dosage as a ratio.
      a. Example: 50 mg. per ml. is written as 50 mg.:1 ml.
      b. Example: A 2-ml. vial labeled 75 mg. is written as 75 mg.:2 ml.
   2. Read the physician's order to determine *amount of drug* to be given the patient.
      a. Example: Physician's order reads "35

mg. of Demerol." This tells you the amount of drug in milligrams, but does not tell you the amount of solution or *volume* to give the patient.
3. Substitute X for the amount of volume to give. The letter X is used to indicate an unknown amount.
4. Write out all four terms of the proportion.

	(physician's order)	(volume to give)
(label) 50 mg.:1 ml. =	35 mg.:	X ml.

NOTE: When setting up a proportion, *always* arrange the same units of measure in the same order. If the first ratio of a proportion expresses a relationship between mg. and ml., then the second ratio must also compare mg. to ml.
If the dosage on hand is not expressed in the same units of measure as the dosage ordered, then you must "translate" the units ordered into the units on hand. Example: The physician orders 500 mg. of a drug and the container label reads "1 Gm. per ml". The 500 mg. must be translated as 0.5 Gm. before the proportion can be written correctly.

G. Solving for X—determining the amount of *volume* (milliliters, tablets, drops, etc.) to give the patient.
1. Multiply the extremes *or* the means. The first multiplication should include the term containing the X or unknown amount.
Example: 50 mg.:1 ml = 35 mg.:X ml. Multiply the extremes because one of them contains the X. After multiplying 50 times X you have 50 X.
2. Write the product of the multiplication to the *left* of an equal sign.
Thus far you have written:
50 mg.:1 ml. = 35 mg.:X ml.
50 X =
3. Multiply the remaining terms. Using the above example, you would multiply 1 times 35.
Now you have:
50 mg.:1 ml. = 35 mg.:X ml.
50 X = 35
NOTE: The product containing the X is *always* written to the *left* of the equal sign.
4. Determine X by dividing 35 by 50. That is, the expression 50 X = 35 means 35 divided by 50. Now you have
50 mg.:1 ml. = 35 mg.:X ml.
50 X = 35
X = 0.7

The X represents ml.; therefore, the answer is 0.7 ml.
H. Proving the answer. If you wish to determine whether the above answer is correct, simply multiply the means and the extremes. The proportion is 50 mg.:1 ml. = 35 mg.:0.7 ml. Fifty times 0.7 is 35 and 1 times 35 is 35. Thus you have a true proportion, since 35 equals 35.
I. Sample situations.
1. The physician orders 75 mg. of a drug. The dosage on hand is a vial labeled 50 mg./ml.
50 mg.:1 ml. = 75 mg.:X ml.
50 X = 75
X = 75 ÷ 50
X = 1.5 ml.
2. The physician orders 6 mg. of a drug. The drug on hand is in a vial labeled 25 mg. per ml.
25 mg.:1 ml. = 6 mg.:X ml.
25 X = 6
X = 6 ÷ 25
X = 0.24 ml.
3. The physician orders 0.16 mg. of atropine. The drug on hand is in a vial labeled 0.4 mg. per 0.5 ml.
0.4 mg.:0.5 ml. = 0.16 mg.:X ml.
0.4 X = 0.80
X = 2 ml.

Questions

1. Drugs are obtained from several sources. These include:
   a. plants
   b. animal products
   c. synthetic chemical compounds
   d. food elements
      1. all but d
      2. b and c
      3. a and d
      4. all of these
2. The reference book that is most useful in the standardization of drugs because it contains a list of approved drugs and includes their sources, composition, and directions for compounding is called the:
   1. Physician's Desk Reference
   2. United States Pharmacopeia
   3. National Formulary
   4. Index of Pharmacology
3. The reference book which would be most helpful when looking up a drug under its *trade name* is the:
   1. National Formulary
   2. List of Nonofficial Drugs
   3. United States Pharmacopeia
   4. Physician's Desk Reference
4. Tinctures and elixirs are both solutions which contain:
   1. sugar and water
   2. alcohol and water
   3. fat globules and water
   4 alcohol and ether

5. Two characteristics common to all liniments are that they:
   1. are taken internally and relax muscle spasms
   2. should be applied externally and provide a sensation of warmth to the area
   3. are applied locally to the skin and mucous membranes and stimulate muscular contractions
   4. always contain alcohol and are applied to the extremities
6. A medication that consists of a suspension of fat globules and water is classified as:
   1. an emulsion
   2. an ointment
   3. a tincture
   4. an elixir
7. Pills that are classified as enteric-coated are:
   1. absorbed by the skin
   2. dissolved by intestinal juices and absorbed through the intestinal wall
   3. administered rectally
   4. held in the mouth until dissolved
8. *All* suppositories:
   1. are administered rectally
   2. produce evacuation of the bowel
   3. are soothing to mucous membranes
   4. have a base which melts at body temperature
9. A drug that is absorbed into the blood and carried to specific organs or tissues is said to have:
   1. a systemic effect
   2. a local effect
   3. side effects
   4. untoward effects
10. Bacteriostatic agents are substances which:
    1. slow down or inhibit the growth of bacteria
    2. kill bacteria
    3. aid in the multiplication of helpful bacteria
    4. destroy all living microorganisms
11. Which of the following is most important in the use of Zephiran as an anti-infective agent?
    1. It should never be used in strengths of 1:2000.
    2. The area being irrigated with Zephiran must be completely free of soap or detergent before irrigation is begun.
    3. A strength of 1:200 is the only effective strength for removal of infectious agents.
    4. The nurse should always cleanse the area with pHisohex before irrigating with Zephiran.
12. Gentian violet is primarily used for:
    1. viral infections
    2. streptococcal infections
    3. fungal infections
    4. gonorrheal infections
13. Which of the following vitamin preparations would lead to a decrease in the blood calcium level if given in excessive doses?
    1. Hykinone
    2. Aquasol-A
    3. riboflavin
    4. Dical-D
14. Vitamin B_{12}, also known as the extrinsic factor, is given specifically for the treatment of:
    1. scurvy
    2. pernicious anemia
    3. rickets
    4. night blindness

15. Vitamin B$_{12}$ usually is given:
   1. intramuscularly
   2. intradermally
   3. orally
   4. sublingually
16. Drugs which relieve pain are classified as:
   1. sedatives
   2. hypnotics
   3. analgesics
   4. antipyretics
17. The drug most commonly used for relief of arthritic pain is:
   1. phenobarbital
   2. aspirin
   3. morphine sulfate
   4. codeine sulfate
18. Adrenalin (epinephrine) is classified as a heart stimulant because it:
   1. strengthens the heartbeat
   2. speeds up the action of the heart
   3. increases respirations
   4. produces hypotension
19. Vasoconstrictors are sometimes used to combat shock because their principal action is to produce:
   1. narrowing of the blood vessels and elevation of the blood pressure
   2. an increase in the pulse rate and respirations
   3. slowing and strengthening of the heartbeat
   4. an increase in the size of blood vessels and elevation of the blood pressure
20. Digitalis preparations are examples of heart tonics which:
   1. increase the heartbeat
   2. raise the blood pressure
   3. quicken the action of the heart
   4. slow and strengthen the heartbeat
21. Before giving any type of digitalis preparation the nurse should always:
   1. check the patient's blood pressure
   2. determine the patient's prothrombin time
   3. count the patient's pulse
   4. count the patient's respirations
22. Dicumarol and Coumadin are anticoagulant drugs which may be given to:
   1. raise the blood pressure when a patient is in shock
   2. relieve the pain during a heart attack
   3. delay the clotting time of the blood
   4. hasten the destruction of red blood cells
23. The most serious complication that may arise from the administration of either of the two drugs just mentioned is:
   1. rapid fall in blood pressure
   2. formation of clots within a major blood vessel
   3. hemorrhage
   4. infection
24. Nitroglycerin is frequently given to patients who have angina pectoris because this drug:
   1. dilates the blood vessels and increases circulation of blood
   2. depresses the pain centers located in the brain
   3. relaxes voluntary muscles and relieves muscular spasms
   4. produces sleep
25. The most common route of administration for nitroglycerin is:
   1. subcutaneous
   2. intramuscular
   3. intravenous
   4. sublingual

26. Iron preparations should be administered:
    1. at bedtime
    2. before meals
    3. after meals
    4. between meals

27. Carbon dioxide is:
    1. a gas that increases the rate and depth of respiration
    2. a liquid that stimulates respiration
    3. a gas that produces a mild anesthesia
    4. a liquid that depresses respiration

28. Morphine sulfate should be withheld and the physician notified if a patient's:
    1. pulse rate is above 60 per minute
    2. pulse rate is below 60 per minute
    3. respirations are above 20 per minute
    4. respirations are below 12 per minute

29. Aminophylline is often used to treat patients having an attack of asthma because this drug:
    1. lowers the blood pressure
    2. stimulates respiration
    3. relaxes the bronchial muscles and dilates the bronchi
    4. dries up bronchial secretions, making it easier for the patient to breathe

30. When giving potassium iodide to a patient, the nurse should know that this drug:
    1. frequently causes a severe allergic reaction
    2. discolors the teeth and should be given diluted in water and taken through a straw
    3. produces thirst because it dries up secretions from mucous membranes
    4. must always be given with a glass of milk

31. One type of medication that is most effective when taken without water is:
    1. a sedative cough mixture
    2. a urinary antiseptic
    3. a laxative
    4. an iron preparation

32. Potassium iodide is an example of:
    1. a sedative cough mixture
    2. a narcotic cough mixture
    3. an expectorant cough mixture
    4. a cough mixture containing syrup, which decreases irritation of the bronchial mucosa

33. Expectorant cough mixtures are those which:
    1. depress the cough reflex in the brain
    2. increase bronchial secretions, making it easier for the patient to cough up these secretions
    3. dry up bronchial secretions, thereby reducing the desire to cough
    4. contain some form of narcotic which prevents coughing

34. Tubercle bacilli are resistant to almost all of the antibiotics. One drug which has been found to be effective in destroying the tubercle bacillus is:
    1. penicillin
    2. sulfadiazine
    3. tetracycline
    4. streptomycin

35. Milk of magnesia and Amphojel are examples of antacids which can be used to:
    1. coat the intestinal tract for x-ray filming
    2. replace acids normally found in the stomach
    3. counteract or neutralize gastric acid
    4. aid digestion by stimulating the secretion of gastric acids

36. A drug that may be given to relieve a deficiency of the acid essential in the proper digestion of food is:
    1. hydrochloric acid
    2. sulfuric acid
    3. acetic acid
    4. nitric acid

37. The acid just mentioned should be administered:
    1. diluted and taken through a straw
    2. in concentrated doses to improve its effectiveness
    3. in a glass of milk
    4. with baking soda
38. The chief action of Kaopectate is that of:
    1. stimulating peristalsis
    2. providing bulk to relieve constipation
    3. soothing the intestinal tract and relieving diarrhea
    4. neutralizing the acids normally found in the colon
39. The nurse should know that any person having severe abdominal pain that has not yet been diagnosed should not be given:
    1. aspirin or other pain relievers
    2. laxatives without a doctor's order
    3. any form of medicine containing an antacid
    4. barbiturates such as Seconal and phenobarbital
40. Cathartics are given primarily for the purpose of:
    1. emptying the colon
    2. relieving diarrhea
    3. aiding digestion
    4. inducing vomiting
41. Drugs which have a local action in the urinary tract and are often used to treat minor infections of this tract are called:
    1. diuretics
    2. antidiuretics
    3. urinary antiseptics
    4. urinary hormones
42. Ergonovine maleate (Ergotrate) is classified as an ecbolic and is sometimes used to control uterine hemorrhage, chiefly because it:
    1. raises the blood pressure and decreases the pulse rate
    2. relaxes the uterine muscles
    3. stimulates contractions of the uterine muscles
    4. speeds up the coagulation of blood
43. Caffeine sodium benzoate is a:
    1. stimulant which affects the central nervous system
    2. narcotic which produces sleep
    3. analgesic which affects the spinal cord
    4. hypnotic which is non-narcotic
44. Barbiturates such as Seconal and phenobarbital are classified as:
    1. anesthetics which produce loss of sensitivity to pain
    2. narcotics which produce sleep
    3. analgesics which affect the voluntary muscles
    4. hypnotics which produce sleep
45. A drug that has been found to be useful in controlling convulsive seizures in an epileptic is:
    1. Dilantin
    2. morphine
    3. Dilaudid
    4. atropine
46. The chemical substances called *hormones* are produced by the:
    1. cortex of the brain
    2. endocrine glands
    3. pancreas and liver
    4. tissue of all organs of the body
47. The anti-inflammatory agents such as cortisone and hydrocortisone are hormones which are produced by the:
    1. pancreas
    2. pituitary gland
    3. cortex of the adrenal glands
    4. thyroid gland

48. A hormone that is secreted by the medulla of the adrenal gland is:
    1. insulin
    2. pituitrin
    3. thyroxin
    4. adrenalin
49. Regular insulin is different from other types of insulin in that it:
    1. is longer acting
    2. usually must be given only once daily
    3. acts more rapidly after injection
    4. is a more concentrated solution and requires smaller doses
50. If a patient receives 20 units of regular insulin at 7:30 A.M., when would be the most likely time for the patient to experience an insulin reaction?
    1. at 8:00 A.M.
    2. at 7:30 P.M.
    3. during the night
    4. between 10:00 A.M. and lunch
51. A patient receiving NPH insulin at 7:00 A.M. should be checked frequently for a possible insulin reaction:
    1. around midnight
    2. immediately after breakfast
    3. before lunch
    4. from 3 P.M. to dinner
52. When would the nurse observe the above patient for signs of diabetic coma?
    1. before lunch
    2. immediately after dinner
    3. around midnight
    4. from 3:00 P.M. to dinner
53. One-half ml. of U80 insulin contains:
    1. 80 units of insulin
    2. one-half unit of insulin
    3. 40 units of insulin
    4. 160 units of insulin
54. Orinase and Diabinase are best described as:
    1. oral insulin
    2. drugs which lower the blood sugar
    3. synthetic preparations of insulin
    4. drugs which are more effective than insulin in treating juvenile diabetics
55. Two liquids which are recommended as safe for irrigating the eye are:
    1. atropine solution and alcohol
    2. hydrogen peroxide and alcohol
    3. boric acid solution and normal saline
    4. Pontocaine and glycerine
56. Atropine eye drops have the effect of:
    1. desensitizing the eye
    2. relieving pain following injury to the eye
    3. dilating the pupil of the eye
    4. constricting the pupil of the eye
57. Pontocaine is often used to:
    1. treat infections of the eye
    2. desensitize the eye during painful treatments or examination
    3. dilate the pupil of the eye
    4. treat glaucoma
58. Pilocarpine is classified as a myotic because it:
    1. inhibits the growth of bacteria
    2. constricts the pupil of the eye
    3. provides local anesthesia
    4. often produces allergic reactions in sensitive individuals
59. Drugs which help relieve the symptoms of an allergic reaction are called:
    1. antihistamines
    2. antibiotics
    3. sulfonamides
    4. analgesics

60. The drugs just described help relieve the symptoms of an allergic reaction chiefly by:
1. drying up excessive secretions
2. producing drowsiness
3. relaxing the involuntary muscles
4. constricting the blood vessels

61. Antibiotics are substances produced by living cells. These particular substances are capable of:
1. destroying all kinds of bacteria
2. killing certain microorganisms without harming human cells
3. curing only minor infections
4. curing all types of viral and bacterial infections

62. A broad-spectrum antibiotic is best described as one that:
1. is effective against many types of organisms
2. destroys only gram-negative organisms
3. has a prolonged effect over a period of several weeks
4. has a delayed reaction that cannot be predicted

63. An antibiotic that is particularly effective against gram-negative bacteria, especially the tubercle bacillus, is:
1. penicillin
2. streptomycin
3. griseofulvin
4. erythromycin

64. When sulfonamides are prescribed for a patient, the nurse must be especially careful to:
1. give the drug on an empty stomach to prevent nausea and vomiting
2. restrict the intake of fluids so the drug will not be eliminated through the urinary tract too rapidly
3. inject the drug deep into the muscle tissue to increase absorption
4. force fluids and measure the patient's intake and output

65. Tranquilizers such as Equanil are used primarily to:
1. produce sleep
2. depress the central nervous system
3. calm the emotions without depressing the central nervous system
4. relieve postoperative pain

66. Antidepressants such as Tofranil are used primarily to:
1. produce sleep and relaxation
2. help overcome severe mental depression
3. stimulate the central nervous system and relieve lethargy
4. eliminate drowsiness following anesthesia

67. When administering medications, the nurse's CHIEF concern should be:
1. securing the patient's cooperation
2. administration of an average dose for every patient
3. complete accuracy in measuring and giving the medications
4. the qualifications of the physician ordering the medications

68. To be sure that the correct medication is being poured for a patient it is most important to:
1. read the physician's written order three times
2. read the label on the container three times
3. glance at the label on the container just before the medicine is poured
4. always have the nurse in charge supervise the pouring of medications

69. If a label on a medicine bottle is difficult to read it is best to:
1. ask the pharmacist to replace it with a clean label
2. withhold the medication and chart that it could not be given
3. make out a new label, using adhesive tape and being sure that the label is easily read
4. pour the medication only if you are familiar with the drug and are fairly sure it is the correct medication to give

70. When there is a change in the color, consistency, or odor of a drug, the nurse should know that:
    1. this frequently occurs in some drugs and is of no significance
    2. the drug may be given, but the changes in its appearance should be charted to relieve the nurse of any responsibility for possible untoward reactions
    3. only the pharmacist is responsible for the medications kept in the cabinet and he must remove it if it is unsafe or spoiled
    4. the drug must not be given and should be returned to the pharmacy in exchange for a fresh supply

71. Which of the following would be considered the safest rule to follow in preparing and giving medications?
    1. Do not give a medication that is likely to produce some unexpected reaction in a patient.
    2. Do not administer a drug until you have checked the name on the patient's identification bracelet.
    3. Always ask the patient his name before giving a medication to him.
    4. If a patient questions you about a drug you are about to give him, reassure him and administer the medication without checking his chart.

72. To be sure that a patient receives the medications ordered for him, it is best for the nurse to:
    1. stay with the patient until he has taken the medication she has prepared for him
    2. ask another patient to observe the patient and notify her if he does not take his medicine
    3. remind the patient that for his own sake he must take the medication she leaves for him when he is out of the room
    4. ask a member of the patient's family to accept the responsibility for administering the medications if she is too busy to give them to the patient

73. When pouring a liquid medication, the container should be held so that the:
    1. label is toward the medicine glass
    2. medication can be poured quickly
    3. thumb is against the label
    4. label is toward the palm of the hand

74. The reason for holding the container in the described manner is:
    1. to avoid soiling the label with the medication
    2. to prevent contamination of the medicine glass
    3. to assure the pouring of an accurate amount
    4. to avoid shaking the medication and forming bubbles of air

75. As a liquid drug is being poured into a medicine glass, the glass is:
    1. placed on a shelf to avoid spilling
    2. placed on the medicine tray
    3. held at waist level to assure proper measurement
    4. held at eye level to assure accurate measurement

76. A medication may be left in a patient's room under which of the following circumstances:
    1. on the physician's specific written order
    2. if the patient is eating at the time the medications are distributed
    3. if the patient is receiving a treatment
    4. if the patient is out of the room when the medication is taken to him and his wife says that she will give it to him when he returns

77. Which of the following solid forms of drugs may be broken in half to administer a smaller dosage?
    1. capsule
    2. pill or tablet
    3. scored tablet
    4. all of these

78. 4 cc. of a liquid can be measured most accurately in a:
    1. small paper cup
    2. teaspoon
    3. tablespoon
    4. minim glass or calibrated syringe

79. The symbol ℥ is read as:
    1. ounce
    2. tablespoon
    3. teaspoon
    4. dram

80. ℥ is equal to approximately:
    1. 15 ml. (cc.)
    2. 20 ml.
    3. 30 ml.
    4. 60 ml.

81. 1 pint is equal to approximately:
    1. 500 ml. (cc.)
    2. 32 ounces
    3. ¼ gallon
    4. 300 ml.

82. 1 ml. is equal to:
    1. 1 ounce
    2. 1 drop
    3. 1 dram
    4. 1 cc.

83. 2000 cc. is equal to approximately:
    1. 1 quart
    2. 1 pint
    3. ½ gallon
    4. 1 gallon

84. The physician orders 0.5 Gm. of Diamox. You have 250-mg. tablets on hand. The patient should receive:
    1. 4 tablets
    2. 1 tablet
    3. 2 tablets
    4. ½ tablet

85. The physician orders Seconal gr. iss. The drug on hand is labeled 0.1 Gm. per capsule. The patient should receive:
    1. 1 capsule
    2. 2 capsules
    3. 1 and ½ capsules
    4. ½ capsule

86. The physician orders chloral hydrate gr. viiss. The drug on hand is labeled 0.5 Gm. per capsule. The patient should receive:
    1. ½ capsule
    2. 1 capsule
    3. 2 capsules
    4. 3 capsules

87. Subcutaneous injections must be given so that the drug is deposited:
    1. under all layers of the skin
    2. between the layers of the skin
    3. into the muscle tissue
    4. directly into the vein

88. A hypodermic injection is given in exactly the same manner as:
    1. an intradermal injection
    2. a subcutaneous injection
    3. an intramuscular injection
    4. an intravenous injection

89. The usual sites for subcutaneous injections include the:
    1. inner aspect of either arm, at the elbow
    2. upper outer arm, or the thigh
    3. gluteal or deltoid muscle
    4. abdominal muscles, or the buttocks

90. The amount to be given by hypodermic injection should not exceed:
    1. 0.5 ml.
    2. 1 ml.
    3. 2 ml.
    4. 3 ml.
91. To administer a hypodermic injection properly, the needle should be held at:
    1. a 90-degree angle to the skin
    2. a 60-degree angle to the skin
    3. a 10- to 15-degree angle to the skin
    4. a 45-degree angle to the skin
92. The parts of a syringe which must NOT be contaminated while preparing an injection are:
    a. the tip
    b. the inside of the barrel
    c. the outside of the barrel
    d. the plunger
    e. the round "handle" of the plunger

    1. all of these
    2. all but b
    3. a, b, and d
    4. b and e
93. An intradermal injection is given:
    1. just under the uppermost layer of the skin
    2. into the muscle tissues
    3. into a vein
    4. between the skin and subcutaneous tissue
94. The most common site for an intradermal injection is:
    1. the thigh
    2. the upper arm
    3. the inner aspect of the lower arm
    4. the buttock
95. Intradermal injections are most often used to administer:
    1. certain substances for skin tests
    2. preparations that contain oil
    3. large amounts of fluids that cannot be given by vein
    4. drugs that are irritating to muscle tissue
96. When administering an intradermal injection, the needle is held so that it is at a:
    1. 90-degree angle to the skin
    2. 45-degree angle to the skin
    3. 40-degree angle to the skin
    4. 10- to 15-degree angle to the skin
97. After an intradermal injection has been administered, the site of injection:
    1. must be covered with a sterile dressing
    2. is gently massaged to distribute the drug
    3. is not massaged
    4. is held with moderate pressure to prevent leakage of blood into the surrounding tissues
98. If possible, the proper positioning of a patient for an intramuscular injection into the buttock is:
    1. on the side with the knees flexed
    2. prone with the knees drawn up
    3. supine with the knees flexed
    4. prone with the toes turned in
99. To penetrate the skin and deposit the drug into muscular tissue, the needle must be held at an angle of:
    1. 45 degrees to the skin
    2. 180 degrees to the skin
    3. 25 degrees to the skin
    4. 90 degrees to the skin
100. The most appropriate size needle for an intramuscular injection is:
    1. 1 inch (25 mm.), 25 gauge
    2. ½ inch (13 mm.), 25 gauge
    3. 1½ inch (38 mm.), 16 gauge
    4. 1½ inch (38 mm.), 22 or 23 gauge

101. Immediately after an intramuscular injection, the area is massaged gently with a cotton pledget to:
   1. prevent bruising
   2. increase the absorption of the medication
   3. relieve pain
   4. prevent bleeding at the site

102. Whenever a needle is inserted for an intramuscular injection or a subcutaneous injection, the nurse should:
   1. apply a tourniquet before giving the injection
   2. pull back on the plunger to see if blood is aspirated into the syringe before injecting the medication
   3. tell the patient to tense his muscles to make insertion of the needle easier
   4. change the angle of the needle after it is inserted

103. The chief danger in giving an intramuscular injection into the wrong area of the buttock is:
   1. poor absorption of the drug
   2. formation of an abscess resulting from contamination of the needle
   3. damage to the sciatic nerve or penetration of a large blood vessel
   4. damage to the underlying bony tissue

104. Local administration of medications refers to:
   1. giving the drug into the spinal cavity
   2. applying the medication directly onto the skin or mucous membranes
   3. injecting the drug into a surface blood vessel
   4. giving the drug by mouth

105. When a drug is administered sublingually, the patient is instructed to:
   1. hold the medication under his tongue until it is dissolved
   2. drink a full glass of water after swallowing the medication
   3. keep the medication at the bedside and use it as needed
   4. rinse his mouth with the medication but not swallow it

106. Drugs that are given by inhalation are usually administered as treatment of diseases of the:
   1. respiratory system
   2. digestive system
   3. nervous system
   4. urinary system

107. When administering medications to the eye the nurse must be sure to apply the medication to the correct eye. If the physician writes O.D. on the order sheet, he wishes the medication to be given in:
   1. the left eye
   2. the right eye
   3. both eyes
   4. the eye which appears to be infected

108. To avoid transfer of microorganisms from an infected eye to a normal eye, the nurse should:
   1. medicate the infected eye first and then proceed to the normal eye
   2. use a sterile dropper for the normal eye only
   3. use a separate dropper for each eye
   4. wipe the dropper with alcohol after treating the infected eye

109. When medications are being administered to the eye, the liquid or ointment is applied to the:
   1. upper lid
   2. lower lid
   3. inner corner only
   4. outer corner only

110. After eye drops are instilled, the patient is instructed to:
   1. keep his eye open without blinking for 2 to 3 minutes
   2. close his eye slowly and rotate the eyeball to spread the medication evenly
   3. squeeze the eyelids closed several times to remove the excess medication
   4. use a tissue and rub his eye vigorously

111. Medications for the ear should be:
    1. refrigerated and applied without heating to avoid chemical changes in the drug
    2. warmed to body temperature
    3. heated to 115 to 120° F. (46 to 49° C.) to sterilize the medication
    4. warmed only if directions to do so are written on the label
112. While ear drops are being instilled, the patient should be:
    1. lying face down on the bed
    2. sitting up with the head tilted forward
    3. sitting up or lying down with the head turned so that the affected ear is uppermost
    4. sitting up with the head tilted back
113. To straighten the ear canal during the administration of ear drops to an adult patient, the ear lobe is gently pulled:
    1. upward and back
    2. upward and forward
    3. downward and back
    4. downward and forward
114. Which of the following medications may be taken with milk or diary products?
    1. prednisone
    2. potassium chloride
    3. the tetracyclines
    4. Dulcolax
115. Alcholic beverages are prohibited when which of the following drugs are being taken?
    1. erythromycin, reserpine
    2. antihistamine, Antivert, Flagyl
    3. the tetracyclines
    4. Diuril and Hydrodiuril
116. Which of the following drugs should be taken on an empty stomach (2–3 hours a.c.)?
    1. potassium iodide and potassium chloride
    2. prednisone and prednisolone
    3. the tetracyclines, except Declomycin
    4. Furadantin and Macrodantin
117. Which of the following drugs may not be taken with fruit juices?
    1. ampicillin, penicillin G, and erythromycin
    2. Lomotil and Antivert
    3. prednisone and prednisolone
    4. rauwolfia and its alkaloids
118. The primary unit of solid measure in the metric system is the:
    1. milligram
    2. gram
    3. milliliter
    4. liter
119. The primary unit of liquid measure (volume) in the metric system is the:
    1. milligram
    2. gram
    3. milliliter
    4. liter
120. If a milligram equals 0.001 Gm., then there are how many milligrams in a gram?
    1. one-tenth
    2. one hundred
    3. one thousand
    4. one-thousandth
121. The label on a container of medication reads "0.5-Gm. tablets." The proper ratio to express the dosage is:
    1. 0.5 Gm.:X ml.
    2. 0.5 Gm.:2 tablets
    3. 500 mg.:X tablets
    4. 0.5 Gm.:1 tablet

122. The physician has ordered 0.75 mg. of a certain drug. The dosage on hand is a vial labeled "1 mg./ml." Which of the following statements best describes the problem you must solve?
    1. You need to determine how many grams to give the patient.
    2. You must find out how many milligrams to give the patient.
    3. You need to know how many ml. to give the patient.
    4. You need to know how many milligrams are in a gram.

123. A patient is to receive 45 mg. of a drug. The label on the container reads "30-mg. tablets." The correct proportion to solve for X is:
    1. 45 mg.:30 = 1 mg.:X
    2. 30 mg.:1 tab. = 45 mg.:X tab.
    3. 30:1 = 45 mg.:X
    4. 45:30 = X:1

124. A patient is to receive 750 mg. of a drug. The dosage on hand is 1 Gm. per ml. The correct proportion to solve for X is:
    1. 1 Gm.:1 ml. = 750 mg.:X ml.
    2. 1 Gm.:1 ml. = 75. mg.:X ml.
    3. 1000 mg.:1 ml. = 750 mg.:X ml.
    4. 1000 mg.:1 ml. = 0.75 mg.:X ml.

125. In the next step of solving the above problem, you would:
    1. multiply 1 times X
    2. divide 750 by 1000
    3. multiply 1000 times X
    4. divide 750 by 1

126. If your proportion is 25 mg.:2 ml. = 17.5 mg.:X ml., the next step is written as:
    1. 25 X = 35
    2. 2 X = 35
    3. 2 X = 437.5
    4. 25 X = 437.5

127. When you write 15 X = 40, this means:
    1. 40 times 15
    2. 40 divided by 15
    3. 15 divided by 40
    4. 15 divided by X

128. You are to give a patient 65 mg. of a drug. The dosage on hand is 50 mg. per ml. The correct amount to give is:
    1. 5/6 ml.
    2. 6.5 ml.
    3. 3.2 ml.
    4. 1.3 ml.

129. A patient is to receive 1.25 mg. of a drug. The container on the label reads "4 ml. contain 0.625 mg." You should give the patient:
    1. 0.19 ml.
    2. 0.8 ml.
    3. 1.9 ml.
    4. 8 ml.

130. A patient is to receive ¼ grain of medication. The drug is available in a vial labeled "30 mg. per ml." You know that 60 mg. are approximately equal to 1 grain. Your proportion should be:
    1. 30 mg.:1 ml. = ¼ grain:X ml.
    2. 30 mg.:X ml. = ¼ grain:60 mg.
    3. 30 mg.:1 ml. = 15 mg.:X ml.
    4. 30 mg.:60 mg. = ¼ grain:X ml.

Part VII

NURSING THE ADULT PATIENT

UNIT 1   THE SURGICAL PATIENT

I. **Introduction**
A. Preoperative care deals with care of the patient before surgery.
  1. Responsibility of the entire health team.
  2. Admission of the patient to the hospital for surgery a critical time when attitudes are formed which will affect the patient's physical and emotional well-being. Patient should be made to feel welcome and every effort made to relieve his anxiety.
  3. Diagnostic tests often done. Nurse may need to explain the need for these tests and help prepare the patient for them.
  4. Physical preparation usually includes surgical preparation of the skin, withholding of fluids, and limitation of the patient's diet.
    a. Surgical preparation of the skin usually includes shaving the operative area because hair harbors bacteria.
    b. Skin cannot be rendered sterile; washing with a bactericidal agent removes only surface bacteria.
    c. Fluids and food are withheld in order to decrease vomiting and the danger of aspiration of vomitus.
  5. Immediate care before surgery
    a. Patient should be wearing hospital gown.
    b. Hairpins removed from hair and head covered.
    c. Valuables, such as watch and rings, are removed and placed in hospital vault or given to a member of the family. If patient refuses to remove a ring it may be left on and secured

with a strip of cotton tape or anchored to the wrist with a bandage.
    d. Dentures removed unless anesthesiologist requests that they be left in the mouth. Some types of anesthesia are administered more easily if dentures are left in.
    e. Patient should void immediately before surgery unless a catheter has been inserted. Bladder is emptied to:
      1. lessen danger of injury to the bladder during surgery;
      2. avoid involuntary urination and contamination of the sterile field during surgery.
    f. Legal forms, such as permission to operate, etc. must be completed and signed before patient is sent to the operating room.
B. Anesthesia
  1. Provides decreased sensitivity to pain and produces muscle relaxation.
  2. Types of anesthesia
    a. Local—drug is injected into area and produces a local loss of sensation. Some types are applied to mucous membranes of nose, throat, eyes, etc.
    b. Spinal—drug is injected into spinal cavity. Nerve impulses are blocked and there is a loss of sensation below the site of injection.
    c. General anesthesia—drug is administered by inhalation or intravenous injection. Produces loss of consciousness and is used most often in major surgery.

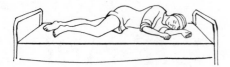

FIGURE 31.

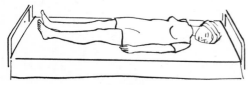

FIGURE 32.

FIGURES 31 AND 32. Preventing aspiration of vomitus. (Sutton: *Bedside Nursing Techniques.* 2nd ed.)

C. Postoperative care deals with care of the patient after surgery.
  1. Immediate postoperative care
    a. Careful observation necessary until patient has reacted from anesthesia.
    b. Head is kept turned to one side when patient is vomiting to prevent aspiration of vomitus into lungs (Figs. 31 and 32).

c. Airway MUST BE MAINTAINED. Suction used to remove mucus as necessary.
d. Vital signs checked frequently. Changes in color, difficulty in breathing, etc. reported immediately.
e. Dressings watched for signs of excessive drainage or hemorrhage.
f. Tubes and catheters checked and connected to drainage bottles, gastric suction, closed drainage, etc. as necessary.
  2. Preparation of the patient's unit
    a. Bed is made so that patient can be transferred from stretcher to bed easily and gently.
    b. Warmth needed only to maintain normal body temperature.
    c. Equipment for checking and recording vital signs should be at the bedside.
  3. After patient has reacted
    a. Food and fluids allowed only as ordered by physician.
    b. Urinary output is carefully checked.
    c. Deep breathing and frequent turning of the patient necessary to prevent pulmonary and circulatory complications.
    d. Early ambulation helps patient avoid formation of blood clots and development of hypostatic pneumonia.
  4. Complications to be avoided (Table 11)
    a. Shock—can be fatal if not treated.

Table 11. Postoperative Care

Control of pain	Nursing measures to provide maximum comfort and reassurance of the patient
	Analgesic drugs
Maintenance of drainage	Urinary catheters
	Gastric suction
	Thoracic drainage
	Bile drainage
	Drainage from surgical wounds
Maintenance of fluid and electrolyte balance	Intravenous fluids and minerals
	Oral intake
	Observation and recording of output
Relief of abdominal distension, nausea, and vomiting	Rectal tube
	Gastric suction
	Ice collar
	Antiemetic drugs
Prevention of complications:	
Shock	Close observation for signs of shock and hemorrhage
Hemorrhage	
Blood clots in vascular system	Frequent turning
	Early ambulation
Hypostatic pneumonia	Encourage coughing and deep breathing and turn frequently
Decubitus ulcers	Frequent turning
	Skin care
Contractures	Proper positioning
	Exercise

Symptoms—skin cold and clammy, pulse rapid and weak, respirations rapid, blood pressure lowered, patient pale and apprehensive.
b. Hemorrhage—bleeding may not be obvious. Symptoms—restlessness,

increased pulse and respiratory rate, bright red blood visible, blood pressure falls as patient goes into shock.
c. Wound infection—prevented by adherence to basic principles of surgical asepsis.

Questions

Mrs. Gibson, age 45, is admitted to the hospital's surgical unit. She has had a gastric ulcer for several years and recently began having episodes of nausea with emesis of bright red blood. The morning after admission to the hospital, Mrs. Gibson is scheduled for x-ray studies of the intestinal tract.

1. Diagnostic tests such as x-ray studies are:
    1. usually not done during the preoperative period
    2. ordered by the physician only when he is not familiar with the patient's history
    3. frequently done during the preoperative period to firmly establish a diagnosis
    4. not helpful in the detection of a gastric ulcer
2. Mrs. Gibson's physician scheduled her for surgery 2 days after her admission. The evening before surgery the operative area was shaved, primarily because:
    1. hair on the skin prevents proper application of surgical dressings
    2. hairs harbor bacteria and predispose the patient to infection
    3. only the skin that has had all hairs removed can be sterilized
    4. it is more difficult to remove adhesive tape from skin that has not been shaven
3. The evening before surgery, Mrs. Gibson asks why she cannot have a bedtime snack since she always sleeps better if she has something to eat each night. What is the best answer to this question?
    1. Hospital policy forbids giving patients bedtime snacks.
    2. The hospital kitchen is closed but you can have a snack if your family will get it for you.
    3. Food and fluids are withheld to avoid nausea and vomiting immediately after surgery.
    4. Any foods or fluids taken before surgery will cause improper absorption of the anesthetic during surgery.
4. Mrs. Gibson does not wish to have her wedding band removed before surgery. In this case it would be best to:
    1. remind the patient that you cannot be held responsible for its loss
    2. tell her that surgery will be cancelled if she arrives in the operating room with any kind of jewelry on
    3. notify the physician of the patient's refusal to cooperate with the hospital policy
    4. put a loop of cotton tape through the ring and anchor it to her wrist so the ring will not be lost if it slips off her finger
5. The anesthesiologist has requested that Mrs. Gibson's dentures be left in her mouth when she is sent to the operating room. He most likely has made this request because:
    1. Mrs. Gibson did not want to remove her dentures for cosmetic reasons
    2. there is really no sound reason for removing the dentures before a general anesthetic is administered
    3. some forms of anesthesia can be administered more easily if the dentures are left in the mouth
    4. there is less danger of misplacing the dentures if they are never removed from the patient's mouth during her hospital stay

6. During general anesthesia there is usually a loss of voluntary control of the sphincter muscles. For this reason the nurse would:
   1. always insert a urinary catheter into the bladder before the patient is sent to the operating room
   2. offer a bedpan or urinal to the patient just before he is sent to the operating room
   3. force fluids several hours before surgery to avoid urinary retention post-operatively
   4. awaken the patient several times during the night before surgery and ask him to void so the bladder will be empty during surgery

7. For spinal anesthesia the drug is injected into the:
   1. lower part of the spinal cord
   2. nerve leading to the operative area
   3. spinal cavity
   4. upper part of the spinal cord

8. Immediately after surgery, Mrs. Gibson was taken to the recovery room. When her family asks how long she will remain there before returning to her room, what should the nurse answer?
   1. About an hour.
   2. Until the surgeon can get around to checking her.
   3. Just a little while unless she develops some serious complication.
   4. Until she has reacted from the anesthetic and it is safe to move her to her room.

9. If Mrs. Gibson began vomiting before she had fully reacted from the anesthetic it would be best to:
   1. place a pillow under her head to reduce gagging
   2. turn her head to the side to prevent aspiration of vomitus
   3. place a cool cloth on her head to reduce the nausea
   4. insert an airway to help maintain good respiration

10. When a patient returns from the operating room with a retention catheter in the bladder, the nurse is responsible for:
    1. removing the catheter immediately
    2. attaching the catheter to a drainage bottle and observing the patient's output
    3. irrigating the catheter every 15 minutes to be sure it is open and draining well
    4. attaching the catheter to an electric suction machine

11. All postoperative patients must be watched carefully for signs of shock. The symptoms of shock include:
    1. high blood pressure, flushed skin, bounding pulse
    2. low blood pressure, rapid pulse, cold clammy skin
    3. sudden drop in blood pressure, decreased respiratory rate
    4. high blood pressure, weak and thready pulse

12. When checking Mrs. Gibson's surgical dressings after surgery it would be most important to:
    1. change the dressings every hour
    2. wear sterile gloves
    3. report any signs of excessive drainage or bright red blood
    4. remove all dressings each time they are checked

13. If Mrs. Gibson complains of feeling chilly after returning to her room, the nurse should:
    1. apply several hot water bottles and extra blankets
    2. recognize this as a definite symptom of shock and notify the physician
    3. realize that Mrs. Gibson is probably hemorrhaging internally
    4. provide additional warmth so that the normal body temperature is maintained

14. Mrs. Gibson should be encouraged to breathe deeply during the first 24 hours after surgery. The main purpose of deep breathing is to:
    1. prevent shock
    2. eliminate the danger of thrombosis
    3. avoid oxygen deficiency
    4. prevent pulmonary complications such as hypostatic pneumonia

15. One of the nurse's main responsibilities in helping maintain a normal fluid and electrolyte balance in a postoperative patient is:
    1. ordering a daily laboratory test of electrolytes
    2. encouraging the patient to eat properly
    3. carefully measuring and recording the patient's intake and output
    4. forcing fluids by mouth

16. Mrs. Gibson's surgeon wished for her to be out of bed the first postoperative day. A very serious complication that is frequently avoided by early ambulation is:
    1. thrombophlebitis
    2. nausea
    3. ankylosis
    4. muscle spasm

17. Abdominal distention during the postoperative period can often be relieved by which of the following simple nursing measures?
    1. high, hot enema
    2. insertion of a rectal tube
    3. drugs which reduce nausea
    4. administration of an analgesic such as morphine

UNIT 2   THE PATIENT WITH CANCER

I. Introduction
A. Cancer is a neoplastic disease, characterized by a new growth of malignant cells. It is a type of tumor.
B. Classification of tumors
  1. Benign—encapsulated; do not spread to other parts of the body.
  2. Malignant—not encapsulated; cells grow rapidly, spread easily; referred to as cancerous.
C. Metastasis
  1. Spreading of malignant cells to other parts of the body.
  2. Routes by which metastasis occurs
    a. By direct extension to neighboring tissues.
    b. Via lymphatic vessels.
    c. By embolism through lymphatic vessels or blood.
    d. Invasion of fluid within a body cavity.

II. Cause of Cancer
A. Specific cause unknown; probably multiple
B. Predisposing cause
  1. Chronic irritations.
  2. Benign tumor which has become malignant.
  3. Other factors such as sex, age, familial tendency.

III. Seven Danger Signals of Cancer
A. Listed by the American Cancer Society
B. Any one of these symptoms that persists beyond several weeks should be reported to a physician.
  1. Any unusual bleeding or discharge.
  2. A lump or thickening in the breast or elsewhere.
  3. A sore that does not heal.
  4. Hoarseness or cough.
  5. A change in bowel or bladder habits.
  6. Indigestion or difficulty in swallowing.
  7. Any change in wart or mole.

IV. Diagnosis
A. Early diagnosis important in successful treatment.
B. Special diagnostic tests
  1. Biopsy—removal of a sample of living cells from the growth.
  2. Papanicolaou smear—technique for collecting samples of body secretions and examining them for malignant cells. Especially helpful in early diagnosis of cancer of the cervix.

V. Treatment
A. Surgical removal—works well for tumors which are readily accessible. Adjacent tissue and lymph nodes and vessels must also be removed or treated with radiation.
B. Radiation therapy—the use of radiation to penetrate and destroy malignant tissue.
  1. Methods of radiation therapy:
    a. X-ray therapy—high voltage x-ray machines are used to aim the beam of radiation directly at the tumor. Done in a series of treatments.
    b. Teletherapy—a radioactive element serves as the source of radiation. It is housed in a shielded unit that is located at a distance from the patient.
    c. Interstitial therapy—placement of a radioactive substance directly into the tissues of a malignant growth.
  2. Radiation protection
    a. Amount of radiation that a nurse might receive from x-rays or radioactive substances will depend on
      1. Distance between nurse and source of radiation,
      2. Amount of time spent in actual proximity to the source of radiation,
      3. Degree of shielding provided.
    b. Nurse must always be aware of the dangers of overexposure to radiation and take necessary precautions.
  3. Effects of radiation
    a. Short-term effects of radiation exposure include localized skin burns, fever, hemorrhage due to destruction of bone marrow, diarrhea, and central nervous system disorders.
    b. Long-term effects (appear years after exposure) include shortening of the life span, predisposition to leukemia and other malignancies, and development of cataracts. When the radiation is directed at the gonads, genetic mutations may arise.
  4. Radiation sickness—a generalized systemic reaction to radiation
    a. Symptoms are temporary and may

vary from mild discomfort and malaise to severe nausea, vomiting, and headache.

   b. Nursing measures include providing adequate rest, encouraging small, frequent feedings rather than large meals, reassurance that the condition is temporary.

C. Chemotherapy—use of drugs which delay growth of malignant cells and thereby prolong the life of the patient.

D. These methods of treatment may be used separately or in combination. The word "cure" as used in relation to cancer means that the patient has been free from cancer for 5 years after treatment.

VI. Nursing Care

A. Emotional aspects play a very important part in providing comfort and feeling of well-being for the patient.

   1. Nurse should know whether or not patient has been told he has cancer before she accepts responsibility for his care.

   2. Some individuals accept this illness well, others never learn to accept it.

B. Physical aspects

   1. Nursing care of patient being treated surgically is essentially the same as for other surgical patients.

   2. Not all types of cancer are accompanied by breakdown of tissue and necrosis. When necrosis does occur, nursing care is aimed at reducing odor and making the patient socially acceptable.

     a. Cleanliness and frequent changing of dressings imperative.

     b. Frequent irrigations with copious amounts of water very helpful in preventing odors and unpleasantness for the patient.

   3. Care of the patient having x-ray therapy requires special attention to the skin.

     a. Avoid using the terms "x-ray burn" or "radium burn" when referring to areas unavoidably affected by x-rays.

     b. Use extreme care in handling areas of entry (called "ports"). Skin should *not* be washed. Constricting clothes removed from this area. Dusting with powder or starch will help relieve itching. Patient should be told to avoid lying on the "ports" whenever possible.

   4. Patients with implants of a radioactive element can serve as sources of radiation to those in close contact with them. Nurses must know and strictly adhere to rules and regulations of the hospital or clinic in regard to the care of these patients.

Questions

  1. Which of the following would least accurately describe cancer?
    1. tumor
    2. new growth
    3. malignant disease
    4. incurable

  2. A malignant tumor differs from a benign tumor in that the malignant tumor:
    1. grows more slowly
    2. spreads more easily
    3. is very easily removed by surgery
    4. is always enclosed in a capsule

  3. The word metastasis is best defined as:
    1. the spread of a new growth to other parts of the body
    2. a medium-sized tumor
    3. a clot in the circulation
    4. the terminal stage of cancer

  4. Cancer may be spread by:
    1. the lymphatic system or by direct extension into adjacent tissues
    2. indirect contact with contaminated articles
    3. direct exposure to a person who has cancer
    4. exposure to radiation

  5. Research has shown that the cause of cancer is:
    1. chronic irritation of the skin
    2. a result of toxins produced by bacteria
    3. a result of malignant changes in a benign tumor
    4. not fully understood and may be the combination of several factors

6. Which of the following may be an early symptom of cancer?
   1. severe hemorrhage
   2. severe pain
   3. any sore that does not heal
   4. necrosis of tissue

7. Women over the age of 30 are encouraged to have a Papanicolaou smear done every 6 months because this is especially helpful in the early diagnosis of:
   1. cancer of the breast
   2. cancer of the cervix
   3. malignant moles
   4. malignancy of the bones

8. Removal of a sample of living cells for the purpose of microscopic examination is referred to as:
   1. a biopsy
   2. a culture
   3. an incision and drainage
   4. a bacteriological study

9. Early diagnosis of cancer is especially important because it:
   1. prevents the spread of the disease to other persons
   2. eliminates the need for surgery
   3. guarantees cure of the disease
   4. helps prevent the spread of the malignancy to other parts of the body

10. In the treatment of cancer the word "cure" means that the patient:
    1. will never have cancer again
    2. has been free of cancer for at least 5 years
    3. can expect to have a malignancy develop in another part of the body within 6 months
    4. will have cancer again in about 2 years

11. Cancer may be treated by all but which one of the following methods:
    1. insertions of radioactive element into the malignant tissue
    2. exposure of malignant cells to x-ray
    3. administration of certain chemicals
    4. administration of immune vaccines that destroy malignant cells

12. Before caring for a patient whose condition has been diagnosed as cancer, it is most important for the nurse to know:
    1. his financial situation
    2. the most recent experimental drugs used in the treatment of cancer
    3. whether or not the patient knows he has cancer
    4. the procedure used for insertion of radium

13. In the nursing care of a patient receiving x-ray therapy for a malignancy, the nurse must remember to:
    1. vigorously scrub the areas of entry or "ports" marked by the radiologist
    2. apply some form of ointment with a metallic base to the area of entry each time the patient goes to x-ray
    3. instruct the patient to avoid irritating the "ports" by not lying on that part of the body or wearing constricting clothing
    4. isolate the patient so he will not expose others to radiation

14. If a patient asks you why the area of skin where the x-ray is beamed into her body appears red and irritated, it would be best to answer her by saying:
    1. "Well, I suppose that is a burn from the extremely high dosage of x-ray you are receiving."
    2. "I don't know. You probably are lying on that area more than any other and are developing a bed sore."
    3. "The reddened area is a result of exposure to the x-rays. It is very much like the redness you notice when you have been out in the sunlight a little too long. It will eventually fade away."
    4. "The reddened area is something like a sunburn and it will get a little worse each time you go to x-ray. Why don't you ask the radiologist? He may want to reduce the amount of x-ray you are receiving."

15. Which of the following is *not* of primary importance in considering how much protection one has when exposed to a source of radiation?
    1. distance between source and person
    2. degree of shielding provided
    3. type of malignancy being treated
    4. amount of time spent in close contact with source
16. The odor frequently noticed around patients with terminal cancer is caused by:
    1. hemorrhage
    2. incontinence
    3. death of the tissues
    4. the malignant cells which have a characteristic odor
17. Nursing care to prevent these odors chiefly consists of:
    1. use of room deodorizers
    2. cleanliness and frequent irrigation of the necrotic area
    3. surgical removal of the necrotic area
    4. use of thick bandages over the area

UNIT 3   THE AGED AND CHRONICALLY ILL

I. Introduction
A. Geriatrics—the branch of medicine concerned with care and service to the elderly.
B. Gerontology—study of the problems and needs of the aged.
C. Aged—usually refers to those who are over the age of 65. However, each person must be considered as an individual because some persons age more rapidly than others.
D. Senile—pertains to aging or growing old. Does NOT necessarily mean mentally and physically incompetent.

II. Needs of the Aged
A. Need to feel that they are loved and wanted.
B. Physical needs include adequate housing and proper nutrition.
C. Should be encouraged to pursue hobbies and find ways to make their lives useful and interesting.

III. Basic Principles of Geriatric Nursing
A. The main objective of nursing care for an elderly person who is ill is restoring the patient to a life-style that is normal for his age. Aged persons are, first of all, *persons*, individuals who happen to be older in years. It is unwise to preface any statement with "all aged persons." Each elderly person must be considered as an individual.
B. Everyone should prepare himself for old age and increased leisure time by developing hobbies and interests that will help keep him active throughout his life.
C. The nurse should examine her own attitudes toward growing old and determine whether she has certain prejudices or biases toward elderly persons.
D. The geriatric nurse must be careful to maintain the human dignity and self-esteem of all elderly patients, no matter what their disabilities may be.
E. One must strive to combine sincere respect for the elderly patient with considerate helpfulness.
F. The nurse's activities should be aimed at motivating the patient to help himself within the limits of his abilities.

IV. Physical Changes in the Aged
A. Skin and hair
1. Oil and sweat glands less active. Skin drier, hair and nails more brittle.
2. Daily bath often aggravates drying and leads to scaling and irritation of the skin.
3. Oils and lotions needed to protect skin and prevent cracking.
4. Nails should be softened with warm oil before cutting.
5. Cosmetics usually not harmful; are beneficial in raising the patient's morale.
B. Digestion
1. Somewhat impaired due to decrease in amount of hydrochloric acid secreted and slowing down of peristalsis.
2. Caloric needs often decreased with age as metabolic rate decreases and physical activity lessens.
3. Poor dietary habits often a problem. May result from economic problems, inability to chew, superstition, or ignorance of food values.
C. Musculoskeletal system
1. Bones are more brittle in the aged and fractures are more likely to occur. Bones become decalcified.
2. Muscles not as elastic; joints become stiff.
D. Sleep and rest
1. The need for sleep varies in individuals. Most aged persons do not sleep soundly for long periods of time. They take short naps and then become restless. Periods of sleep and activity alternate throughout day and night.
2. Moderate amount of physical activity of some kind helps muscles relax and aids the body in eliminating waste products.
E. Incontinence
1. Getting patient up out of bed helps in the control of incontinence.
2. Regular routine for offering bedpan and urinal often prevents accidental wetting or soiling of the bed.

V. Mental Changes in the Aged

A. Mental deterioration is NOT necessarily a part of the aging process.

B. There may be some loss of memory for recent events but companionship and someone to talk with help keep the mind alert.

C. Physical activity, recreation, and a variety of interests help preserve mental competence.

D. Disorientation as to time and place is most likely to occur when elderly patients are isolated and do not have access to clocks, calendars, or radios and are deprived of conversation with others who are well oriented. The nurse should take every available opportunity to reinforce the patient's knowledge of where he is, the time of year, the time of day. She may need to help him periodically re-establish acquaintances with other patients and nursing personnel. Disorientation also occurs temporarily in many older patients who suffer an acute illness or serious accident.

VI. Prevention of Accidents

A. Provide a safe environment that permits the aged person freedom in moving about.

B. Must take into consideration dimness of vision, diminished reflexes, and inability to move about quickly when removing safety hazards from their environment.

VII. Chronic Illness

A. Characterized by gradual beginning with vague symptoms that become progressively more severe.

B. Progress of the disease and accompanying degenerative changes vary with each patient.

C. Acute flare-ups (exacerbations) often alternate with periods of remission during which the patient has few symptoms.

D. Main categories of chronic illness
1. Circulatory disorders (heart and blood vessels).
2. Metabolic disorders (diabetes, etc.).
3. Malignant new growths (cancer).
4. Arthritides (arthritis).

E. Nursing care
1. During acute stage the patient is cared for in the same manner as any patient with a serious illness.

2. Convalescent stage is usually longer than for acute illness and patient is likely to become discouraged and depressed. Special care must be used to avoid complications which might permanently handicap the patient or aggravate his condition.

3. Rehabilitation—begins as soon as the patient is admitted and his condition diagnosed.
   a. Rehabilitation is the restoration of the patient to as near normal as possible considering his illness and limitations.
   b. Patient is directed toward the goal of helping himself and becoming as independent as possible.
   c. Adjustment to a new way of life and learning to live with his illness may be very difficult for the patient.
   d. Nurse must consider diversional activities and ways in which the patient can lead a happy and useful life.

VIII. Effects of Immobility

A. Chronic illness frequently imposes some degree of immobility.

B. The human body is designed for motion; therefore complications will develop if measures are not taken to combat inactivity.

C. Complications that may arise include:
1. Circulatory stasis and development of blood clots within the blood vessels.
2. Accumulations of secretions within respiratory tract and disturbance in balance between CO_2 and O_2.
3. Digestive disturbances that produce diarrhea, constipation, distention, and indigestion.
4. Loss of muscle tone, contractures, and osteoporosis.
5. Decubitus ulcers.
6. Urinary stasis with formation of stones and development of infection.

D. Nursing measures to combat complications of immobility.
1. Getting patient up in chair whenever possible.
2. Proper positioning of patient
3. Adequate diet and fluid intake, use of stool-softeners.
4. Range of motion exercises. (See Fig. 33). These can be done while a patient is being given a bed bath.

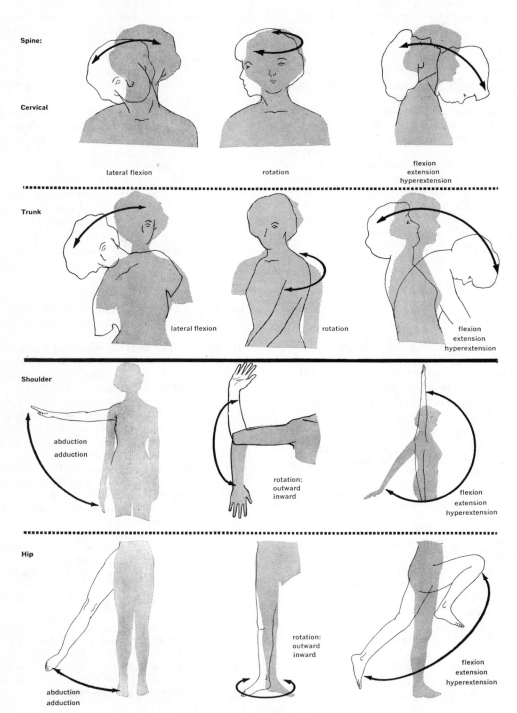

FIGURE 33.   Ranges of motion. All exercises can be performed from the supine position in bed except hyper-extension of the spine, hips, and shoulders and flexion of the knees, for which the person must lie prone or on his side. (Kelly, M. M.: *American Journal of Nursing*, 66:2209, 1966.)

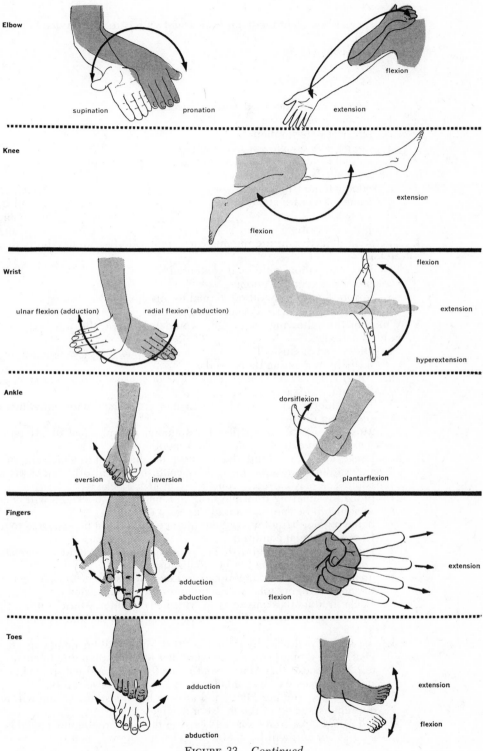

FIGURE 33. *Continued.*

Questions

1. The special branch of medicine concerned with care and service to the elderly is called:
    1. gynecology
    2. geriatrics
    3. pediatrics
    4. orthopedics
2. In its proper usage the word *senility* pertains to:
    1. mental deterioration
    2. physical deterioration
    3. the process of aging or growing old
    4. mental illness and confusion
3. The basic needs of the aged include:
    a. adequate housing
    b. someone to care about them
    c. recreation
    d. proper nutrition

    1. all of these
    2. all but c
    3. b and d
    4. c and d
4. The *main* objective in the nursing care of an elderly patient who is ill should be to:
    1. keep the patient quiet and contented
    2. prevent all complications
    3. restore him to a condition normal for his age
    4. prevent accidents and injury
5. Which of the following statements would best serve the nurse caring for an elderly patient?
    1. Older persons usually are very childlike and prefer to depend on others for help in meeting their needs.
    2. All elderly persons suffer from a loss of sensory perception such as sight, hearing, taste, and feeling.
    3. Each elderly patient should be treated as a person with individual needs, likes, and dislikes.
    4. Most elderly persons suffer from mental and physical deterioration that makes them extremely dependent on others.
6. Mrs. Locke, age 78, is admitted to the hospital after a fall in which she sustained a fracture of the femur. She seems very confused and disoriented at the time of admission. You may correctly conclude that Mrs. Locke is:
    1. probably suffering from physical and emotional shock and will need time to adjust to her new surroundings
    2. behaving normally for a patient her age and cannot be expected to recover from her mental condition
    3. going to be very childish in her behavior and would appreciate your "babying" her during her hospitalization
    4. unable to control her emotional and mental disorders and can be expected to continue being totally dependent on the nursing staff
7. Mrs. Locke frequently confuses you with her daughter, Marie, during the first few days of hospitalization. When she calls you by her daughter's name it would be best to:
    1. reassure Mrs. Locke by telling her that Marie will be along very soon for a visit, even though you are not sure that Marie is planning to come
    2. tell Mrs. Locke that Marie went home for a rest and will probably return, but the nurses will take good care of her until Marie returns
    3. pretend that you are Marie and answer her questions so she will not feel apprehensive and in the midst of strangers
    4. tell Mrs. Locke your name and explain that you are the nurse who is taking care of her and will be glad to help her in any way you can

8. Mrs. Locke often apologizes for being so much trouble to the nurses and says "If only I hadn't broken my hip, I could take care of myself, instead of asking you to do things for me." The practical nurse should realize that Mrs. Locke most probably is:
   1. expressing a desire to become more dependent
   2. regressing into senility and childishness
   3. anxious that she is losing her self-esteem and independence
   4. expressing guilt about her carelessness that caused her accident.

9. A complete bath daily may sometimes be considered undesirable for elderly patients because:
   1. they are less active than younger persons
   2. their sweat and oil glands are no longer as active
   3. most elderly patients do not like to bathe
   4. most elderly patients are free from body odor

10. The nails of an elderly patient are different from those of a younger person in that they:
    1. are more brittle and thicker
    2. do not continue to grow
    3. are more thin and fragile
    4. usually require the attention of a physician

11. Cosmetics and attractive clothing for the elderly patient are:
    1. a waste of time since she is usually unaware of her appearance
    2. not necessary, especially since the cosmetics will damage the skin
    3. important because they improve his attitude toward himself and others
    4. too expensive for the value received from them

12. The diet of an elderly person should include:
    1. fewer calories as he becomes less active
    2. more calories as he becomes less active
    3. high fat content to aid in controlling digestive disturbances
    4. less protein because protein foods are more difficult to digest

13. Malnutrition is present in most persons over the age of 60. Factors which contribute to this include:

    a. chewing difficulties and digestive difficulties
    b. lack of money for purchase of food
    c. poor eating habits
    d. ignorance of food values

    1. all but a
    2. all but b
    3. a and b
    4. all of these

14. The prevention of accidents and fractures in the elderly should be based on:
    1. placing them in homes specially designed for the elderly
    2. providing a safe environment for them
    3. keeping them inactive
    4. confining them to bed

15. Fractures are very common in the aged because:
    1. they usually have a serious loss of vision
    2. their bones are more brittle due to decalcification
    3. their bones are completely infiltrated with calcium
    4. they often indulge in physical activities that are too strenuous for persons of their age

16. An elderly person living with a young family will probably be most contented if he is:
    1. made the center of attention
    2. ignored and encouraged to live apart from the rest of the family
    3. allowed to feel independent and given simple but useful chores to perform
    4. given the responsibility of caring for the younger children

17. In planning the nursing care for an elderly person, the nurse should bear in mind that an elderly person usually:
    1. needs less sleep than younger, more active persons
    2. sleeps at short intervals during the day and night
    3. needs at least 12 hours of sleep each night
    4. sleeps well during the night but is restless during the day

18. Constipation in the elderly is usually the result of:
    1. inactivity and poor eating habits
    2. failure to take a laxative daily
    3. too much bulk in the diet
    4. absence of peristalsis
19. A simple nursing measure that often can be used to control urinary incontinence in elderly patients is:
    1. keeping a urinal in place at all times
    2. inserting a retention catheter
    3. using disposable diapers to prevent wetting the bed
    4. offering the bedpan at regular intervals and getting them up out of bed as much as possible
20. In regard to mental changes in the elderly, which of the following would be most correct to say?
    1. Elderly patients are individuals and some regress more rapidly than others.
    2. All elderly persons are stupid and forgetful.
    3. Mental deterioration is inevitable in persons over 60 years of age.
    4. There is a steady decline in mental and physical ability after 50 years of age.
21. Which of the following would be the best action to take when a elderly patient asks for his breakfast at 5:00 P.M.?
    1. Give him his supper tray when it arrives and tell him it is his breakfast
    2. Give him his supper tray and say nothing since he will only become more confused if you try to explain that it is supper.
    3. Tell him it is a little late for breakfast but you'll see what can be done.
    4. Tell him it is 5:00 in the evening and you will help him prepare for his supper if he wishes.
22. A person who is forced to retire at age 65 will adjust to his retirement better if he has:
    1. a large family with which to live
    2. arranged to live in a community built for "senior citizens"
    3. developed some hobby or vocation that will occupy his time
    4. adequate social security plus an income of at least 400 dollars a month
23. When a person is forced to live in a nursing home he should be provided with:
    1. uniform clothing so he won't be different from the other patients
    2. a wheel chair to conserve his energy
    3. his own private place for keeping his personal belongings
    4. a television set at his bedside
24. Rehabilitation is best described as:
    1. helping the patient to help himself
    2. restoring the patient to health and complete normalcy
    3. a return to normal functions
    4. treatment of complications that have resulted from disease
25. Rehabilitation is best accomplished by:
    1. the physician
    2. nursing personnel
    3. physical therapists
    4. a group of individuals working together
26. The success of rehabilitation PRIMARILY depends on the:
    1. desire of the patient to overcome his handicaps
    2. type of medical care the patient receives
    3. types of nursing care the patient receives
    4. financial resources of the patient
27. Rehabilitation should begin:
    1. as soon as complications develop
    2. with the admission of the patient to the hospital
    3. when the patient is discharged from the hospital
    4. as soon as funds are available to pay for it

28. An illness which has a gradual onset and requires prolonged treatment is classified as:
    1. an acute illness
    2. a critical condition
    3. a chronic or long-term illness
    4. a convalescent illness
29. A phase of prolonged illness in which the patient experiences a temporary relief of symptoms is called the period of:
    1. remission
    2. flare-up
    3. temporary cure
    4. regression
30. Which of the following is true concerning chronic illness?
    1. Patients with a chronic illness are totally incapacitated.
    2. Those who suffer from chronic illness cannot be expected to assist in their financial support.
    3. All chronic illnesses terminate in death within 2 to 3 years of the onset.
    4. Progress of a chronic illness varies with each patient.
31. Complications arise from inactivity and lack of exercise chiefly because:
    1. each body system acts independently from the others
    2. the body is designed for motion and activity
    3. muscles and bones deteriorate rapidly from disuse
    4. lack of motion places an added strain on the heart and circulatory system
32. Immobility can lead to respiratory complications chiefly because:
    1. secretions accumulate in the respiratory tract and interfere with exchange of oxygen and carbon dioxide
    2. the lungs cannot fully expand when a patient is lying on his back.
    3. the exchange of carbon dioxide and oxygen is decreased proportionately as the metabolic rate is decreased
    4. gravity flow of secretions in the respiratory tract is impeded by a prone position
33. Which of the following is most advisable in preventing constipation in an active elderly patient?
    1. All-bran cereals and other foods high in cellulose and roughage.
    2. Administration of a strong laxative at least once a week.
    3. Adequate fluid intake and administration of stool-softening agents.
    4. Administration of a retention enema every other day.
34. Osteoporosis is a condition resulting from immobility and affects the:
    1. muscles
    2. bones
    3. urinary tract
    4. digestive tract
35. Two complications that are most likely to develop in the urinary tract as a result of immobility are:
    1. hematuria and dysuria
    2. incontinence and retention
    3. renal stones and infection
    4. overdistention of the bladder and enuresis

UNIT 4   DISEASES OF THE SKIN

I. Diagnostic Tests and Examinations
  A. Visual examination
    1. Physician examines lesions under a strong light and palpates lesions to determine whether they are raised or nodular.
    2. Classification of skin lesions (Table 12)
  B. History
    1. Must know when the individual noticed a change in the skin.
    2. Where the lesions first appeared on the body.
    3. Whether or not the patient has had these lesions before.
    4. Under what conditions the lesions appeared; for example, every time a certain soap was used.
  C. Skin tests
    1. Definition—test of individual's sensitivity to specific substances.
    2. Methods
      a. Skin is scratched slightly and a sample of pollen, food, etc. is applied to the scratch.
      b. The sample is injected just below the first layer of skin.
    3. Reaction—a small dime-sized wheal appears at the site of contact.
  D. Culture and sensitivity tests—used in cases of infectious diseases, especially boils, carbuncles.

II. Prevention of Skin Disease
  A. Cleanliness

    1. Delicate skin requires special care to prevent dryness and irritation.
    2. Individual with oily skin will need to clean the skin frequently.
  B. Diet
    1. Adequate intake of vitamins and minerals.
    2. Well-balanced diet.
  C. Factors to be avoided in the environment
    1. Prolonged exposure to chemicals.
    2. Excessive drying of the skin.
    3. Excessive burning of the skin by strong sunlight.

III. General Nursing Care
  A. Definitions
    1. Dermatology—specialized study of diseases of the skin.
    2. Dermatologist—one who specializes in treatment of disorders of the skin.
  B. General rules in care of patients with skin diseases
    1. Bathing with soap and water is usually contraindicated.
    2. Dressings should not be removed without an order to do so.
    3. Do not attempt to remove crust and scales without specific order to do so.
    4. Observe skin carefully and record observations.
    5. Avoid excessive rubbing of the skin.
    6. Lotions should not be applied without an order.
    7. Ask before acting.

Table 12.   Classification of Skin Lesions

NAME OF LESION	EXAMPLE	DESCRIPTION
Macule	Freckle, purpura	A discolored spot or patch on the skin. Usually is not elevated or depressed and cannot be felt.
Papule	Present in measles	A solid elevation of skin. May vary from size of a pinhead to that of a pea. Usually red, resembling small pimples without pus.
Pustule	Acne, smallpox	A small elevation of the skin or pimple filled with pus.
Vesicle	Blister	A small sac containing serous fluid.
Bleb	Common in pemphigus	A large elevation of the skin filled with fluid.
Excoriation	Friction burn, chemical burn	An injury caused by scraping or rubbing away a portion of the skin.
Wheal	Insect sting, hives, nettle rash	An area of local swelling, usually accompanied by itching.

C. Colloid baths
   1. Definition—special bath prepared by adding soothing agents to the bath water.
   2. Purpose—to relieve pruritus; have soothing effect.
   3. Substances used
      a. Starch.
      b. Oatmeal.
      c. Sodium bicarbonate.
   4. Precautions
      a. Protect from chilling; patients have less resistance to heat and cold.
      b. Dry patient by patting him rather than by rubbing.

IV. Drugs Affecting the Skin and Mucous Membrane
A. Emollients—have soothing effect. Examples: cold cream, lanolin, petrolatum.
B. Demulcents—act to relieve irritation. Examples—starch, cream, milk, gums, and mucilages (acacia).
C. Astringents—used to arrest minor bleeding, promote healing, and toughen skin. Examples—salts of aluminum, zinc (as in zinc oxide ointment), and other heavy metals; tannins, alcohols.
D. Local anesthetics—available in ointments, sprays, aerosols. Also injectable form. Examples—cocaine, procaine (Novocaine), Nupercaine, benzocaine.

V. Disorders
A. Herpes simplex
   1. Definition—fever blisters.
   2. Cause—virus.
   3. Symptoms—vesicles on the lips and inside the mouth.
   4. Treatment—warm compresses, spirits of camphor, tincture of benzoin
B. Herpes zoster
   1. Definition—shingles.
   2. Cause—virus.
   3. Symptoms—groups of vesicles that appear on the skin in the area of the spinal cord and along nerve pathways; accompanied by pain and itching.
   4. Treatment—nonspecific.
C. Impetigo contagiosa
   1. Definition—highly contagious disease of the skin.
   2. Cause—staphylococcus or streptococcus.
   3. Symptoms—small vesicles which rupture and exude a pustular, honey-colored material that dries and forms a crust.
   4. Treatment—antibiotics.
D. Contact dermatitis (eczema)
   1. Definition—inflammation of the skin resulting from contact with a given substance.
   2. Cause—a substance in the environment.
   3. Symptoms—redness, vesicles, pruritus.
   4. Treatment
      a. Removal of substance from environment.
      b. Desensitization—exposing patient to small amounts of the substance until he has built up an immunity.
E. Acne vulgaris
   1. Definition—inflammatory disease of the sebaceous glands, especially of face and back.
   2. Symptoms—raised pustules.
   3. Cause—increased hormonal activity blocks pores of skin, forms blackheads, which become infected with bacteria.
   4. Treatment—varies with the individual.
F. Ringworm
   1. Definition—fungus infection of the skin, usually on face or scalp.
   2. Cause—fungus.
   3. Symptoms—red papules which spread in a circular pattern.
   4. Treatment—antifungal drugs.
G. Epidermophytosis
   1. Definition—athlete's foot.
   2. Cause—fungus.
   3. Symptoms—lesions usually begin between the fourth and fifth toes; may involve the entire foot; cracking and peeling of the skin.
   4. Treatment—antifungal ointments.
H. Burns
   1. Definition—injury to the skin caused by extreme heat or chemicals.
   2. Classification according to degree.
      a. First—redness, tenderness, pain; involves only epidermis.
      b. Second—blisters; involves both layers of skin.
      c. Third—involves both layers and underlying tissues; surface may appear charred or white and lifeless.
   3. Classification according to depth.
      a. Partial-thickness—epithelializing elements remain intact.
      b. Full-thickness—all epithelializing elements and those lining the sweat glands, hair follicles, and sebaceous glands are destroyed.
      c. Deep thermal burn—has white, waxy appearance of a full-thickness burn, but is a deep partial-thickness burn.
   4. Classification according to extent; Rule of Nines (Table 13).
   5. Emergency treatment
      a. Cover in cold packs.
      b. Wrap in clean white material.
   6. Measures by physician to combat shock

Table 13. Rules of Nines

AREA OF BODY	PERCENTAGE OF BODY SURFACE
Head and neck	9
Anterior trunk	18
Posterior trunk	18
Upper limbs	18
Lower limbs	36
Genitalia and perineum	1

a. Replacement of fluids lost.
b. Relief of pain.
7. Measures by nurse in emergency room
a. Gentle handling of patient and as little as possible to
1. Reduce pain.
2. Prevent infection.
8. Methods of treating the wound
a. Open—wound is thoroughly cleansed and left uncovered and exposed to air.
1. Nursing precautions—guard against infection, use sterile sheets, gowns, masks, and gloves.

2. Special unit is desirable.
b. Closed—area is cleansed, covered with Furacin or some other type of medication, and then wrapped in pressure dressings.
9. Record of intake and output. Important because physician uses this information to determine need for additional fluids.
10. Diet—should be high in protein.
11. Complications
a. Infection.
b. Contractures—may be prevented by proper positioning and adequate exercise.

Questions

Mrs. Ballard is admitted to the hospital with a diagnosis of severe contact dermatitis.
1. The nurse admitting Mrs. Ballard observes that the patient's hands, arms, and lower legs are inflamed and covered with small vesicles. A vesicle is:
   1. an elevation of the skin filled with pus
   2. a small round area of discoloration
   3. a small blister-like lesion of the skin filled with serous fluid
   4. a dime-sized area of swelling on the skin
2. When a patient is admitted to the hospital with a disease of the skin the nurse should:
   1. scrub the affected areas well with soap and water to remove the unsightly crust and exudate
   2. remove all dressings and bandages and apply dry sterile compresses to the skin lesions
   3. give the patient a tub bath using a mild disinfectant solution in the bath water
   4. observe the patient's skin very carefully and record these observations
3. Mrs. Ballard's contact dermatitis is most likely the result of:
   1. bathing too frequently
   2. sensitivity to a substance in her environment
   3. an infection she has caught from someone with a similar disease
   4. failure to keep her skin clean
4. Most patients with contact dermatitis suffer from pruritus. This is a condition in which the patient has:
   1. severe itching
   2. areas of excoriation due to scratching
   3. excessive scaling of the skin
   4. an inflammation of the skin

5. The dermatologist caring for Mrs. Ballard orders colloid baths b.i.d. This means that the bath should be given:
   1. once a day
   2. twice a day
   3. three times a day
   4. each night at bedtime
6. A colloid bath is:
   1. a special bath using some form of saline
   2. usually prepared by adding starch, sodium bicarbonate, or a cereal to the bath water
   3. a special preparation of an antiseptic solution
   4. a cool tap water bath given to cool the inflamed skin
7. The purpose of giving a colloid bath is to:
   1. cleanse the skin
   2. soothe the skin
   3. eliminate odors
   4. prevent infection
8. The patient receiving a colloid bath must be protected from chilling because:
   1. the bath usually lasts 1 to 2 hours and the patient can become chilled easily
   2. the temperature of the bath water must be less than 80° F. (27° C.)
   3. patients with skin diseases have less resistance to cold and heat
   4. the room must be well ventilated during the bath
9. When drying the patient after a colloid bath the nurse should:
   1. rub the skin vigorously to remove the old crusts and scales
   2. pat the skin dry
   3. allow the bath water to dry by evaporation so that the medication is not removed
   4. use sterile cotton balls to dry the affected areas of skin
10. Mrs. Ballard warns you not to get the fluid from her skin lesions on your hands because you may catch the disease. You should tell her that:
    1. this fluid does not contain any bacteria
    2. the fluid from the lesions of the contact dermatitis is not contagious
    3. you have had dermatitis before and are immune
    4. you will wash your hands carefully after caring for her

Tom Dawson is a teen-age neighbor of yours. He frequently talks with you about his problems and within the past few months he has had trouble with the appearance of acne on his face and back.

11. Tom has probably developed this condition because:
    1. he does not clean his face as thoroughly as he should
    2. he has reached the age at which there is increased hormonal activity
    3. he has been eating too much chocolate and sweets
    4. he has caught the disease from one of his classmates
12. Acne results when oil glands in the skin become overactive and their secretions block the pores of the skin. The oil glands are called:
    1. sebaceous glands
    2. sweat glands
    3. ceruminous glands
    4. ciliary glands
13. Which of the following is true concerning the treatment of acne?
    1. The disease can be cured by administering large doses of sulfur.
    2. Antibiotics are the drugs of choice for this disease.
    3. Each case must be treated on an individual basis.
    4. Deep x-ray therapy is the only positive cure.
14. When Tom confides in you about his problem with acne you should:
    1. tell him that everyone has problems of one kind or another
    2. remind him of all the good things he has to be thankful for
    3. realize that he is going through a difficult period of adjustment and needs your help
    4. try to get his mind off the subject because there is nothing that can be done for acne

Mr. White, age 40, is admitted to the hospital with second- and third-degree burns of the right shoulder, arm, and hand.

15. A person who is severely burned is very likely to suffer from shock at the time of the injury. To combat this condition the nurse might expect the physician to:
    1. administer intravenous fluids
    2. order a platelet transfusion
    3. place the patient in Trendelenburg position
    4. order hot water bottles and a heat cradle to replace body heat that is lost

16. When assisting in the emergency care of Mr. White, the practical nurse is responsible for:
    1. administering intravenous medication to relieve pain
    2. careful handling of the patient to reduce the danger of contaminating the wound
    3. scrubbing the burned area with an antiseptic soap to destroy the bacteria in the wound
    4. applying sterile dressings to the area

17. Mr. White's physician chose the open method of treatment for him. This means that:
    1. the wound is thoroughly cleaned and then left uncovered
    2. the wound is covered with petrolatum and a light dressing is applied
    3. the burned area is covered with a special type of material that allows circulation of air to the wound
    4. the burned area is wrapped in Ace bandages

18. Before Mr. White is transferred to his room, the following preparation must be made:
    1. making the bed with sterile sheets and obtaining a supply of sterile masks, gowns, and gloves to be used by nurses caring for the patient
    2. removing the hospital bed and replacing it with a Stryker frame which is always used for burned patients
    3. "fogging" the room with a disinfectant solution
    4. securing a supply of sterile dressings

19. One of the most important aspects of nursing Mr. White will be to accurately measure his urinary output. Extreme care should be used in measuring the output because:
    1. the physician will use the urinary output as a guide for ordering fluids to replace those lost
    2. there is always kidney damage with a burn
    3. a burn patient usually receives intravenous fluids
    4. the skin is an excretory organ and since it is damaged the kidneys will not function normally

20. One of the most common complications in a severely burned patient that usually can be avoided by good nursing care is:
    1. malnutrition
    2. contractures
    3. heart failure
    4. pulmonary edema

21. Mr. White's entire right arm has been burned. To prevent a permanent deformity of the arm the nurse should:
    1. encourage Mr. White to exercise his arms several times a day
    2. realize that extending the arm is painful and postpone exercises until the burn has healed
    3. place the arm in a sling to help support its weight
    4. keep the arm extended at all times

22. The physician has ordered a high-protein diet for Mr. White. The high-protein diet is given because protein:
    1. replaces sodium lost through the burned area
    2. replaces lost body fat
    3. builds and repairs body tissues
    4. provides a source of quick energy

23. Which of the following foods would be highest in complete protein?
    1. dried beans and peas
    2. eggs and cheese
    3. fresh vegetables
    4. cooked cereals, such as oatmeal
24. If all the following liquids are available for bedtime nourishment, which would you choose for Mr. White?
    1. orange juice
    2. lemonade
    3. ginger ale
    4. milkshake
25. Mr. White's sister wishes to bring a meal from home to encourage the patient to eat. She asks your advice on the menu. To provide the largest amount of protein the meal should include:
    1. beef bouillon, pork chops, potatoes, lime sherbet
    2. cream of tomato soup, roast beef, lima beans, carrots, chocolate custard
    3. fried chicken, rice, cole slaw, and ice cream
    4. barbecued ribs, tossed green salad, hot rolls with butter, and lemon pie

UNIT 5   DISEASES OF THE MUSCULOSKELETAL SYSTEM

I. Special Diagnostic Tests
A. X-ray films—used to determine abnormal changes in contour, size, and density of bone.
B. Culture—samples of infected bone are used to grow cultures and thereby determine the causative organism in an infection of the bone.
C. Biopsy—samples of bone cells are taken and studied for diagnosis of various bone tumors.

II. General Nursing Care
A. Lifting and turning patient
  1. Nurse must use good body mechanics to protect herself and her patient.
  2. All movements by the nurse should be gentle and firm.
  3. Frequent turning and altering the patient's position in bed are important in the prevention of deformities.
    a. Contracture—a shortening of the skeletal muscle and permanent loss of elasticity of the muscles.
    b. Loss of muscle tone—muscle becomes flabby and loses its state of partial contraction; is no longer able to produce motion by contracting.
    c. Ankylosis—permanent fixation of a joint with loss of motion.
  4. Changing joint positions necessary to prevent deformities listed.
  5. Exercises to maintain motion and muscle tone.
    a. Each joint should be put through its full range of motion at least once daily.
    b. Active exercises are those done by the patient.
    c. Passive exercises are done for the patient by the nurse or physical therapist.

III. Drugs Used in Disorders of the Musculoskeletal System
A. Antirheumatics—used to relieve pain and reduce inflammation and swelling of the joints.
  1. Examples: the salicylates such as aspirin and sodium salicylate.
  2. Symptoms of toxicity—headache, ringing in ears, gastrointestinal disorders; rarely, heart depression and skin eruptions.
B. Skeletal muscle relaxants—used to relieve discomfort of sprains or strains, back pain, traumatic injuries.
  1. Examples: Soma, Rela, Trancopal, Isomeprobamate.
  2. Side-effects include drowsiness, skin rash, nausea, and voiding difficulties.

IV. Nursing Care of the Patient in a Cast
A. Types of casts
  1. Long-leg or short-leg casts cover all or part of the lower limb.
  2. Walking casts have extra material added to the sole for weight bearing.
  3. A spica covers the trunk and one or more extremities.
B. Preparations for application of cast
  1. Skin is washed thoroughly with soap and water, and rinsed well.
  2. Shaving of the area is not necessary unless orthopedic surgery is done before the cast is applied.
  3. Mattress and pillows covered with a waterproof material until the cast is completely dry.
C. Care of fresh plaster cast
  1. Patient is placed in bed gently; be sure there is sufficient help available to avoid rough handling of the patient or the cast.
  2. Wet cast should always be handled with the palm of the hand, NEVER with the fingertips.
  3. Curves of the cast are supported with pillows to prevent flattening of the cast and distortion of its original shape (Fig. 34).
  4. Patients in a spica are more comfortable if a pillow is not placed under the head.
D. Drying cast
  1. Cast dryer may be used to increase circulation around the cast. Avoid the

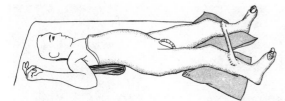

FIGURE 34. Good cast support. (Wiebe, A. M.: *Orthopedics in Nursing,* Philadelphia, W. B. Saunders Co., 1961.)

use of heat, as this may burn the skin under the cast.

2. Frequent turning helps the cast dry evenly.

3. Cast should remain uncovered until it is completely dry. Bed cradles trap moisture and hinder drying of the cast.

E. Important observations for possible complications

1. Sharp localized pain may indicate excessive pressure under the cast.

2. Observe protruding fingers or toes for cyanosis, coldness to the touch, or failure of the skin to blanch and then return to normal color after pressure is released.

3. Elevation of temperature or foul smell may indicate the development of an infection.

4. Support the cast so that there is no undue pressure on any part of the body over a period of time.

F. Daily care

1. Give special attention to the skin around the edges of the cast.

2. Avoid wetting the cast with bath water.

3. Elevate the head of the bed slightly when placing a patient in a spica on the bedpan. The perineal area must be cleansed thoroughly each time the bedpan is used. Covering the edge of the cast around the perineal area will prevent soiling of the cast.

4. When the cast is removed the underlying skin will be dry and scaly. The skin should be gently cleansed with soap and water and massaged with lotion or oil.

V. Nursing Care of the Patient in Traction

A. Types of traction

1. Skeletal traction in which the pull is exerted directly on the bone. Example, traction on Crutchfield tongs which have been inserted into the skull.

2. Skin traction uses moleskin or some other type of adhesive bandage to cover the affected limb, and traction is applied to the bandage.

B. Purpose of traction is to exert a constant pull on a certain part of the body in order to straighten the part and hold it in a fixed position.

C. Uses—in the treatment of fractures and contracture deformities, and to relieve muscle spasm due to strain.

D. General nursing care

1. Special back care necessary to prevent breakdown of skin.

2. When changing the linen, the bottom sheets are changed starting on the unaffected side. Or they may be changed from head to foot. The limb in traction may be covered with a small blanket in case the limb becomes cold.

3. Trapeze bar may be installed over the bed to allow the patient to lift himself and move about in bed. The patient is instructed to lift himself straight up toward the trapeze (Fig. 35).

4. Special observations

a. Be sure the weights are always hanging free and exerting pull.

b. Check to see if the patient's weight is counteracting the pull of the weights.

c. Observe bony prominences for signs of pressure.

d. Position patient so that body is in good alignment.

VI. Disorders of the Musculoskeletal System

A. Fractures

1. Definition—a break or interruption in the continuity of a bone.

2. Types

a. Comminuted—one in which the bone is broken and shattered into fragments.

b. Closed (simple)—one in which there is no break in the skin.

c. Open (compound)—one in which there is a break in the skin with fragments of bone protruding.

d. Greenstick—one in which the bone is partially bent and partially broken; common in children.

3. Treatment—aimed at establishing a sturdy union between the broken ends of bone so that healing will restore the bone to its former state of continuity.

a. Reduction—procedure for bringing the two fragments of a broken bone into proper alignment.

b. Three methods of reducing a fracture

1. Closed reduction—manual alignment of the bone; accomplished without a surgical incision.

2. Open reduction—bone is reduced after a surgical incision has exposed the site of the fracture.

3. Internal fixation—pins, screws,

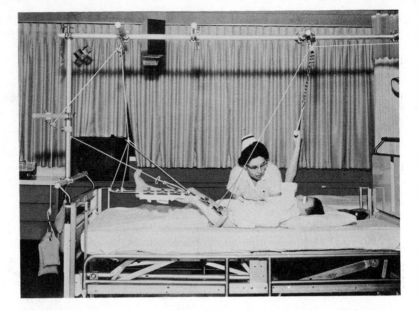

FIGURE 35. Skeletal traction, Thomas splint with a Pearson attachment. (Wiebe: *Orthopedics in Nursing.*)

plates, are used to stabilize the position of the broken ends of bone.

    4. Nursing care

      a. Emergency treatment consists of prevention of shock and hemorrhage and immediate splinting of the affected part to avoid damage to the soft tissues adjacent to the fracture.

      b. Reduction usually relieves severe pain. Care of patient in traction, cast, as outlined.

B. Sprain

    1. Definition—stretching of the ligaments around a joint so that there is a rupture of these fibers.

    2. Symptoms—pain, bruising, and swelling.

    3. Treatment—rest, adequate support of the part with elastic bandages. elevation of the part to reduce swelling, local applications of heat and cold.

C. Dislocation

    1. Definition—stretching and tearing of the ligaments of a joint with complete separation of the bones which make up the joint.

    2. Symptoms—severe pain on motion of the joint; muscle spasm; an abnormal appearance of the joint.

    3. Treatment—reduction with replacement of the bones to their normal position; immobilization of the joint by bandage or cast.

D. Osteomyelitis

    1. Definition—bacterial infection of the bone. Causative organism is most often *Staphylococcus aureus,* which also causes boils and furuncles.

    2. Symptoms—sudden onset with chills and fever; severe pain and swelling at the site of infection.

    3. Treatment—antibiotics, complete rest of the part, general supportive measures to improve patient's physical condition. Surgical incision and drainage may be necessary.

E. Arthritis

    1. Definition—a broad term used to cover all inflammatory diseases of the joints.

    2. Cause—specific cause not known. Predisposing causes include

      a. Infection elsewhere in the body.

      b. Overweight; poor posture or other injury to the joint.

      c. Emotional or physical strain.

      d. Heredity.

    3. Symptoms—depend on the type.

      a. Rheumatoid arthritis is the most crippling form. Onset is sudden with joint pain, elevated temperature, elevated white count.

      b. Other types may have more gradual onset, with weight loss, malaise, and pain in the affected joints.

    4. Treatment and nursing care

      a. Drugs include aspirin (acetylsalicylic acid) and other salicylates to relieve pain. Steroids act as anti-inflammatory agents to relieve symptoms of inflammation.

      b. Two most important factors are rest and moderate exercise.

      c. Good position of the joints of primary importance in the prevention of deformities.

    5. Osteoarthritis

a. A degenerative form of arthritis, commonly found in elderly persons.
b. Treatment aimed at preventing injury to the joints and avoiding undue strain.

VII. Amputation
  A. Definition — surgical removal of a limb or part of a limb because of severe physical trauma, malignancy, or gangrene.
  B. Preoperative care may involve plans for fitting a prosthesis and rehabilitation. Phys-

ical preparation of the limb is usually an orthopedic preparation.
  C. Postoperative care
    1. Stump is elevated on pillows protected with plastic.
    2. Observe carefully for signs of hemorrhage — large tourniquet is kept at bedside in event sudden hemorrhage occurs.
    3. Stump must be kept in good alignment; encourage patient to lie on abdomen as much as possible.
    4. "Phantom" pains may be relieved by pressure on stump.

Questions

Mrs. Smith is brought to the hospital emergency room after falling at her home. She is 67 years old and was in fairly good health before her accident. She has experienced pain in her right leg since the accident.
  1. When transporting Mrs. Smith from the scene of the accident to the hospital, it is most important to:
    1. immobilize the injured leg before attempting to move Mrs. Smith
    2. move Mrs. Smith into the house and improvise some kind of splint for the leg
    3. apply hot compresses to the leg to relieve the pain
    4. apply traction or a steady pull to the lower part of the injured leg to reduce the fracture, and then apply a splint
  2. A diagnostic test that the nurse might expect to be done as soon as Mrs. Smith arrives at the hospital would be:
    1. culture from the injured part
    2. biopsy of the injured bone
    3. sensitivity test
    4. x-ray study
  3. Mrs. Smith sustained a closed fracture. This means that:
    1. the bone was broken and shattered into many fragments
    2. the bone was broken but there was no protrusion of fragments through the skin
    3. the bone was partially bent and partially broken
    4. there was no evidence of injury to the bone
  4. The fracture was located in the bone of the upper leg. This bone is called the:
    1. femur
    2. radius
    3. tibia
    4. fibula
  5. The ulna is an example of a long bone. The cavity in the *shafts* of long bones is filled with:
    1. red marrow
    2. yellow marrow
    3. blood vessels and lymph vessels
    4. strong fibrous tissue
  6. At each end of a long bone there is a knob-like enlargement of the bone. These ends are called:
    1. epiphyses
    2. diaphyses
    3. articular cartilage
    4. medullary cavities

7. The ends of long bones contain a spongy material called:
   1. yellow marrow
   2. adipose tissue
   3. red marrow
   4. cartilage

8. The skeletal system supports and gives shape to the body. In addition to these functions the bones of the skeletal system also:
   a. protect some of the internal organs
   b. manufacture red blood cells in the red bone marrow
   c. provide the body with its supply of calcium and other salts necessary for life
   d. serve as levers for the muscles that are attached to them

   1. all of these
   2. a, b, and c
   3. a, c, and d
   4. all but c

9. Mrs. Smith complained of severe pain after her fall. Fractures are accompanied by pain because:
   1. bones contain many nerve endings
   2. there are spasms of the muscles attached to the bone that is broken and damage to the surrounding soft tissues
   3. there is always severe hemorrhage with a fracture
   4. the skin is broken whenever there is a fracture and the nerve endings are exposed

10. The surgical procedure used to treat Mrs. Smith's fracture was *open reduction* of the fracture and internal fixation. Reduction of a fracture means:
    1. making the bone smaller by removing the bone fragments
    2. manual manipulation of the broken bone and surrounding muscles
    3. surgical removal of bone tissue
    4. bringing the two ends of bone into proper alignment

11. Internal fixation means that:
    1. the joint of the bone is immobilized in a fixed position
    2. a surgical incision was necessary to treat the fracture
    3. the broken bone has been permanently attached to a stronger bone
    4. a support such as a metal plate, pins, or screws has been applied to stabilize the bone

12. Postoperatively, Mrs. Smith was to be turned every 2 hours. This changing of position is necessary to prevent:
    1. hypostatic pneumonia and circulatory stasis
    2. excessive nausea and vomiting
    3. spasms of the muscles resulting from being in one position too long
    4. postoperative shock

13. When turning Mrs. Smith onto her side it is very important to:
    1. remember to use the drawsheet to turn her
    2. place pillows between the legs to support the entire uppermost leg
    3. flex the knee of the affected leg before attempting to turn her
    4. turn her torso first and then position the lower extremities

14. When Mrs. Smith's fracture had healed sufficiently the physician ordered Mrs. Smith to use a wheel chair twice a day. While Mrs. Smith is in the chair she would probably be most satisfied to stay:
    1. in her room and out of the nurses' way
    2. in the hospital solarium where other convalescing patients gather
    3. out in the hall so she can enjoy watching people go by
    4. downstairs in the hospital lobby

15. Like many elderly persons, Mrs. Smith does not want to drink milk. Her refusal to drink milk may lead to a deficiency in calcium which is important in the:
    1. formation of bone tissue and maintenance of strong bones in the body
    2. building of hemoglobin
    3. regulation of the body's acid-base balance
    4. prevention of stiffness of the joints

Maria is a 19-year-old college student who suffered a fractured femur in an automobile accident. The fracture was reduced and the patient was placed in a cast that covered the trunk of the body and the affected leg.

16. A cast that covers the trunk of the body and one extremity or more is called a:
    1. spica
    2. long-leg cast
    3. walking iron
    4. Stryker cast
17. A cast is most often applied for the purpose of:
    1. immobilizing the part to allow it to rest for a period of time
    2. protecting the skin and soft tissues of the body
    3. preventing contamination of a wound
    4. preventing fractures
18. A newly applied cast is usually not dry for a number of hours. When transferring the patient in a wet cast from the stretcher to his bed:
    1. there should be enough personnel available to lift the patient onto the bed with ease
    2. the cast should be grasped firmly with the fingertips to eliminate the danger of dropping the patient
    3. the crossbar between the extremities should be used to lift the patient
    4. the patient should always be placed on his abdomen
19. When lifting the patient from the stretcher to the bed, there will be less strain on the body of the patient and the backs of those lifting if:
    1. all personnel lifting the patient will hold their knees straight
    2. one person will count and all lift in unison
    3. those lifting will stand on opposite sides of the stretcher
    4. at least five persons are available to help lift the patient
20. While the cast is wet:
    1. pillows should be used to support the curves of the cast
    2. the patient in a body cast must have a pillow under his head and shoulders
    3. a heat cradle should be used to support the weight of the top covers and hasten drying of the cast
    4. the cast must be covered with at least two cotton blankets
21. As long as a cast is wet its shape can be changed by prolonged pressure in one area. To avoid altering the shape of the cast it is important to:
    1. apply heat so that it dries quickly
    2. support the cast properly and avoid changing the patient's position
    3. place the patient on a very soft mattress until the cast is dry
    4. support the cast properly and change the patient's position frequently
22. The nurse may expect the patient to have some swelling under the cast soon after it is applied, but an excessive amount of swelling may impair circulation. Signs of impaired circulation are:
    a. bluish gray discoloration of the skin   1. a and d
    b. excessive redness of the skin   2. b and d
    c. the skin feels cold to the touch   3. a and c
    d. the skin feels hot and looks inflamed   4. c and d
23. If Maria complains of numbness or a tingling sensation under the cast the nurse should realize that:
    1. this will subside as soon as she gets used to wearing the cast
    2. there is always some numbness and tingling of the skin under a cast
    3. these may be signs of pressure on the nerves and should be reported immediately to the nurse in charge or to the physician
    4. as soon as the cast dries these symptoms will disappear
24. When placing the patient in a body cast on a bedpan the nurse should:
    a. support the small of the back with a small pillow or folded towel   1. a and c
    b. elevate the head of the bed *slightly*   2. b and d
    c. protect the perineal area with some waterproof material   3. all but d
    d. cleanse the perineum thoroughly after the bedpan is removed   4. all of these

25. While giving Maria her daily bath, the nurse should:
    1. avoid wetting the cast with bath water
    2. clean the cast with warm soapy water and rinse well
    3. place Maria in a semi-Fowler position and encourage her to take her own bath
    4. remember that the skin around the edges of the cast cannot be washed
26. Maria had been a very active person before her injury and she quickly became despondent when she realized that she would have to remain in the cast until her leg healed. When she asked the practical nurse how long it would be before she could walk again, what would the best reply have been?
    1. Don't worry about that now because there is nothing you can do about it.
    2. I don't know, but I am sure you wouldn't want to get up too soon and be crippled for life.
    3. Why don't you ask the doctor when he comes? I've never taken care of a patient in this kind of cast before and I don't know anything about it.
    4. You have many things in your favor—good health, youth, and the desire to get well. It won't be easy for you to stay in the cast, but I am sure the doctor will let you up as soon as it is safe.
27. Since time will certainly drag for Maria if she has nothing to do but lie in bed and stare at the ceiling, the nurse could help her by:
    1. showing interest in Maria's schoolwork and encouraging her to continue her studies while in the cast
    2. making an exception to hospital rules and allowing unrestricted visiting privileges for Maria's friends
    3. advising Maria's parents that she will become mentally ill if they don't find something for her to do to pass away the time
    4. tell Maria that she will have to stop acting like a child and learn to accept her illness without complaint
28. Assuming that Maria is in a fairly large hospital, which department could be most helpful in solving Maria's problem of boredom?
    1. diet therapy
    2. physical therapy
    3. social service
    4. occupational therapy
29. When Maria's cast was removed the skin under it was very dry and scaly. Which of the following nursing measures should be taken to relieve this condition?
    1. rubbing the skin with alcohol to remove any bacteria that may cause an infection
    2. applying lotion or oil to the skin after bathing the area
    3. applying continuous warm saline compresses to the area
    4. scrubbing the skin vigorously to remove the scales
30. The day Maria was dismissed from the hospital her parents expressed their appreciation for the care given their daughter and offered you a tip for your services. The best action in this situation would be to:
    1. refuse the tip, saying that it is beneath your dignity to accept any gift or tip
    2. accept the tip and then split it evenly among the other personnel who helped care for Maria
    3. refuse the tip, saying that it was a pleasure to care for her and seeing her recover from the accident was reward enough
    4. tell them that only the head nurses are allowed to accept tips from patients or their families

Walter Wilson is a young man who was injured while working on the construction of a building. He suffered a fracture of the large bone in his lower leg. The fracture was reduced and traction was applied.

31. The large bone in the lower leg is called the:
    1. fibula
    2. tibia
    3. radius
    4. humerus

32. Traction was applied to Mr. Wilson's leg for the purpose of:
    1. exerting pressure on the muscles of the leg
    2. elevating the injured leg
    3. removing any weight-bearing on the injured leg
    4. exerting a pull on the limb to hold it in a certain position
33. Two general types of traction are:
    1. skeletal and muscular
    2. skeletal and skin
    3. skin and muscular
    4. cervical and skin
34. Weights from Mr. Wilson's traction apparatus may be removed:
    a. when he goes to x-ray   1. all of these
    b. if he complains of pain   2. none of these
    c. at mealtime so he can sit up and eat   3. all but c
    d. while his bed is being made   4. b and d only
35. A trapeze bar was installed over Mr. Wilson's bed to facilitate his moving about in bed. When Mr. Wilson uses the trapeze to lift himself he should:
    1. wait until the weights have been removed from the traction apparatus
    2. be able to get onto the bedpan without assistance
    3. be told that he must not change position unless supervised by the nurse or physician
    4. be instructed to lift himself straight up toward the trapeze to avoid altering the amount of pull exerted on the fractured leg
36. To avoid disturbing the leg in traction any more than necessary when making Mr. Wilson's bed, it would be best for the nurse to:
    1. change the bottom sheet by starting at the head of the bed or on the affected side
    2. eliminate all top covers except for a bath blanket
    3. change only the cotton draw-sheet, leaving the bottom sheet unchanged until traction is discontinued
    4. change only the top sheet, using it to cover the leg in traction as well as the rest of Mr. Wilson's body
37. Mr. Wilson complained that his foot and leg in traction were cold. To provide warmth for the limb it would be best to:
    1. apply several hot water bottles
    2. wrap the leg in a wool blanket
    3. use a heat cradle with a 100-watt bulb
    4. place a small blanket over the limb

Mrs. Wood is a 45-year-old woman who was admitted with rheumatoid arthritis.

38. Arthritis is best defined as:
    1. an infection of the bone
    2. an allergic reaction to certain substances
    3. an inflammation of the joints
    4. a disease of the muscles and tendons which makes motion very painful
39. The most crippling type of arthritis is:
    1. rheumatoid arthritis
    2. osteoarthritis
    3. traumatic arthritis
    4. gouty arthritis
40. The symptoms of arthritis include:
    1. pain and tenderness of the joints
    2. discoloration and swelling of the joints and muscles
    3. elevated blood pressure and dizziness
    4. permanent fixation of all the joints
41. A complication that frequently results from inactivity of a person with arthritis is ankylosis, which may be defined as:
    1. brittleness of the bones
    2. permanent fixation of a joint
    3. overstretching of the muscles around a joint
    4. permanent contraction of the muscles of the ankle

42. To prevent crippling deformities while the arthritis patient is confined to bed, the nurse must help the patient maintain good body position and proper alignment. This means:
   1. keeping the patient flat on his back at all times
   2. providing active exercises to promote good circulation
   3. maintaining good posture in bed
   4. keeping the patient comfortable in the position he chooses

43. In positioning Mrs. Wood's feet, the practical nurse should know that:
   1. the soles of the feet should rest on the mattress
   2. the soles of the feet are kept at right angles to the mattress
   3. the toes are extended toward the foot of the bed
   4. the ankles are relaxed so that the sides of the feet rest on the mattress

44. Mrs. Wood's arthritis involves the cervical vertebrae. These vertebrae are located:
   1. in the lower back
   2. in the lower end of the spine
   3. in the neck
   4. parallel with the ribs

45. Mrs. Wood sometimes objected to having her position changed so frequently. This is probably because:
   1. motion of the affected joints is painful for the person with arthritis
   2. she could be comfortable in only one position
   3. she was reading or otherwise occupied and did not want to be disturbed
   4. most arthritis patients are very stubborn and difficult to get along with

46. Those who suffer from arthritis frequently turn to patent medicines for relief. Most of those medicines are:
   1. dangerous to the general health of the patient
   2. effective in curing only a few cases of arthritis
   3. not effective in severe cases
   4. mild pain relievers that delay the person's receiving adequate medical care

47. Acetylsalicylic acid is frequently used in the treatment of arthritis. The common name for this drug is:
   1. A.P.C.
   2. Empirin compound
   3. codeine
   4. aspirin

48. Since large doses of this drug are administered to the arthritic patient, the practical nurse should know the symptoms of a toxic reaction to the drug. These include:
   1. ringing in the ears, headache
   2. severe dehydration, hypotension
   3. diarrhea, vomiting
   4. headache and blurred vision

49. ACTH and cortisone are sometimes used in the treatment of arthritis. These drugs are examples of:
   1. antibiotics
   2. analgesics
   3. sedatives
   4. steroids

50. It has been found that patients with arthritis do best when they follow a regimen of:
   1. absolute bed rest until all symptoms subside
   2. strenuous exercises
   3. a daily balance between mild exercise and rest
   4. periods of absolute bed rest for several weeks followed by several weeks of strenuous exercises

51. Which of the following statements is true in regard to prevention of arthritis?
   1. It is an inherited disease which cannot be prevented or cured.
   2. People who keep very active are léss likely to develop arthritis than those who do not indulge in strenuous exercises.
   3. Eating a low-protein diet will prevent arthritis.
   4. Avoiding strain, fatigue, and worry will lessen one's chance of developing arthritis.

52. The type of arthritis seen most commonly in elderly persons is:
    1. acute rheumatoid arthritis
    2. traumatic arthritis
    3. osteoarthritis
    4. gouty arthritis
53. Mrs. Wood has had difficulty with obesity since adolescence. Obesity is most often caused by:
    1. glandular disturbances
    2. heredity
    3. anxiety or depression
    4. eating more than the body needs
54. Because she has arthritis, Mrs. Wood's diet should consist of:
    1. only the foods which will cure the disease
    2. a well-balanced diet that will not produce overweight
    3. a low-sodium diet
    4. a low-protein diet
55. Mrs. Wood is placed on a 1000-calorie diet to help her lose weight. Which of the following meals would be characteristic of this type of diet?
    1. pork chops, creamed potatoes, green beans, plain Jello, and black coffee
    2. roast beef, small baked potato, tossed salad, skim milk, and sherbet
    3. sliced ham, corn pudding, carrots, Jello, and iced tea
    4. fried chicken, rice and gravy, baked apple, chocolate pudding, and black coffee
56. Osteomyelitis is:
    1. a progressive degeneration of the bone
    2. a condition in which the bones become decalcified
    3. an infection of the bone
    4. a congenital deformity of the bones
57. The primary cause of osteomyelitis is:
    1. *Staphylococcus aureus* organisms which also cause boils and carbuncles
    2. the tubercle bacillus
    3. a virus
    4. the pneumococcus
58. In the immediate postoperative care of a patient who has had amputation of an extremity, the nurse must know that:
    1. the patient's intake and output must be measured very carefully.
    2. the patient is to be placed in semi-Fowler's position with the stump below the level of the body.
    3. the stump is elevated on pillows which have been covered with plastic or other protective covering.
    4. the patient is allowed to lie on the unaffected side only
59. Which of the following should be at the bedside of a recent amputee?
    1. a tracheotomy set
    2. oxygen tank and mask
    3. a large tourniquet
    4. suction apparatus for nasopharyngeal suction
60. Drugs such as Soma, Trancopal, and Isomeprobamate are sometimes used to relieve the discomfort of sprains, strains, or back pain. These drugs are classified as:
    1. central nervous system depressants
    2. antihistamines
    3. skeletal muscle relaxants
    4. antirheumatics
61. Side-effects of these drugs include:
    1. severely decreased body temperature
    2. drowsiness and skin rash
    3. depressed respiration and pulse rate
    4. elevated blood pressure and headache

UNIT 6   DISEASES OF THE DIGESTIVE TRACT

I. Special Diagnostic Tests

A. X-ray examination—accomplished by using a radiopaque substance, such as barium, to fill the hollow organs so that they can be visualized by x-ray.
 1. Gastrointestinal series (G.I. series)—x-ray examination of the esophagus, stomach, and small intestine.
  a. Preparation
   1. Explain procedure to patient.
   2. Withhold fluids and food 6 to 9 hours prior to examination.
  b. Procedure
   1. Patient drinks barium suspension which outlines hollow organs as it passes through.
   2. X-ray films and fluoroscopic examinations are done.
  c. Purpose—useful in diagnosing obstructions, ulcers, and growths.
 2. Barium enema—x-ray examination of the lower intestine.
  a. Preparation
   1. Explain procedure to the patient.
   2. Laxative the night before examination.
   3. Enemas until clear the morning of the examination.
   4. Restriction of fluids and foods depends on wishes of radiologist.
  b. Procedure
   1. Barium suspension is instilled into the rectum.
   2. Barium is retained while x-ray films are taken.
  c. Purposes—useful in diagnosis of tumors, ulcerations, obstructions, and abnormalities in the structure of the intestinal walls.
B. Gastroscopy and esophagoscopy
 1. Gastroscopy—visual examination of the interior of the stomach by means of a special instrument.
C. Proctoscopy and sigmoidoscopy
 1. Both are examinations of the interior walls of the rectum and lower intestinal tract.
 2. Tumors, ulcerations, or obstructions

may be seen and examined, and biopsy may be taken.
D. Gastric analysis
 1. Definition—laboratory examination of the fasting contents of the stomach.
 2. Preparation
  a. Levin tube is passed into stomach.
  b. Sample of the gastric juice is taken.
  c. A substance (usually histamine) is given to stimulate the flow of gastric juices.
  d. More specimens are taken of the gastric juices.
  e. Specimens are tested for the amount of hydrochloric acid present.
 3. Value—determining presence of gastric malignancy, pernicious anemia, or peptic ulcer.
E. Tubeless gastric analysis
 1. Definition—test to determine the presence or absence of hydrochloric acid in the gastric juice.
 2. Procedure
  a. Patient is given special granules in water.
  b. At prescribed intervals, urine specimens are collected.
  c. If hydrochloric acid is present the urine will be blue; if not, it will remain straw-colored.
 3. Value—useful as a screening technique for detection of absence of hydrochloric acid.
F. Stool specimen—laboratory examination for abnormal constituents.
 1. Occult blood (hidden blood)—no obvious bleeding.
 2. Parasites.

II. Drugs Used for Disorders of Digestive System

A. Antiemetics—used to relieve nausea and vomiting.
 1. Examples include Dramamine, Torecan, and Tigan. Side-effects include drowsiness, dry mouth.
 2. Thorazine and Sparine, both tranquilizers, may also be used as anti-

emetics. Patients should be watched for hypotension and signs of overdepression.

B. Antacids—for neutralization of gastric acidity. Used almost exclusively in treatment of peptic ulcer. Given between or before meals or may be alternated hourly with milk and cream.
  1. Examples—aluminum hydroxide gel (Amphojel, Creamalin, Gelusil). Other aluminum antacids include Alzinox, Robalate, Riopan.
  2. Sodium bicarbonate—used mainly as systemic alkalizer; can produce alkalosis if taken in excessive amounts.
C. Digestants—aid digestion
  1. Bile and bile salts—used to aid fat digestion and as substitute for natural bile salts.
  2. Dilute hydrochloric acid—aids gastric digestion when HCl is insufficient.
D. Antispasmodics—decrease gastric motility—act as depressants to parasympathetic nervous system.
  1. Pro-Banthine reduces both motility and hyperacidity.
  2. Belladonna and hyoscyamine decrease secretions and relax smooth muscle tissue.
E. Antidiarrheics—control diarrhea
  1. Kaolin (incorporated in Kaopectate) and pectin.
  2. Paregoric—camphorated tincture of opium. Interferes with peristalsis, slows movement of wastes through intestines.
  3. Lomotil—contains atropine—structurally similar to meperidine but has little or no addicting liabilities.
F. Fecal softeners—emulsify and soften feces.
  1. Surfak, Colace, Doxinate, Magcyl, and Polykol are examples.
G. Laxatives
  1. Bulk-increasing laxatives used frequently by elderly patients to promote regularity of bowel movements. Examples include: agoral, petrogalar, Metamucil, Casyllium.
  2. Lubricant laxatives—mineral oil, olive oil.
H. Saline cathartics—used when rapid evacuation is desired. Examples include milk of magnesia, Epsom salt, citrate of magnesia.
I. Irritant cathartics—stimulate peristalsis by local irritation of the intestinal mucosa. Examples include castor oil, cascara, Dulcolax.

III. Inflammatory Diseases
A. Gastritis
  1. Definition—inflammation of the mucous membrane lining of the stomach.
  2. Symptoms
    a. Nausea and vomiting.
    b. Pain and tenderness in the stomach region.
    c. Diarrhea in some cases.
  3. Treatment and nursing care
    a. Acute gastritis
      1. Withhold fluids by mouth.
      2. Administer I.V. fluids for dehydration.
      3. Drugs to decrease peristalsis.
    b. Chronic gastritis
      1. Diet therapy—frequent feedings of bland foods.
      2. Medications to coat the gastric mucosa.
      3. Antispasmodic drugs.
B. Ulcerative colitis
  1. Definition—inflammation of the colon with ulceration of the mucous membrane.
  2. Cause
    a. Specific cause is unknown.
    b. Predisposing causes
      1. Acute infections.
      2. Emotional tension.
  3. Symptoms
    a. Diarrhea—stool consists of bits of mucus, blood, and pus.
    b. Nausea and vomiting.
    c. Dehydration.
    d. Malnutrition.
  4. Treatment and nursing care
    a. Supportive measures
      1. Blood transfusions.
      2. High-protein, high-calorie, high-vitamin diet.
      3. Rest and freedom from anxiety.
    b. Constant reassurance from family and nurses.
    c. Antidiarrheic drugs.
    d. Careful observation of
      1. Number of stools.
      2. Character of stools.
  5. Surgical removal of the affected part.
C. Appendicitis
  1. Definition—inflammation of the veriform appendix.
  2. Cause—bacteria in the intestinal tract.
  3. Symptoms
    a. Pain in the right side.
    b. Elevated temperature.
    c. Nausea and vomiting.
    d. Increased WBC.
  4. Treatment—surgical removal.
  5. Preoperative nursing care
    a. Withhold food and fluids.
    b. Ice bag to abdomen.
    c. Routine preoperative orders.
  6. Postoperative nursing care
    a. Early ambulation.
    b. Fluids by mouth as soon as tolerated.

IV. Peptic Ulcer

A. Definitions

1. Peptic ulcer—open lesion on the mucous membrane lining of the stomach or small intestine.
2. Gastric ulcer—peptic ulcer located in the stomach.
3. Duodenal ulcer—peptic ulcer located in the duodenum.

B. Causes

1. Exact cause is not known.
2. Predisposing causes
   a. Personality characterized by anxiety and fear.
   b. Increased secretion of hydrochloric acid.
   c. Poor eating habits.

C. Symptoms

1. Burning and gnawing pain in the stomach region.
2. Nausea.
3. Frequent belching.
4. Vomiting food or blood.

D. Complications

1. Hemorrhage.
2. Perforation.
3. Obstruction.

E. Medical treatment

1. Rest
2. Diet therapy
   a. Designed according to individual needs of patient.
   b. Small frequent feedings of bland foods.
   c. Special diets—usually restrict only those foods that the patient has found will produce symptoms.
3. Drug therapy
   a. Antacids which neutralize the gastric juice.
   b. Antispasmodics—reduce muscle spasms and gastric secretions.
   c. Sedatives—reduce emotional tension.

F. Education of patient

1. Regulate types of foods he eats and manner in which he eats them.
2. Rest after meals.
3. Should learn to take several swallows of water every hour.
4. Use moderation in smoking.
5. Avoid anxiety.
6. Remain under medical supervision.

G. Surgical treatment of peptic ulcer

1. Indications for surgery
   a. Chronic ulcer which fails to respond to medical treatment.
   b. Perforation.
   c. Hemorrhage.
   d. Obstruction.
2. Types of surgical procedures
   a. Plastic repair of perforation—per-
forated area in stomach is sutured and the area reinforced with a graft.
   b. Subtotal gastrectomy (gastric resection)—removal of part of the stomach.
   c. Total gastrectomy—removal of all of the stomach.
   d. Vagotomy—cutting of the vagus nerve to prevent transmission of impulses to the glands of the stomach.
3. Nursing care of a patient undergoing gastric surgery
   a. Preoperative care
      1. Diagnostic tests.
      2. Routine preparation that is necessary for all abdominal surgery.
      3. Enemas to empty the colon.
      4. Insertion of a Levin tube.
   b. Postoperative care
      1. Semi-Fowler's position to promote drainage via Levin tube.
      2. Nothing by mouth for about 24 hours.
      3. Administration of I.V. fluids.
      4. Maintain gastric decompression, observe drainage for bright red blood and signs of excessive drainage. Avoid tension on the nasal tube.
      5. Frequent mouth and nasal care.
      6. Encourage coughing and deep breathing.
      7. Keep accurate output record.
      8. After the tube is removed, the patient is given small amounts of liquids. These are gradually increased according to the patient's tolerance.

V. Tumors of the Alimentary Tract

A. Cancer of stomach

1. Definition—a malignant growth within the stomach.
2. Symptoms
   a. Similar to those of a gastric ulcer.
   b. Symptoms may not be recognized until growth has reached the advanced stages.
3. Treatment—surgical removal of all or part of the stomach.

B. Cancer of large intestine

1. Definition—malignant growth within the large intestine.
2. Symptoms
   a. Change in bowel habits—alternate between diarrhea and constipation.
   b. Change in shape of stool.
   c. Rectal bleeding.
3. Treatment—surgical removal of the affected part.

VI. Intestinal Obstructions

A. Definition—blocking of the intestinal tract

which prevents normal passage of gastrointestinal contents through the intestines.

B. Causes
  1. Strangulated hernia.
  2. Cancer.
  3. Twisting of the bowel (volvulus).
  4. Telescoping of one part of the bowel into another (intussusception).
  5. Interference of the flow of nerve impulses to the bowel.

C. Symptoms
  1. Severe pain.
  2. Abdominal distention.
  3. Nausea and vomiting.
  4. Foul-smelling emesis.

D. Treatment — surgery.

VII. **Nursing Care of Patients Undergoing Surgery of Lower Intestine**
A. Types of surgical procedures
  1. Colectomy (colon resection) — surgical removal of the diseased portion of the colon.
  2. Colostomy — surgical formation of an artificial anus through an abdominal incision.
  3. Abdominoperineal resection — surgical removal of part of the colon and the entire rectum and anus.

B. Preoperative nursing care
  1. Restricted diet
    a. Low-residue diet 7 to 10 days before surgery.
    b. Liquid diet 24 to 72 hours prior to surgery.
    c. Withhold food and fluids 8 hours prior to surgery.
  2. Administer vitamin and mineral supplements.
  3. Laxatives and enemas to cleanse the intestinal tract.
  4. Emotional preparation by the doctor and nurse.
  5. Insertion of a gastric or intestinal tube.
  6. Routine preoperative surgical care.

C. Postoperative nursing care
  1. Watch closely for shock.
  2. Administer I.V. fluids and blood if necessary.
  3. Turn frequently.
  4. Encourage coughing and deep breathing.
  5. Record intake and output.
  6. Maintain gastric or intestinal suction.
  7. Nothing by mouth first 24 hours.
  8. Progression of diet depends on the individual case.

D. Special aspects in nursing care of patient using colostomy
  1. Emotional preparation is extremely important.

a. Doctor should explain what a colostomy is and how it works.
b. Nurse should be prepared to supply additional information.
c. Sometimes helpful to have another person with a colostomy talk to the patient.
d. Patient needs to know that he can lead a normal life with a colostomy.

  2. Teaching aspects
    a. Restriction of diet
      1. Avoid foods that cause diarrhea.
      2. Low-residue diet until the patient can control bowel movements.
      3. Avoid foods that cause flatus.
    b. Special appliances available for use, and procedure for irrigating colostomy.
    c. Irrigation of colostomy to establish a regular pattern for evacuation of the bowel.
      1. Irrigate at the same time each day.
      2. Allow approximately 1 hour for evacuation.
      3. Amount of solution varies.
      4. Evacuation is more nearly normal if the patient sits on the toilet.
      5. Patient should gradually assume all responsibility for care of the colostomy if physically able to do so.

VIII. **Hernia**
A. Definitions
  1. Hernia — protrusion of a loop of tissue or organ through a defect in the muscular wall.
  2. Reducible hernia — protruding tissue or organ can be replaced by pressure on the organ.
  3. Irreducible or incarcerated hernia — protrusion cannot be pushed back through the opening.
  4. Strangulated hernia — blood supply to the protruding part is cut off.

B. Causes
  1. Congenital weakness.
  2. Surgical incision.
  3. Injury to the part.

C. Common sites
  1. Umbilicus.
  2. Groin.
  3. Old abdominal incision.

D. Symptoms
  1. Lump or local swelling at the site.
  2. Pain.
  3. If the hernia becomes strangulated, the patient will have symptoms of an intestinal obstruction.

E. Treatment
  1. Surgery — herniorrhaphy.

2. Use of appliances such as a truss for support—useful for individuals who are poor surgical risks.

IX. Hemorrhoids
A. Definition—varicose veins of the rectum.
B. Predisposing causes
1. Constipation.
2. Prolonged standing or sitting.
3. Pregnancy.
C. Symptoms
1. Local pain.
2. Itching.
3. Bleeding from the rectum.
D. Treatment
1. Correction of constipation.
2. Local application of heat or cold.
3. Sitz baths.
4. Ointments which provide local anesthesia.
5. Surgical removal.
E. Nursing care of patient following hemorrhoidectomy
1. Rubber ring to relieve pressure on the area.
2. Warm sitz baths.
3. Wet dressings such as tucks.
4. Administer medications to soften the stool.

UNIT 7   DISEASES OF THE ACCESSORY ORGANS OF DIGESTION

I. Special Diagnostic Tests and Examinations
  A. X-ray examinations
   1. The gallbladder and ducts that carry bile may be visualized by x-ray if an opaque dye is used.
   2. Cholecystogram, gallbladder studies, and cholangiogram are terms used to describe x-ray examination of the gallbladder.
   3. Preparation of the patient requires administration of cathartics and enemas until return is clear.
   4. The dye is administered by the radiologist.
  B. Bilirubin test—bilirubin is a pigment normally found in the blood and removed by the liver. When the liver is diseased the bilirubin accumulates in the blood and produces jaundice.
  C. Bromsulphalein test—Bromsulphalein is a dye that is removed from the blood by the liver. If the liver is not functioning normally, the dye remains in the blood.

II. Jaundice
  A. Definition—jaundice refers to a group of symptoms rather than a disease. It is an indication that there are excessive amounts of the bile pigment in the blood.
  B. Types of jaundice
   1. Obstructive jaundice—caused by plugging of the bile ducts.
   2. Nonobstructive jaundice—associated with damage to the liver cells.
   3. Hemolytic jaundice. Hemolysis means destruction of the red blood cells. When large numbers of red blood cells are destroyed their pigment is released into blood, and jaundice develops.
  C. Nursing care
   1. Relief of itching of the skin—soda baths; mild lotions; frequent changing of bed linens.
   2. Indigestion due to blockage of the flow of bile into the intestinal tract—low-fat diet; relief of constipation.
   3. Close observation of the color of the urine and stools. The urine may be dark due to excretion of bile by the kidneys.

Stools may be light (clay-colored) because of lack of bile.
   4. Observation of the patient for signs of bleeding, because the liver manufactures prothrombin, which plays an important role in the clotting of blood.

III. Viral Hepatitis
  A. Definition—an inflammation of the liver caused by a virus.
  B. Types
   1. Epidemic hepatitis or catarrhal jaundice—transmitted through human excreta and direct personal contact.
   2. Serum hepatitis—contracted through use of contaminated needles or syringes.
  C. Symptoms—early symptoms similar to those of an upper respiratory infection; later, there is local tenderness over the liver, and the appearance of jaundice.
  D. Treatment and nursing care
   1. Bed rest.
   2. Isolation to prevent contamination of others. Special care must be used in handling all body secretions.
   3. High-calorie and high-protein diet.

IV. Cirrhosis of the Liver
  A. Definition—a chronic disease characterized by degeneration of the liver cells.
  B. Cause—specific cause unknown; associated with vitamin deficiency.
  C. Symptoms
   1. Early symptoms are the same as those of acute hepatitis.
   2. Later there is congestion of the blood vessels that drain the digestive organs and transport the blood to the liver (the portal circulation). This leads to an accumulation of fluid within the intestines and eventually into the abdominal cavity.
   3. Ascites—excess of fluid within the abdominal cavity. This condition is relieved by withdrawing the fluid from the cavity (paracentesis).
   4. Other symptoms include edema, jaundice, and small hemorrhages under the skin.

183

D. Treatment and nursing care—no known cure for cirrhosis, treatment is symptomatic.
  1. Rest in bed—best position is with head and shoulders elevated if the patient has ascites.
  2. Weigh patient daily.
  3. Low-salt diet for edema relief.
  4. Care of the skin important.
  5. Be alert for signs of bleeding internally.
  6. Dietary treatment consists of a high-protein, low-sodium, low-fat diet.
  7. Mental changes can be expected in the last stages. Delirium, convulsions, or coma must be watched for.

V. **Cholecystitis**
  A. Definition—an inflammation of the gallbladder. Cause is unknown.
  B. Symptoms—abdominal distention, indigestion; in acute inflammation, severe pain in upper right quadrant, chills, fever, nausea, and vomiting.
  C. Treatment
    1. May be conservative or surgical, depending on the case. In acute inflammation, the symptoms are relieved until the inflammation subsides and surgery can be performed.
    2. Surgical treatment—cholecystectomy, surgical removal of the gallbladder; cholecystostomy, surgical opening of the gallbladder for the purpose of drainage.

VI. **Cholelithiasis**
  A. Definition—the presence of gallstones within the gallbladder or the bile ducts.
  B. Symptoms—severe pain in the gallbladder region. Nausea and vomiting and a history of intolerance to fatty foods.
  C. Treatment and nursing care
    1. Surgical correction of the condition necessary.
    2. Relief of symptoms; restriction of fats in the diet.

VII. **Nursing Care of the Patient Undergoing Surgery of the Gallbladder**
  A. Preoperative care
    1. Assist with diagnostic tests. Vitamin K may be given if jaundice is present and the level of prothrombin is low.
    2. Levin tube may be inserted before surgery.
    3. Routine preparation as for any abdominal surgery.
  B. Postoperative care
    1. Semi-Fowler's position after patient has reacted from anesthetic.
    2. Proper care of drains or tubes which may have been inserted.
      a. Drains may be used to remove purulent material from infected gallbladder. Dressings must be changed frequently.
      b. T tube may be inserted to drain bile. This tube is to be kept open at all times and should be connected to a bedside bottle.
      c. Avoid tension on the tubes or drains.
      d. Use Montgomery straps for holding the dressings in place.
    3. Carefully observe color of stools and urine.
    4. Deep breathing and coughing may be painful because suture line is near the diaphragm.

Questions

Mr. Kent is admitted to the hospital for diagnostic studies of the digestive tract. He has had repeated attacks of indigestion, nausea, and vomiting, and a burning sensation in the epigastric region.

  1. The first test performed on Mr. Kent was an x-ray examination of the esophagus, stomach, and small intestine. This test is referred to as a:
    1. gastroscopy
    2. barium enema
    3. gastrointestinal series
    4. gastric resection
  2. Prior to the x-ray examination of the upper intestinal tract it is necessary for the patient to:
    1. take a strong laxative for several days
    2. refrain from eating or drinking for 6 to 8 hours before the examination
    3. receive an intravenous injection of a special dye
    4. receive a medication which slows down peristalsis

3. If Mr. Kent asks you what will be done to him when the x-rays of his stomach are taken, what would be best to tell him?
    1. You will be asleep through the whole procedure so there is no need to worry.
    2. I haven't any idea, but most patients are very sick after the test is done.
    3. You will be given a solution of barium to drink and then x-ray films will be taken. The barium is harmless and not too unpleasant to take.
    4. Don't worry about it. It is just exactly like having an x-ray of your chest.

4. A series of gastrointestinal x-rays would be most helpful in diagnosing:
    1. obstructions and ulcerations of the upper intestinal tract
    2. inflammations of the gastric mucosa
    3. obstructions in the bile ducts
    4. ulcerative colitis

5. Another test ordered for Mr. Kent was a gastric analysis. In this test:
    1. stool specimens must be collected daily for 3 days
    2. specimens of the contents of the patient's stomach are removed after he has fasted for 8 hours
    3. a special instrument called the gastroscope is used to examine the interior of the stomach
    4. a small section of the stomach wall is removed and examined under a microscope

6. Mr. Kent's illness was eventually diagnosed as gastric ulcer. This condition is best described as:
    1. an inflammation of the stomach wall
    2. an ulceration involving the small intestine
    3. an open lesion in the mucous membrane of the stomach
    4. a perforation through the wall of the small intestine

7. The acid that is normally present in the stomach, and which aids in the digestion of certain foods, is:
    1. sulfuric acid
    2. nitric acid
    3. tannic acid
    4. hydrochloric acid

8. Patients who have gastric ulcers are often treated with drugs which contain aluminum hydroxide. These drugs are classified as antacids and their chief action is to:
    1. increase the flow of gastric acid
    2. render excess gastric acid neutral
    3. coat the lining of the intestinal tract
    4. reduce the patient's appetite

9. There are several diets which may be used in the treatment of a gastric ulcer. Generally speaking, all these diets consist of:
    1. liquids only
    2. foods containing a large amount of sodium to inhibit the flow of gastric juices
    3. only one meal a day so as to avoid stimulation of the flow of gastric juices
    4. small frequent feedings of bland foods and liquids

10. Which of the following foods would not be allowed on Mr. Kent's tray as long as his ulcer is being treated medically?
    1. butter and cream
    2. sugar and butter
    3. pepper or vinegar
    4. citrus fruit juices

11. Most physicians restrict from an ulcer patient's diet:
    1. only those foods that produce symptoms in the patient.
    2. all foods that are high in fat content and likely to cause weight gain
    3. all acid-ash foods
    4. foods that contain carbohydrates and are therefore likely to irritate the stomach

12. Mr. Kent responded well to his treatment and was discharged with special instructions regarding his diet. In addition to remaining within the limits of his diet, it is also important for Mr. Kent to:

   a. eat slowly and avoid strenuous exercise immediately after meals
   b. return to the outpatient clinic weekly for an x-ray of his stomach
   c. try to avoid mental anxiety and tension at work and at home
   d. restrict his intake of water because it stimulates the flow of gastric juices

   1. all of these
   2. a and c
   3. b and d
   4. all but b

Several weeks after his discharge, Mr. Kent was brought to the emergency room. While at work, he had experienced a sudden, severe pain in his epigastric region. He had become very weak and pale and was apparently in shock.

13. Mr. Kent's emergency condition was diagnosed as perforated ulcer. This means that:
   1. the ulcer had become larger and had spread to cover the entire stomach wall
   2. he had an obstruction which prohibited the passage of food through the stomach
   3. the ulcer had become malignant and spread to other parts of the intestinal tract
   4. the ulcer had deepened and penetrated the wall of the stomach

14. Mr. Kent was immediately prepared for a gastric resection. This procedure involves surgical removal of:
   1. the entire stomach
   2. a loop of small intestine
   3. part of the large intestine
   4. part of the stomach

15. When Mr. Kent returned from surgery he had a Levin tube in his stomach. It was attached to a Gomco suction apparatus. The purpose of this tube is to provide:
   1. for adequate drainage of fluids and gases collecting in the stomach
   2. a means for feeding the patient until he is able to eat solid foods again
   3. an airtight drainage system for the intestinal tract
   4. a means for administering fluids to combat dehydration

16. In the nursing care of this patient during the immediate postoperative period it is most important for the nurse to:

   a. irrigate the Levin tube with boric acid solution every 5 minutes to prevent infection of the operative site
   b. observe the drainage frequently for signs of excessive amounts of bloody drainage
   c. give the patient sips of water frequently to combat dehydration
   d. check the Levin tube and suction apparatus frequently to be sure the tube is open and draining freely

   1. all of these
   2. a and c
   3. b and d
   4. all but a

17. Mouth care is important for Mr. Kent while the Levin tube is in place because:
   1. poor oral hygiene will affect his appetite
   2. the tube causes irritation and excoriation of the lips
   3. he will not be eating or drinking and his mouth will be very dry
   4. most patients develop fever blisters soon after a Levin tube is inserted

18. After the Levin tube was removed the physician ordered a bland liquid diet for Mr. Kent. The purpose of this diet is to:
   1. provide only alkaline foods which will not be irritating to the stomach
   2. stimulate peristalsis and prevent constipation
   3. provide small feedings which are easily digested and are not irritating to the gastric mucosa
   4. provide sterile feedings to avoid infection of the operative site

19. As Mr. Kent improved, his diet was changed to a soft bland diet. Which of the following foods would not be allowed on this diet?
    1. cottage cheese
    2. eggs
    3. smoked fish
    4. creamed soups

20. Whole cereals and raw fruits and vegetables are not allowed on a bland diet because they are:
    1. too high in acid content
    2. mechanically irritating to the intestinal mucosa
    3. chemical stimulants
    4. too low in fat content

21. Which of the following would not be allowed on a convalescent ulcer diet?
a. extremely hot or cold foods		1.	all of these
b. eggs and rice		2.	a and c
c. strong tea and coffee		3.	b and d
d. fish and ground meat		4.	all but b

22. During his convalescent period Mr. Kent received phenobarbital gr. 1/4 three times a day. The chief purpose of administering this drug in this dosage is to:
    1. allow the patient to have a good night's sleep
    2. relieve pain
    3. reduce nausea and vomiting
    4. reduce emotional tension and relax the patient

Mrs. Bird is a middle-aged woman who comes regularly to the outpatient department for treatment of ulcerative colitis. She is a very thin, nervous little woman who complains of being tired all the time.

23. Ulcerative colitis is best defined as:
    1. chronic constipation due to a spastic colon
    2. inflammation and ulceration of the mucous membranes of the colon
    3. chronic diarrhea due to improper diet
    4. inflammation of the lining of the stomach

24. Although the exact cause of ulcerative colitis is not known, a predisposing cause is thought to be:
    1. intake of too much bulk in the diet
    2. daily enemas
    3. overdependence on laxatives
    4. nervousness and emotional tension

25. Mrs. Bird is quite disturbed by the changes in bowel habits that are symptomatic of ulcerative colitis. The stools of these patients are characteristically:
    1. hard and constipated
    2. frequent and watery, containing mucus and blood
    3. frequent but of a very hard consistency
    4. tarry and of a watery consistency

26. Mrs. Bird's chronic fatigue is most likely due to:
    1. anemia and malnutrition due to poor absorption of the food elements
    2. her lack of interest in things outside her home
    3. lack of appetite produced by constipation
    4. failure to follow the diet prescribed by her physician

27. The type of diet recommended for patients with ulcerative colitis would include:
    1. foods containing bulk or roughage to combat diarrhea
    2. high-protein, high-vitamin foods to combat malnutrition due to chronic diarrhea
    3. restriction of liquids to decrease the number of watery stools
    4. restriction of citrus fruits to avoid irritation of the mucous membrane of the colon

28. Which of the following nursing measures is contraindicated in acute appendicitis?
    1. alcohol back rub to relax the patient
    2. application of an ice collar to relieve nausea
    3. alcohol sponge to reduce body temperature
    4. application of a hot water bottle to the abdomen to relieve pain

29. The most serious complication to develop from a ruptured appendix is:
    1. inflammation of the peritoneum
    2. intestinal obstruction
    3. hemorrhage
    4. ulceration of the ileum

Miss Tillman, a 60-year-old librarian, is assigned to your care while she is in the hospital. Her diagnosis is possible cancer of the colon.

30. The colon is:
    1. located just below the stomach in the digestive tract
    2. another name for the small intestine
    3. the large intestine
    4. the lower part of the anal canal
31. A diagnostic test that would be most helpful in determining the presence of an obstruction or growth in the colon would be:
    1. a barium enema
    2. an upper gastrointestinal series of x-rays
    3. a complete blood count
    4. an icterus index
32. Miss Tillman's physician requested that a stool specimen be sent to the laboratory for testing for occult blood. This test is done to determine:
    1. the presence of parasites in the intestinal tract
    2. whether there is an ulceration in the digestive tract
    3. the presence of "hidden" blood in the stools when there are no obvious signs of bleeding from the digestive tract
    4. a special type of blood cell that may be present in the stool
33. Cleansing the lower colon is necessary before x-ray studies of this area are made because:
    1. barium causes diarrhea if the colon is not free of fecal material when the test is done
    2. gas and fecal material in the colon produce confusing shadows on the x-ray and prevent proper filling of the colon with barium
    3. the patient is less likely to be nauseated if he has had cleansing enemas prior to the test
    4. most patients with disorders of the colon suffer from chronic constipation, and enemas are necessary to relieve this condition
34. Which of the following symptoms is considered to be a possible sign of cancer of the colon?
    1. persistent diarrhea with bright red blood
    2. clay-colored stools
    3. hemorrhage from the rectum
    4. changes in bowel habits, alternating between constipation and diarrhea
35. Miss Tillman's surgeon told her that surgical treatment would be necessary. He explained that the surgical procedure would be a colostomy. This procedure is best defined as:
    1. surgical removal of the stomach
    2. insertion of a tube into the stomach for the purpose of feeding a patient with an obstruction in the digestive tract
    3. surgical removal of the affected portion of the colon and creation of an artificial anus through the abdominal incision
    4. removal of the entire lower part of the intestinal tract and creation of an artificial anus through the abdomen
36. Miss Tillman's physician placed her on a low-residue diet for 1 week prior to surgery. In this case, the purpose of this diet would be to:
    1. relieve diarrhea
    2. decrease the amount of waste excreted through the colon
    3. relieve a fecal impaction
    4. increase peristalsis and thereby avoid irritation of the colon

37. Miss Tillman refused to look at her colostomy for the first few days after surgery. Her reaction should be considered:
    1. not unusual, and must be handled with patience and understanding
    2. childish and a result of an inability to face any of life's problems
    3. absurd, and indicates her lack of appreciation for everything that has been done for her during her illness
    4. very serious because she can never be taught to care for her own colostomy
38. While caring for Miss Tillman's colostomy it is especially important to care for the skin around the stoma. This special care includes:
    1. rinsing the area with normal saline and applying fresh bandages
    2. gently washing the area with soap and water, drying and covering with a protective ointment or paste
    3. pouring peroxide over the stoma and rubbing vigorously to remove hardened fecal material
    4. submerging the area in warm water and rinsing with alcohol
39. As soon as Miss Tillman is able to be out of bed, it would be best to irrigate her colostomy while she is:
    1. lying in the bathtub
    2. up in a chair in her room
    3. standing beside the bathroom sink
    4. sitting on the commode in the bathroom
40. The chief purpose of irrigating a colostomy is to:
    1. cleanse the small intestine and prevent fecal impaction
    2. prevent absorption of wastes from the intestinal tract
    3. establish a regular pattern for evacuation of the bowel
    4. prevent collections of gas in the lower intestine
41. When teaching a patient to irrigate his own colostomy, it is most important to:
    1. use equipment such as that available in the hospital
    2. irrigate the colostomy at the same time each day
    3. have the patient lie down in a comfortable position during the irrigation
    4. use at least 4 quarts of fluid for each irrigation
42. Miss Tillman adjusted well to her colostomy and eventually learned to irrigate and dress it herself. When she asks you about appliances and other dressings that may be needed to prevent soiling of her clothes it would be best to tell her:
    1. that there is really no way she can avoid soiling her clothes as long as she has a colostomy
    2. special appliances are very expensive and she will need special instruction in their use
    3. most colostomy patients need only a small square of gauze to cover the stoma once they have established a regular routine for irrigation and evacuation
    4. she will have to ask someone who has had a colostomy and knows the best type of appliance to use
43. Miss Tillman will need to make some alterations in her diet as long as she has the colostomy. These alterations would include:
    1. eliminating all seasonings and spices from her diet
    2. avoiding foods that are natural laxatives or likely to cause diarrhea or flatus
    3. decreasing the intake of protein foods
    4. increasing the intake of sweets and other foods which provide quick energy

The following questions refer to various disorders of the digestive tract.
44. The most common sites for development of hernia are:
    1. the groin and chest wall
    2. at the site of an old abdominal incision and in the groin
    3. over the umbilicus or upper abdomen
    4. between the ribs
45. An irreducible hernia is one in which the:
    1. protruding tissue or organ cannot be pushed back into place
    2. hernia continues to enlarge
    3. patient experiences little or no pain with the swelling
    4. blood supply to the protruding part is cut off

46. The most serious complication of a strangulated hernia is:
    1. hemorrhage
    2. shock
    3. intestinal obstruction
    4. gangrene
47. When an individual with a hernia cannot be treated surgically, an appliance for support of the weakened area may be worn to relieve the symptoms. This appliance is often referred to as a:
    1. brace
    2. halter
    3. binder
    4. truss
48. The medical term for varicose veins of the rectum is:
    1. hernia
    2. thrombosis
    3. hemorrhoids
    4. rectal prolapse
49. Following a hemorrhoidectomy, the dressings can be held in place best by using a:
    1. T binder
    2. abdominal binder
    3. pair of Montgomery straps
    4. scultetus binder
50. Sitz baths are often given following a hemorrhoidectomy. The main purpose of these baths is to:
    1. prevent hemorrhage
    2. relieve pain and promote healing
    3. prevent infection of the operative area
    4. relieve constipation

Mrs. Marino is a 48-year-old woman who has been suffering from nausea, vomiting, and indigestion for several weeks. Her physician has admitted her for diagnostic studies, although he suspects that she has gallstones.

51. If Mrs. Marino's gallbladder is affected she would most likely experience abdominal pain in the:
    1. upper left quadrant
    2. lower left quadrant
    3. upper right quadrant
    4. lower right quadrant
52. Mrs. Marino's indigestion would most likely be associated with eating:
    1. sweets and other carbohydrates
    2. fatty foods
    3. protein foods
    4. highly spiced foods
53. Mrs. Marino's physician ordered several diagnostic tests for her. One of these tests was a cholangiogram, also known as a gallbladder study. These terms are used to describe:
    1. a test for bile in the blood
    2. laboratory tests for obstruction of the bile ducts
    3. x-ray examination of the gallbladder and bile ducts
    4. a liver function test
54. The function of the gallbladder is to:
    1. produce bile
    2. store bile
    3. secrete bile into the stomach
    4. remove bile pigment from the blood
55. Mrs. Marino was found to have gallstones which were obstructing the flow of bile through the bile ducts. Bile is important in the digestion of fats because it:
    1. emulsifies or breaks down fat globules into smaller particles
    2. changes fat globules chemically, making them more difficult to digest
    3. prevents rapid absorption of fat through the intestinal walls
    4. speeds up elimination of fats through the intestinal tract

56. It was decided that Mrs. Marino's condition would be treated surgically. The correct term for surgical removal of the gallbladder is:
    1. colostomy
    2. cholecystectomy
    3. cholecystostomy
    4. colectomy
57. For several days prior to surgery, Mrs. Marino was given a vitamin K preparation. This vitamin is important in:
    1. digestion of fats
    2. healing of tissues
    3. elimination of bile
    4. clotting of blood
58. After Mrs. Marino returned from the recovery room she was fully awake. The best position for her during the immediate postoperative period would be:
    1. semi-Fowler's to prevent strain on the suture line
    2. on her left side to facilitate drainage from the Levin tube
    3. flat on her back with a pillow under her head to prevent respiratory difficulty
    4. on her abdomen to reduce nausea
59. The nurse who accompanied Mrs. Marino from the recovery room tells you that Mrs. Marino has a T tube and drainage bottle as well as the Levin tube and suction. The T tube was inserted during surgery for the purpose of:
    1. removing serous fluid from the abdominal cavity
    2. providing a means for irrigating the operative area
    3. providing for drainage of bile from the bile ducts
    4. removing excess bile from the intestinal tract
60. Mrs. Marino complained of pain each time she was asked to take deep breaths and coughs. This is most probably because:
    1. Mrs. Marino is very obese
    2. she does not understand the importance of deep breathing and coughing
    3. the Levin tube is irritating her throat
    4. the suture line and operative site are very near the diaphragm
61. Observation of the patient's urine and stool are important whenever there is an obstruction in the flow of bile through the bile ducts. If there is little or no bile passing into the small intestine the stools will be:
    1. tarry
    2. clay-colored
    3. very watery
    4. full of mucus
62. As Mrs. Marino's condition improved she was allowed out of bed even though the T tube was still in place. When getting Mrs. Marino up, it is most important to:
    1. clamp off the T tube even though there may not be a written order to do so
    2. avoid tension or pulling on the tube
    3. keep the drainage bottle above the level of the surgical incision
    4. irrigate the tube before getting her out of bed
63. Before her discharge from the hospital, Mrs. Marino received instructions regarding her diet. The physician wished her to have a limited fat diet. Which of the following foods would be allowed on this type of diet?
    1. chocolate
    2. nuts and avocados
    3. cream cheese
    4. jelly and jam
64. Which of the following foods is highest in fat content?
    1. liver
    2. pork
    3. ground beef
    4. baked chicken

The following questions refer to various disorders of the accessory organs of digestion.

65. Which of the following definitions best describes jaundice?
    1. a group of symptoms indicating excessive amounts of the bile pigment in the blood
    2. a disease which affects the liver and gallbladder
    3. a disease characterized by yellowing of the conjunctiva
    4. a symptom which frequently accompanies anemia

66. Patients who are severely jaundiced frequently suffer from pruritus. This discomfort can best be relieved by:
    1. forcing fluids
    2. rubbing the skin with alcohol
    3. cleansing the skin with a soda solution
    4. restricting the intake of sodium

67. Infectious hepatitis can be transmitted by:
    a. ingestion of contaminated foods or liquids
    b. injection of contaminated whole blood or blood derivatives
    c. careless handling of contaminated syringes and needles
    d. inhalation of the virus into the respiratory tract

    1. all but b
    2. b and d
    3. a and c
    4. all of these

68. When caring for a patient with infectious hepatitis the nurse must be especially careful when handling:
    a. all body secretions from the patient
    b. syringes and needles that have been contaminated by the patient's blood
    c. plates and eating utensils used by the patient
    d. thermometers which have been in the patient's mouth

    1. all but c
    2. a and d
    3. b only
    4. all of these

69. The only way to be absolutely sure that syringes and needles are free from the virus causing hepatitis is to:
    1. soak them for a few minutes in a Lysol solution
    2. boil them for 5 minutes
    3. soak them in Lysol solution and then sterilize in the autoclave
    4. leave in direct sunlight for 6 to 8 hours

70. One very important function of the liver that is impaired when a patient has infectious hepatitis is storage of:
    1. bile
    2. sugar as glycogen
    3. fats for energy
    4. proteins for energy

71. Which of the following foods would be highest in carbohydrate content?
    1. sweetened fruit juices
    2. buttermilk
    3. lean beef
    4. cottage cheese

72. Cirrhosis of the liver is:
    1. caused by a deficiency of an unknown vitamin
    2. associated with malnutrition and vitamin deficiencies
    3. caused by excessive drinking of alcoholic beverages
    4. believed to be a viral infection

73. Patients with cirrhosis of the liver frequently suffer from an accumulation of fluid within the abdominal cavity. This condition is referred to as:
    1. peritonitis
    2. pedal edema
    3. ascites
    4. flatulence

74. The removal of this excess fluid from the abdominal cavity is referred to as a:
    1. thoracentesis
    2. thoracotomy
    3. paracentesis
    4. gastrostomy
75. The normal liver manufactures prothrombin. When the liver is diseased there is a decrease of this substance in the blood, and the patient must be watched carefully for:
    1. cyanosis
    2. elevation of body temperature
    3. a drop in blood pressure
    4. signs of bleeding internally or externally

UNIT 8   DISEASES OF THE CARDIOVASCULAR SYSTEM

SECTION 1   THE BLOOD

I. Special Diagnostic Tests
  A. Complete blood count—determination of the number of red blood cells and white blood cells per cu. mm.
  B. Hemoglobin test—determination of the amount of hemoglobin present in the red blood cells.
  C. Microscopic examination of the blood to determine the size and color of erythrocytes, and types and number of leukocytes.
  D. Sternal puncture—removal of cells from the bone marrow of the sternum.
  E. Blood typing—determination of the blood group to which the individual belongs.

II. Disorders of the Blood
  A. Anemia
    1. Definition—an abnormal reduction in the number of red blood cells circulating in the blood.
    2. Types of anemia may be divided into three main groups:
      a. Resulting from blood loss.
      b. Resulting from impaired production of blood cells.
      c. Associated with excessive destruction of blood cells.
    3. Symptoms—skin pale, chronic fatigue, headache, dizziness, shortness of breath on slightest exertion.
    4. General treatment and nursing care
      a. Rest. Absolute bed rest may be necessary in acute anemia. In other types patient should take periods of rest during the day. Best position is lying flat in bed without a pillow so as to increase flow of blood to the brain.
      b. Warmth. Patients with anemia suffer from lack of warmth due to inadequate circulation. Extra warmth in form of warm clothing and additional blankets preferred to use of hot water bottles or heating pads.
      c. Diet. Consists of foods rich in iron, protein, and vitamins B and C be-

cause these are used in the production of red blood cells.
        1. Patient may need education in food values and the importance of eating a well-balanced diet.
        2. Poor appetite is not unusual in anemic patients. Sore mouth and gums often contribute to anorexia. Highly spiced foods and extremely hot or cold foods should be avoided in these cases.
      d. Special mouth care. Often necessary because of sore gums which bleed easily. Brushing of the teeth may have to be discontinued and the mouth cleansed with cotton-tipped applicators and peroxide or mouthwash.
      e. Drugs
        1. Iron salts may be given by mouth in certain types of anemia. These should be given after meals to avoid irritation of the intestinal mucosa. Symptoms of toxicity include gastritis, constipation, diarrhea. Liquid preparations must be administered through a straw and the mouth thoroughly cleansed after each dose to prevent discoloration of the teeth. These salts produce black tarry stools.
        2. Imferon—an iron preparation that is given deep into the gluteal muscles. Sites are rotated to avoid local inflammation from the drug, which is very irritating to the tissues.
        3. Vitamin C (ascorbic acid)—given with iron because it improves the absorption of iron from the intestinal tract.
        4. Vitamin B_{12} and liver extract—given to patients with pernicious anemia because oral preparations of iron are ineffective in this disease. These injections must be continued as long as the patient lives.

f. Blood transfusions
   1. Used in both acute and chronic anemia. Given to replace or maintain adequate blood elements.
   2. Donor and recipient must be of compatible types.
   3. Nursing care: patient must be carefully observed for signs of a reaction or sensitivity to the blood. Signs include rash, itching, chills and fever; in more serious cases patient may have dyspnea, restlessness, coma; death may result.

B. Leukemia
   1. Definition—classified as a malignant disease of the blood cells. White blood cells increase in number and fail to function normally.
   2. Types—usually classified as acute or chronic.
   3. Symptoms
      a. Acute leukemia has a rapid onset with high fever, extreme pallor, tendency toward hemorrhage, swelling of the lymph nodes. Usually occurs in children.
      b. Chronic leukemia has a more gradual onset, with increase in white cell count, anemia, fatigue, swelling of the lymph nodes; sometimes there is a tendency toward hemorrhage. Usually occurs in persons over 45 years of age.
   4. Treatment and nursing care
      a. There is no known cure for leukemia.

In children the disease progresses rapidly and is fatal. In adults the disease progresses more slowly.
   b. Treatment is aimed at relief of symptoms, prevention of infection, and maintenance of a normal level of blood cells.
   c. Nursing care: protection of the patient from infection; nursing care similar to that of patient with severe anemia; proper positioning important when neck glands are swollen and breathing is difficult.

C. Sickle cell disease
   1. Definition—a group of hereditary disorders related to the presence of sickle hemoglobin (S) in the blood. In sickle cell *trait* only about 35% of the total hemoglobin is affected and most persons with the trait have no symptoms.
   2. Symptoms—caused by clumping of red cells and obstruction of blood flow leading to poor oxygenation of tissues. Anemia is present as are periodic joint pain, swelling of the hands, feet, and abdomen, and jaundice.
   3. Treatment—primarily symptomatic and preventive.
      a. Severe anemia is treated with folic acid and other nutrients essential to the formation of blood elements.
      b. Patient encouraged to drink plenty of fluids to make blood less viscous, to eat a well-balanced diet, and to avoid upper respiratory infections.

SECTION 2   THE HEART

I. **Special Diagnostic Tests and Examinations**
   A. Electrocardiogram—aids in the diagnosis of disturbances in the rhythm of the heartbeat.
   B. X-rays—may reveal abnormal changes in the contour and size of the heart.
   C. Heart catheterization—useful in determining structural defects in the heart.
   D. Angiocardiogram—an x-ray examination of the heart using a special dye which aids in outlining the heart's chambers and large blood vessels leading to and from the heart.

II. **General Nursing Care**
   A. Rest. Patient may be placed on complete bed rest, but most often the physician will

allow the patient to sit up in a reclining chair and to use the bedside commode.
   B. Diet and fluids
      1. Food is usually allowed in small frequent feedings to avoid overtaxation of the heart and circulatory system.
      2. If edema is present fluids may be restricted. Sodium is restricted because it has a tendency to hold fluids in the tissues.
      3. Extremely hot or cold foods and liquids may be restricted because of their effect on the contraction and expansion of the blood vessels.
   C. Positioning and exercise
      1. Dypsnea may be relieved by placing the patient in Fowler's position.

2. Good body position allows for expansion of the chest and adequate circulation of the blood.
3. Mild exercises to avoid circulatory stasis and clot formation in the lower extremities. Elastic stockings used to facilitate venous return and avoid thrombosis.

D. Care of the skin. When edema is present the skin must be watched carefully because edematous tissues break down much more readily than normal tissue. Bed rest demands extra attention to the back and bony prominences.

E. Drugs
1. Digitalis—used to slow and strengthen the heartbeat.
2. Quinidine—a heart depressant used when the heart muscle is quivering and does not function effectively as a pump.
3. Diuretics—administered to remove excess fluid from the tissues.
4. Analgesics—Demerol often used to relieve pain associated with severe heart attacks.

III. Congestive Heart Failure

A. Definition—heart fails to function as a pump and the heart chambers and major blood vessels become congested with blood. This condition is actually a complication of other types of heart diseases.
B. Symptoms—depend on which side of the heart is affected. Usually the left side fails first and then the right side becomes involved.
1. In left-sided failure the symptoms include dyspnea, cough, and eventually pulmonary edema in which the lungs fill with fluid.
2. In right-sided failure there is a damming up of blood in the superior and inferior venae cavae. Symptoms include mental confusion and loss of consciousness, edema of the lower extremities, and an accumulation of fluid in the liver and abdominal organs.
C. Treatment and nursing care
1. Rest is of great importance. Some patients with mild congestive failure may be allowed out of bed but they should avoid any strenuous exercise which will place a strain on the heart.
2. Diet usually includes restriction of sodium to avoid increasing edema. Food may be seasoned with garlic, onion, lemon juice, or vinegar instead of table salt. Sodium bicarbonate (baking soda) must also be restricted. Many patent medicines and preservatives also contain large amounts of sodium.
3. Medications
a. Digitalis given to regulate the heart-

beat; patient may need to take a daily dose for the rest of his life.
b. Diuretics given to relieve edema.

IV. Diseases of the Coronary Arteries

A. Acute myocardial infarction (coronary occlusion; "heart attack")
1. Definition—necrosis of an area of the myocardium resulting from blockage of the blood flow through the coronary arteries which serve that area.
a. Occlusion—a blocking off or obstruction.
b. Thrombus—blood clot which forms inside a blood vessel and is attached to the vessel wall.
c. Embolus—blood clot or any foreign substance circulating in the blood.
2. Symptoms
a. Sudden severe pain in the chest, sometimes confused with acute indigestion.
b. Nausea, vomiting, pallor, and anxiety. Many victims have a feeling of approaching death.
c. After 24 hours there is an elevation in body temperature and white cell count.
d. The levels of the enzymes SGOT and LDH are elevated.
3. Treatment and nursing care
a. Immediate care includes relief of pain with Demerol or morphine sulfate. Oxygen is given to relieve cyanosis and dyspnea.
b. Later care includes
1. Bed rest to avoid strain on the heart. Use of bedside commode. Amount of physical activity gradually increased.
2. Complications to be avoided include formation of a thrombus elsewhere in the body, and "frozen shoulder" which results from the patient's keeping his left arm immobilized against his chest to relieve pain. Both of these can be prevented by frequent changing of position, adequate support of the extremities, and passive exercises as ordered by the physician.
3. Digitalis to regulate the heartbeat.
4. Anticoagulants to impair the clotting mechanism of the blood and discourage the formation of clots within the blood vessels. Examples are Coumadin and Dicumarol.
B. Angina pectoris
1. Definition—severe cramp-like pain in the chest and left arm, produced by gradual obstruction of the blood supply to the heart. Caused by narrowing of the arteries due to atherosclerosis.

2. Symptoms
   a. Dull pain in the chest under the breast bone; pain often radiates down the left arm.
   b. Attacks may last from 3 to 5 minutes or longer. Often brought on by physical exertion or emotional upset.
   c. Other symptoms include pallor or flushing of the face and profuse perspiration.
3. Treatment and nursing care
   a. Aimed at relief of symptoms and avoiding occasions which bring on the attacks.
   b. Drugs used include the vasodilators which expand the blood vessels and increase circulation to the heart muscle. Example, nitroglycerin tablets, which are administered sublingually.
   c. Avoiding exposure to extreme cold also is important in preventing constriction of the blood vessels and diminished supply of blood to the heart muscle.

V. Inflammatory Diseases of the Heart

A. Endocarditis—inflammation of the inner lining of the heart.
B. Pericarditis—inflammation of the sac surrounding the heart.
C. Myocarditis—inflammation of the muscle of the heart.
D. Rheumatic heart disease
   1. Definition—an inflammation involving one or more parts of the heart. Most often affects the endocardium and the heart valves. Follows acute rheumatic fever and occurs most often in children and young adults.
   2. Symptoms—depend on the location of the inflammation in the heart.
      a. Changes in the rate and rhythm of the heartbeat and heart failure may result from myocarditis.
      b. Heart murmurs, fatigue, and hematuria may occur with endocarditis and involvement of the valves.
      c. Pain over the heart, increase in the heart rate (*tachycardia*), and dyspnea are present in pericarditis.
   3. Treatment and nursing care
      a. Aimed at decreasing the workload of the heart and prevention of extensive damage to the heart tissues.
      b. Rest is of primary importance.
      c. Antibiotics are given to prevent bacterial infections and repeated attacks of rheumatic fever.
      d. Well-balanced diet necessary to improve patient's general health.
      e. Surgical repair of damaged mitral valve done in some cases. This procedure is called a *commissurotomy*.

VI. Hypertensive Heart Disease

A. Definition—damage to the heart as a result of high blood pressure.
B. Symptoms—undue fatigue, dyspnea, edema of the extremities, and cyanosis.
C. Treatment and nursing care
   1. Aimed at relief of underlying cause, i.e., high blood pressure.
   2. Hypotensive drugs (those which lower the blood pressure) are given. These include Serpasil and Raudixin. Digitalis may also be given.
   3. Patient is taught to use moderation in everything he does, to avoid elevation of the blood pressure and additional strain on the heart.

VII. Congenital Heart Disease

A. Definition—a defect in the structure of the heart or one or more of the large blood vessels. This condition occurs as a result of improper development of the heart during fetal life and is present at birth.
B. Symptoms—depend on the location and type of defect.
   1. General signs and symptoms include
      a. Dyspnea.
      b. Cyanosis ("blue baby").
      c. Abnormality in pulse rate.
      d. Clubbing of fingers and toes.
      e. Feeding problems in infants and poor physical development.
C. Treatment and nursing care
   1. Supportive measures include prevention of infection and measures to improve and maintain the general health of the child.
   2. Surgical correction through open heart surgery is now possible in many of these cases.

SECTION 3   DISEASE OF THE BLOOD VESSELS

I. Diseases of the Extremities

  A. General treatment and nursing care

    1. Maintenance of adequate warmth important to prevent constriction of the blood vessels and further impairment of circulation.

    2. Avoidance of cold also important. Best to encourage the patient to dress warmly, since these patients have a decreased sensitivity to heat and may very easily burn themselves without knowing it.

    3. Any clothing which impairs circulation should be avoided; e.g., circular garters, tight shoes, etc.

    4. Special care must be given to the feet; toenails must be cut straight across; any sign of blistering, redness, or swelling should be reported to the physician immediately.

    5. Rest and exercises

      a. Patient is instructed to rest periodically during the day, elevating his feet to improve circulation.

      b. Exercises are done on the advice of the physician. Their purpose is to increase circulation to the extremities.

      c. Patients on bed rest are turned frequently; knee rests are used only for very short periods. A bed cradle may be used to prevent pressure of the top covers on the extremities.

      d. Elastic stockings used to support the blood vessels near the surface of the legs.

        1. The hose are applied early in the morning before arising from the bed.

        2. Stockings are held up with supporters rather than garters.

        3. Two pairs are needed for daily washing and drying.

      e. Nicotine is avoided because it constricts the blood vessels.

      f. Diet

        1. If patient is obese he must be placed on a diet to reduce body weight and pressure on the legs.

        2. Increase in fluid intake is believed to improve excretion of waste products in the blood and inhibit the formation of blood clots in the vessels.

      g. Drugs

        1. Vasodilators—to enlarge the size of blood vessels and increase circulation.

        2. Anticoagulants—to discourage the formation of blood clots in the vessels.

    6. Ulcers often form on the legs because of impaired circulation. These are treated in a number of ways.

      a. Special pressure bandages or paste boots may be applied in order to exert an even pressure on the blood vessels and thereby improve circulation, and to protect the ulcer from injury and infection.

      b. Surgical debridement of the ulcer may be necessary before healing can take place.

      c. These ulcers heal very slowly and tend to recur in spite of treatment.

  B. Arteriosclerosis of the extremities

    1. Definition—hardening of the arteries of the extremities. Most often occurs in the lower extremities.

    2. Symptoms

      a. In the early stages the extremities feel cold to the touch. There may also be numbness and tingling.

      b. Fatigue and leg cramps, especially at night.

      c. Ulcers and eventually gangrene if the condition is not treated in time.

    3. Treatment and nursing care

      a. There is no cure at the present time.

      b. Exercising helps improve circulation to the limb.

      c. Other measures such as those listed under general nursing care.

      d. Surgical amputation necessary if limb becomes gangrenous; amputation is surgical removal of a limb or part of a limb.

      e. Preoperative nursing care

        1. Plans for rehabilitation and purchase of a prosthesis are discussed with the patient unless the situation is an emergency.

        2. Surgical preparation of the skin depends on the written order of the physician. Often includes repeated scrubbing of the limb with a special antiseptic and then wrapping the part in sterile towels.

      f. Postoperative nursing care

        1. Stump is elevated on one or more pillows.

        2. Must be observed carefully for signs of hemorrhage. A tourniquet should be kept at the bedside since

sudden hemorrhage is always a possibility.
3. Exercises are often ordered so as to improve the muscular strength of the remaining portion of the limb and prepare it for fitting with a prosthesis.
4. Phantom pains actually are felt and may necessitate further surgery if they persist.

C. Varicose veins
1. Definition—enlargement and distortion of the shape of the veins as a result of inadequate flow of blood through the veins, and stretching of the vein walls.
2. Symptoms
   a. Early symptoms include fatigue, feeling of heaviness in the legs, or swelling of the legs after prolonged standing.
   b. Later there are pains in the legs, itching along the course of the veins, and eventually enlargement of the vein.
3. Treatment and nursing care
   a. Medical treatment consists of relief of symptoms by proper support of the vessels with elastic stockings or pressure bandages, and removal of causative factors.
   b. Surgical treatment involves tying off the affected vein (ligation) or surgical removal of the vein (vein stripping).

D. Thrombophlebitis
1. Definition—inflammation of the vein resulting from decreased circulation which is brought about by the formation of blood clot on the vessel wall.
2. Symptoms
   a. Pain in the calf of the leg that is aggravated by flexing the ankle.
   b. Elevated temperature and increased pulse rate; local area of redness along the affected vein.
3. Treatment and nursing care
   a. Anticoagulants given to prevent enlargement of the clot.
   b. Patient may be placed on bed rest and the affected leg elevated.
   c. UNDER NO CIRCUMSTANCES IS THE LEG TO BE MASSAGED, AS THIS MAY DISLODGE THE CLOT AND CREATE AN EMBOLUS.
   d. Warmth is applied locally.
   e. Patient must avoid straining or physical exertion and take precautions against respiratory infections.

II. Diseases of the Cerebral Vessels
A. Arteriosclerosis
1. Definition—hardening of the arteries leading to the brain.
2. Symptoms—signs of mental deterioration, slowing of the mental processes, and a decrease in intelligence. Emotional changes may also occur.
3. Treatment and nursing care
   a. At present there is very little that can be done to relieve this condition. Vasodilator drugs may be of some help in relieving the symptoms.

B. Cerebrovascular accident (stroke)
1. Definition—obstruction of the flow of blood to a part of the brain. May result from formation of a clot within a cerebral artery, or from rupture of an artery with hemorrhage into the brain tissue.
2. Symptoms—depend on the cause of the stroke and the size and location of the area of brain tissue involved.
   a. In a mild stroke the patient may feel dizzy and experience a severe headache.
   b. Disturbances in speech or momentary loss of consciousness.
   c. Paralysis on one side of the body, inability to speak or swallow, or all of these may occur.
3. Treatment and nursing care
   a. Emergency treatment—loosen all constricting clothing and turn victim's head to the side to prevent obstruction to breathing. Do not try to arouse the victim or move him until an ambulance arrives.
   b. Suctioning may be necessary to remove mucus from the throat. Other measures to maintain an open airway are necessary during the acute phase of the illness.
   c. Fluids may be given intravenously until the patient is able to swallow. Tube feeding is necessary for those who do not improve within a few days.
   d. Proper positioning of the patient is of primary importance. There is no local involvement of the bones and muscles, and they must be kept in good condition until the patient is able to control his muscular activities again.
   e. Passive exercises are usually instituted. Each joint must be put through its full range of motion at least once a day to prevent complications which will cripple the patient for life.
   f. Many stroke victims can recover with a minimum of crippling if they receive good nursing care and complications are prevented.

Questions

Mr. Long is a 47-year-old carpenter who has been suffering from shortness of breath, increased fatigability, dizziness, and headaches. His physician has admitted him to the hospital for diagnostic tests and treatment. His diagnosis on admission is "anemia."

1. Laboratory tests ordered for Mr. Long included a hemoglobin test. Hemoglobin is best defined as the:
   1. substance in the plasma which aids in the formation of red blood cells
   2. pigment in the red blood cells which gives them their color
   3. chief constituent of platelets
   4. substance in white blood cells which destroys bacteria

2. One of the most important characteristics of hemoglobin is its ability to:
   1. aid in the formation of antibodies
   2. assist in the formation of platelets
   3. unite with oxygen and carbon dioxide
   4. manufacture red blood cells

3. The laboratory report showed that Mr. Long's hemoglobin was 6 Gm. per 100 ml. That is:
   1. about average for a man of his age
   2. slightly lower than normal for males
   3. seriously below the normal range
   4. slightly above the normal range

4. In addition to the laboratory tests, Mr. Long was also scheduled for a sternal puncture. The sternum is:
   1. the hip bone
   2. the shoulder blade
   3. the collar bone
   4. the breast bone

5. The purpose of a sternal puncture is to:
   1. aspirate fluid from the chest
   2. obtain a sampling of breast tissue
   3. aspirate blood cells from the bone marrow
   4. allow for drainage of purulent material in the bone

6. Mr. Long had an increasing loss of appetite for several months. The medical term for this condition is:
   1. anoxia
   2. anorexia
   3. cachexia
   4. inertia

7. If Mr. Long complains that he is "always tired," the nurse should understand that:
   1. his anemia is the cause of his fatigue and he should have adequate rest
   2. most of his fatigue is probably the result of boredom
   3. fatigue is a symptom of anemia and there is nothing that can be done about it
   4. his fatigue is a result of a lack of carbohydrates in his diet

8. Frequent "dizzy spells" or fainting is not uncommon in anemic patients, primarily because:
   1. they often receive a large amount of narcotic drugs for relief of their headaches
   2. they habitually refuse to eat an adequate diet
   3. a decrease in the number of red cells leads to a deficiency in oxygen supply to the brain
   4. most of these patients have mental deterioration brought about by loss of blood

9. When Mr. Long requests more heat in his room the nurse should:
    1. realize that he is mentally deranged and is just trying to get attention
    2. tell him that the room must be kept cool for others who are busily working in the area
    3. ignore his complaint because he should be kept in a cool environment
    4. provide him with extra warmth because most anemic persons cannot tolerate cold as well as others

10. While helping Mr. Long to brush his teeth you notice that his gums appear very sore and bleed easily. This is:
    1. an indication that he does not brush his teeth very often
    2. a sign of decaying teeth
    3. a result of brushing the teeth too vigorously
    4. a common condition in patients with severe chronic anemia

11. In providing additional warmth for Mr. Long, it would be best to:
    1. give him additional blankets and slightly raise the temperature in his room
    2. apply several hot water bottles to his feet and legs
    3. allow him to sleep in his robe
    4. place a small electric heater near his bed

12. Special mouth care for Mr. Long should include:
    1. gentle cleansing of the mouth and teeth with cotton applicators dipped in a mild cleansing solution or lubricant
    2. cleansing of the mouth several times a day, using alcohol to destroy bacteria
    3. brushing the teeth several times a day, using a brush with very stiff bristles
    4. using a highly astringent mouthwash to decrease bleeding and stimulate the gums

13. Mr. Long is scheduled to receive a blood transfusion during the day. In planning the nursing care it would be best to:
    1. omit his bath and change of linens that day because the blood transfusion is more important
    2. postpone the bath and bed-making until several hours after the transfusion is completed
    3. give the bath and A.M. care early before the transfusion is started so Mr. Long will be more comfortable during the procedure
    4. wait until the transfusion is started and then give A.M. care to divert his attention from the procedure

14. To avoid serious difficulties that may arise from a blood transfusion, it is most important that:
    1. the blood be warmed to above body temperature before it is administered
    2. a very small gauge needle be used for administration of the blood
    3. the skin at the site of the injection be shaved and scrubbed with pHisoHex solution
    4. the blood of the recipient and donor be of the same type

15. During the transfusion the patient must be watched carefully for signs of a reaction. This condition results from:
    1. infection within the blood
    2. sensitivity of the patient to the blood, or to minerals added to the blood to preserve it
    3. administration of the blood in a vein that is too small
    4. use of transfusion equipment that is defective in some way

16. Symptoms of a transfusion reaction include:
    1. rash, chills, fever, or dyspnea
    2. fall in the blood pressure and pulse rate
    3. hemorrhages under the skin
    4. convulsions and coma

17. Mr. Long's illness was eventually diagnosed as pernicious anemia. This disease is best defined as:
    1. a decrease in red blood cells due to hemorrhage
    2. decreased production of red blood cells due to poor dietary habits
    3. decreased production of red blood cells due to poor absorption of iron and protein from the digestive tract
    4. excessive destruction of red blood cells

18. The treatment of pernicious anemia includes injections of vitamin B_{12}. The practical nurse should know that this medication:
    1. will cure the disease
    2. must be given at regular intervals for the rest of the patient's life
    3. must be given at least once a week for 6 months before it is discontinued
    4. will help only about 50 per cent of the cases of pernicious anemia
19. Special nursing considerations that must be taken into account when Imferon is given include:
    1. giving the drug by deep injection into the gluteal muscle
    2. using the same site each time to insure proper absorption
    3. watching the patient for signs of hemorrhage during the course of the drug
    4. administering vitamin K with each injection of Imferon to prevent hemorrhage

Mrs. Luke is 28 years old and the mother of four small children. She was admitted to the hospital for an emergency appendectomy and the routine laboratory tests done before surgery revealed that she was anemic. Further tests after surgery showed that Mrs. Luke had nutritional anemia.

20. To combat Mrs. Luke's nutritional anemia, the physician ordered an iron preparation by mouth. When giving iron preparations orally the nurse should:
    1. give the liquid preparations through a straw and instruct the patient to rinse her mouth thoroughly after the medication is taken
    2. dilute the iron preparation in a glass of milk to decrease irritation of the gums
    3. always have the patient drink a full glass of water with each dose
    4. count the patient's pulse before each dose is given
21. Oral preparations of iron are given with meals or immediately after meals because concentrated iron salts are:
    1. more readily absorbed from a full stomach
    2. irritating to the gastric mucosa
    3. generally used as an appetizer
    4. helpful in the digestion of foods
22. Iron preparations are given to patients with anemia primarily because this mineral is important in the:
    1. prevention of hemorrhage
    2. manufacture of normal, healthy red blood cells
    3. formation of plasma and antibodies
    4. prevention of infections in the blood
23. Symptoms of toxicity to iron preparations include:
    1. tinnitus and headache
    2. cardiorespiratory difficulties
    3. hemorrhage and anemia
    4. abdominal cramps, diarrhea, and nausea
24. Mrs. Luke tells you that she has had black tarry stools for the past few days and she is worried that this is a sign of cancer. You should tell her that:
    1. this is a symptom of internal hemorrhage in the intestines and she should tell her physician about it
    2. she may be hemorrhaging from the intestines and that is probably why she is anemic
    3. this is a normal color for stools and there is nothing unusual about it
    4. her stools are this color because she is taking an iron preparation by mouth
25. In addition to the iron salts, the physician has also ordered ascorbic acid. This drug is:
    1. vitamin C
    2. vitamin A
    3. liver extract
    4. another type of iron preparation
26. The physician ordered ascorbic acid because it will:
    1. prevent Mrs. Luke from developing an infection
    2. prevent the development of rickets
    3. prevent night blindness
    4. assist in the proper utilization of iron for the formation of red blood cells

27. Since Mrs. Luke's anemia results from poor nutrition, she will need some advice in eating well-balanced meals. While you are discussing nutrition with Mrs. Luke, she tells you that she is sure her children will never become anemic because they drink milk with every meal. What would the best reply to this statement be?
  1. You are right, milk is very rich in iron.
  2. Milk is a good source of protein but it does not contain all the nutrients necessary for good health.
  3. Milk contains many vitamins but no minerals.
  4. The only way to prevent anemia is by taking vitamin and mineral tablets daily.

28. Which of the following foods are richest in iron?
  1. apricots and prunes
  2. cottage cheese and American cheese
  3. whole wheat bread and cereals
  4. lemons and oranges

29. Mrs. Luke needs to rest when she gets home, but with four small children it will be difficult for her to take long naps. Her symptoms of fatigue and dizziness will be relieved most effectively if she will:
  1. sit down as much as possible while doing her household chores
  2. rent a wheel chair until her anemia is cured
  3. lie down without a pillow several times a day, as this position increases the blood supply to the brain
  4. avoid bending over or making sudden movements while she is doing her housework

Miss Lowell is a 55-year-old former schoolteacher who is seriously ill with chronic leukemia. You are assigned to care for this patient while she is in the hospital.

30. Leukemia is:
  1. classified as a malignant disease
  2. characterized by an increase in the red cell count
  3. a disease of the blood vessels
  4. always fatal within 6 months from the onset of symptoms

31. The white blood cells of a leukemic patient do not function like normal white blood cells. Since this is true, the nurse might expect patients with leukemia to have:
  1. malformation of the bone marrow
  2. a lowered resistance to infections
  3. enlargement of the blood vessels
  4. a tendency to develop clots within the blood vessels

32. Which of the following may be signs of internal bleeding and should be reported if they are noticed while you are nursing Miss Lowell?
  a. tarry stools
  b. smoky urine
  c. yellowing of the skin
  d. coffee-colored emesis

  1. all of these
  2. all but c
  3. a and d
  4. b and c

33. At times Miss Lowell is very irritable and difficult to please. As a nurse you should consider this behavior as:
  1. typical of a person of her age and background
  2. an indication that Miss Lowell is very neurotic
  3. a symptom of her illness and one she may not be able to control
  4. the result of a lack of spiritual depth which leaves Miss Lowell unable to accept her illness

34. Mary Long, age 14, has been diagnosed as having sickle cell disease. In order to help avoid the crippling effects of the disease, Mary should:
  1. receive monthly transfusions until she reaches adulthood
  2. eat a well-balanced diet, force fluids, and avoid infections
  3. exercise regularly and limit her fluid intake to control the edema
  4. be fitted for braces so that orthopedic deformities of the joints do not develop

35. Mary's mother has sickle cell trait. She is afraid that she will eventually become crippled and chronically ill. You could advise her that:
1. she should consider moving to a warmer climate where her symptoms will be less severe
2. Mary's physician probably will prescribe for her the same treatment Mary is receiving
3. there is little that can be done to prevent the symptoms of sickle cell trait
4. sickle cell trait usually does not cause symptoms

Mr. Wood, aged 64, is assigned to you for morning care. His diagnosis is congestive failure.

36. Congestive failure is best described as a heart condition in which there is:
1. an abnormality in the structure of the heart
2. a decreased flow of blood through the heart and great vessels resulting from failure of the heart to function as a pump
3. a result of the formation of a blood clot within one of the heart chambers
4. a sudden spasm of the heart muscle due to a decreased blood supply

37. Which of the following would cause less strain on Mr. Wood's heart when he has a bowel movement?
1. getting him up to walk to the bathroom
2. sitting him upright on the bedpan
3. having him lie flat on the bedpan
4. having him use a bedside commode

38. Mild exercises of the legs and the wearing of elastic stockings are prescribed for Mr. Wood. The purpose of these is to:
1. prevent clot formation in the lower extremities
2. reduce circulation to the legs and thereby reduce the work load of the heart
3. prevent edema of the abdomen
4. reduce edema of the extremities

39. Mr. Wood is suffering from severe dyspnea; the position in which he would be most comfortable is:
1. Sims' left lateral
2. Fowler's position
3. Trendelenburg position
4. supine

40. Back care for a cardiac patient is:
1. always contraindicated because the patient must have absolute rest
2. of less importance than for most patients because the edema "pads" the bony prominences of the body
3. of more importance than for most patients because cardiac patients often have edematous tissue which readily breaks down
4. not important unless the patient's skin shows signs of developing ulcerations

41. Cardiac patients are sometimes not allowed to have cold drinks or iced foods because:
1. they act as a stimulant to the heart
2. cold has a constricting effect on blood vessels and may therefore increase the workload of the heart
3. cold increases circulation and overburdens the heart
4. they cause the formation of gas and lead to stomach cramps

42. Mr. Wood was given a low-sodium diet. When edema is present the intake of sodium is restricted because it:
1. slows the heartbeat
2. causes hardening of the arteries
3. increases urinary output
4. holds fluid in the tissues

43. One food substance that contains sodium and is commonly used in the average person's diet is:
1. tea
2. sugar
3. table salt
4. coffee

44. Which of the following foods would you consider to be lowest in sodium content?
    1. citrus fruits
    2. canned meats and fish
    3. milk and milk products
    4. baking soda
45. Many persons may not be aware of the "hidden" sources of sodium. Which of the following should be carefully checked by reading the label to see if sodium is present?
    a. canned or processed foods, such as frozen vegetables
    b. toothpastes and mouthwashes
    c. bakery products
    d. patent medicines

    1. all of these
    2. b and d
    3. a and c
    4. all but b
46. Substances which may be used *freely* as seasonings for foods in a low-sodium diet include:
    1. salt substitutes
    2. garlic salt and celery salt
    3. lemon juice, vinegar, and garlic
    4. butter or other animal fats
47. Mr. Wood's doctor placed him on digitalis. The drug is classified as a:
    1. depressant
    2. heart tonic
    3. coagulant
    4. respiratory stimulant
48. The chief action of digitalis is to:
    1. lower the blood pressure
    2. prevent the formation of blood clots
    3. increase the pulse rate
    4. slow and strengthen the heartbeat
49. Before each dose of digitalis is administered to the patient, the nurse must remember to:
    1. count the patient's pulse
    2. count the patient's respirations
    3. take the patient's blood pressure
    4. check with the laboratory to see if a test of bleeding time has been done
50. Drugs which are sometimes given to increase the urinary output and relieve edema are called:
    1. urinary stimulants
    2. heart stimulants
    3. diuretics
    4. urinary disinfectants
51. The doctor has ordered a check of weight daily for Mr. Wood. The reason for this is to determine loss of:
    1. body fat
    2. appetite
    3. tissue fluid
    4. blood volume
52. When weighing Mr. Wood, you should remember to:
    1. take the patient to the treatment room scales, which are accurate
    2. weigh him in the late afternoon each day
    3. weigh him at the same time every day, on the same scales, and with the same amount of clothing each time
    4. ask the orderly to weigh him because it is difficult to get the patient out of bed

Mr. Brown is brought to the hospital emergency room after having experienced a sudden severe pain in his chest while at work. When he arrived in the emergency room he was very short of breath, was perspiring profusely, and complained of nausea.

53. The doctor ordered morphine sulfate gr. 1/4 to be given intravenously. The morphine was given primarily for the purpose of:
    1. relieving the nausea and vomiting
    2. relieving the severe pain
    3. increasing the circulation of the blood
    4. relieving the shortness of breath

54. Morphine is considered a narcotic because it is a:
    1. central nervous system depressant
    2. dangerous drug
    3. derivative of cocaine
    4. derivative of opium

55. "Digitalization" of a patient is often done when the drug is first begun. This means that:
    1. very small doses are given initially to determine the patient's reaction to digitalis
    2. an intravenous preparation of digitalis is given for the first three doses
    3. a stimulant is administered with digitalis to avoid respiratory failure
    4. the first few doses will be larger than subsequent maintenance doses

56. Which of the following is *not* a digitalis preparation?
    1. Cedilanid
    2. Crystodigin
    3. Lanoxin
    4. Pronestyl

57. Which of the following drugs is used for disorders of cardiac rhythm and requires counting of the pulse before administration?
    1. Serpasil
    2. quinidine sulfate
    3. Dicumarol
    4. Diamox

58. Drugs that are given intravenously have:
    1. a delayed effect
    2. an immediate effect
    3. a local effect on the blood vessels
    4. a more prolonged effect than those given by mouth

59. A deficiency of oxygen in the blood produces a bluish discoloration of the skin. This is called:
    1. pigmentation
    2. apnea
    3. pallor
    4. cyanosis

60. As soon as Mr. Brown entered the emergency room the doctor ordered oxygen by mask. Oxygen is usually administered for the purpose of:
    1. stimulating respiration
    2. reinflating the lungs after respiration has ceased
    3. relieving the symptoms of anoxia
    4. relieving an obstruction of the respiratory tract

61. Mr. Brown was transported from the emergency room to the medical unit by stretcher. Since he was under sedation the nurse should:
    a. have at least three people to transport the patient
    b. secure the patient's arms so they will not protrude over the sides of the stretcher
    c. use straps to hold the patient on the stretcher
    d. wait until the patient is fully conscious before moving him

    1. all of these
    2. b and d
    3. all but b
    4. b and c

62. The correct position for the nurse when transporting a patient on a stretcher is at the:
    1. foot of the stretcher so she can pull it along
    2. head of the stretcher so she can push it along
    3. foot of the stretcher so she can push it along
    4. head of the stretcher so she can pull it along

63. A diagnostic study that was done immediately after Mr. Brown's admission was an electrocardiogram. This test:
    1. measures the strength of the heartbeat
    2. records the activity of the heart muscle
    3. measures the rate at which oxygen is used by the body
    4. records the flow of blood through the heart chambers

64. During his first few days in the hospital, Mr. Brown was extremely apprehensive and expressed the fear that he was going to die. His attitude frightened Mrs. Brown and she asked the nurse why Mr. Brown felt this way. What would the best reply to this question be?
    1. Mr. Brown probably realizes that he had a heart attack and is very seriously ill.
    2. Many people sense that they are dying when they are very near death.
    3. This reaction is not unusual in patients who have had heart attacks, and Mr. Brown needs reassurance that he is getting along all right.
    4. Mr. Brown's heart attack has probably affected his mind because he was without oxygen for so long.

65. Mr. Brown's condition was diagnosed as *coronary occlusion*. The coronary blood vessels are located:
    1. within the chambers of the heart
    2. around the top of the heart with branches reaching down into the heart muscle
    3. in the pericardial sac
    4. just below the aorta

66. The word occlusion means:
    1. an obstruction or closing off
    2. a seizure
    3. a spasm of the muscles
    4. a blood clot

67. Coronary occlusion may result from a thrombus or an embolus. A thrombus is:
    1. a foreign body in the blood
    2. constriction of a blood vessel
    3. an enlargement of a blood vessel in the heart
    4. a stationary blood clot attached to the vessel wall

68. An embolus is:
    1. hardening of the arteries
    2. a deposit on the walls of a blood vessel
    3. a blood clot or foreign body circulating in the blood
    4. weakening of the walls of a blood vessel

69. An occlusion of the coronary arteries leads to death of some of the cells of the myocardium. The myocardium is the:
    1. major blood vessel of the heart
    2. sac surrounding the heart
    3. wall separating the chambers of the heart
    4. muscular tissue of the heart

70. The nurse can best help Mr. Brown relax and rest if she will:
    a. place things within easy reach so he will not have to call her when he needs something
    b. demonstrate a willingness to do everything for Mr. Brown so he will not feel that he is a bother to everyone
    c. explain to Mr. Brown the importance of rest in the treatment of his condition
    d. check frequently to see if Mr. Brown needs anything and try to anticipate his wishes

    1. all of these
    2. all but d
    3. all but a
    4. c and d

71. Mr. Brown is placed in Fowler's position to relieve his dyspnea. Dyspnea is best defined as:
  1. mild discomfort
  2. severe pain
  3. labored or difficult breathing
  4. inability to breathe unless sitting upright

72. Mr. Brown developed the habit of holding his left arm in a fixed position against his chest. The nurse should realize that he is doing this because:
  1. he is attempting to "splint" his chest and relieve the pain around his heart
  2. his left arm is paralyzed as a result of his heart attack
  3. he does not wish to be disturbed for a daily bath and back rub
  4. he is cold and is attempting to conserve his body heat

73. To relieve Mr. Brown's discomfort and avoid complications in the shoulder joint, it would be best for the nurse to:
  1. apply an Ace bandage around the left arm and chest
  2. apply a hot water bottle to the arm and chest
  3. support the left arm on a pillow and change his position frequently
  4. vigorously massage the left arm and chest

74. Each day Mr. Brown's physician requests a prothrombin level and then orders an anticoagulant drug. The chief action of this drug is:
  1. prevention of hemorrhage
  2. stimulation of the heart's action
  3. slowing down the formation of blood clots
  4. prevention of infection in the blood

75. Which of the following drugs is an example of an anticoagulant?
  1. digitalis
  2. Demerol
  3. Diuril
  4. Coumadin

76. Which of the following is *not* a specific nursing measure for a patient receiving an anticoagulant?
  1. shaving must be done with caution
  2. symptoms of bleeding must be reported immediately
  3. catheterization is done every eight hours if the patient is unable to void
  4. all nursing procedures involving introduction of tubes into body orifices must be done with caution

77. To help the physician determine the extent of necrosis present in the myocardium, the nurse's chief responsibility would be:
  1. accurate recording of the patient's intake and output
  2. taking and accurately recording the patient's temperature, pulse, and respirations every 4 hours
  3. conscientious administration of oxygen as needed and recording amount needed by the patient
  4. determination of the patient's hemoglobin level each morning

78. Another indication of damage to the myocardium is:
  1. an increase in the levels of the enzymes SGOT and LDH
  2. a decrease in the rate of the heartbeat
  3. the development of severe cyanosis and dyspnea
  4. the development of edema in the abdomen and chest cavity

The following questions refer to various types of heart disease.

79. Angina pectoris is a type of heart disease in which there is:
  1. an inflammation of the heart muscle
  2. a gradual decrease in the blood supply to the heart muscle
  3. formation of a blood clot in one of the heart's chambers
  4. a sudden increase in the rate of the heartbeat

80. The outstanding symptom of angina pectoris is:
    1. cyanosis
    2. elevation of the blood pressure
    3. pain in the chest radiating down the left arm
    4. acute pain often mistaken for indigestion
81. Angina pectoris is treated with nitroglycerin which has the effect of:
    1. stimulating respirations
    2. relaxing the muscles of the chest
    3. relieving pain by depressing the central nervous system
    4. dilating the blood vessels
82. Nitroglycerin tablets are administered sublingually. This means the tablets are:
    1. dissolved and administered under the skin
    2. held under the tongue until dissolved
    3. taken by mouth with a small amount of water
    4. crushed and dissolved in water and given by teaspoon
83. If nitroglycerine is left at the patient's bedside the nurse should:
    1. realize that she has no responsibility toward the patient in regard to this medication
    2. discourage her patient from taking the drug any more than absolutely necessary because he may become overly dependent on it
    3. check the patient's blood pressure every 4 hours
    4. make a routine check on the number of tablets left in the bottle and record the amount taken by the patient each time
84. Side-effects that occur in some patients taking vasodilators include:
    1. nausea, vomiting, and diarrhea
    2. hypotension, flushing, and tachycardia
    3. decrease in pulse and respiration
    4. sudden elevation in blood pressure, increased pulse rate
85. An inflammation of the sac surrounding the heart is called:
    1. endocarditis
    2. carditis
    3. myocarditis
    4. pericarditis
86. Rheumatic heart disease follows the acute phase of rheumatic fever. When there is involvement of the inner lining of the heart, the patient is said to have:
    1. endocarditis
    2. pericarditis
    3. myocarditis
    4. pancarditis
87. Rheumatic heart disease often affects the valves of the heart. The formation of scar tissue on the heart valves prevents their normal functioning. Surgical correction of the defective valve is called a:
    1. valvectomy
    2. commissurotomy
    3. cardiectomy
    4. myomectomy

Mrs. Carter, age 58, has varicose veins of both lower extremities. She also has an ulceration on the anterior surface of the right leg.

88. Varicose veins are veins which have become:
    1. enlarged and engorged with blood
    2. hardened, and their openings are narrowed
    3. infected by the invasion of bacteria
    4. atrophied because of constriction of the surface blood vessels
89. A condition that makes a person more susceptible to the development of varicose veins is:
    1. deposits of material along the walls of the veins
    2. repeated bacterial infections in the veins
    3. improper functioning of the valves that control the flow of blood through the veins
    4. congenital malformations of the lower extremities in which there is improper circulation

90. Predisposing factors in the development of varicose veins include:
    a. obesity
    b. prolonged sitting or standing in one position
    c. wearing of circular garters or other constricting clothing that impairs circulation to the legs
    d. wearing shoes with high heels

    1. all of these
    2. a and b
    3. c and d
    4. all but d

91. Mrs. Carter is unduly despondent and cries frequently during her hospitalization. The practical nurse should realize that Mrs. Carter's mental attitude is most likely due to:
    1. her confinement to bed
    2. the typical slow healing in the type of ulcer she has
    3. inadequate medical care which has resulted in failure of the ulcer to heal
    4. her financial difficulties

92. Mrs. Carter has an ulcer on her lower leg. Continuous warm moist compresses have been ordered. When administering these compresses it is important to:
    1. explain the procedure to the patient carefully so that she can learn to prepare the compresses for herself
    2. warm at least 1 quart (1 liter) of solution each time because these are continuous compresses
    3. get the patient up in a wheel chair so that the compresses can be applied more easily
    4. check the moisture of these compresses frequently so that they are never allowed to dry

93. After Mrs. Carter's ulcer had healed, the physician recommended elastic stockings. The purpose of these stockings is to:
    1. decrease circulation in the lower limbs
    2. protect the legs from injury
    3. provide warmth for the lower legs
    4. support the surface blood vessels in the leg

94. When instructing Mrs. Carter in the proper use of these stockings, the nurse should tell her that the stocking should be:
    1. worn 24 hours a day
    2. applied early in the morning before arising from bed
    3. held up with circular garters
    4. worn only when she anticipates standing on her feet for long periods of time

95. Some patients with varicose veins cannot be treated successfully by medical means, and surgical correction is necessary. A tying off of the affected vein is referred to as:
    1. phlebotomy
    2. venectomy
    3. vein ligation
    4. phlebectomy

96. Surgical removal of a varicose vein is termed a:
    1. vagotomy
    2. varicosity
    3. vein ligation
    4. vein stripping

Mr. Moore is an outpatient who receives regular treatment for arteriosclerosis of his lower extremities. On one of his visits to the clinic Mr. Moore seems anxious to discuss his condition with you. His first question is, "Why has the doctor told me to stop smoking? How can that affect my condition? It's my legs that bother me, not my lungs."

97. What would the best reply to Mr. Moore's questions be?
    1. The doctor is afraid that your condition may eventually spread and involve your lungs.
    2. Nicotine, which is present in cigarettes, is a drug and it narrows the blood vessels in the body and makes your condition worse.
    3. Smoking dulls the appetite and you are not eating properly. This prevents the healing of your legs.

4. There is really no connection between your smoking and your present illness, but you would feel better if you stopped smoking.

98. While you are talking to Mr. Moore you might take this opportunity to teach him some important facts regarding proper care of his feet and legs. These include:

   a. avoid extreme cold and be sure to wear warm clothing during cold weather
   b. be very careful about applying heat to the feet and legs because you might burn yourself without feeling it
   c. do not elevate your lower extremities above the level of the heart
   d. wear tight shoes and garters because this helps keep the blood from collecting in the lower extremities

   1. all of these
   2. all but c
   3. c and d
   4. a and b

99. In spite of all measures taken to avoid it, an ulcer formed on Mr. Moore's right foot and he was admitted to the hospital for treatment. After several weeks, gangrene developed and an amputation was necessary. Amputation is best defined as:
   1. surgical removal of a limb or part of a limb
   2. removal of necrotic tissue from a sore or ulcer
   3. surgical removal of an entire leg or arm
   4. surgical removal of the bone of a limb

100. A serious complication that must always be considered in the immediate post-operative period following amputation is:
   1. evisceration
   2. hemorrhage
   3. abdominal distention
   4. urinary suppression

101. If Mr. Moore complains of pain in the right foot even after it has been removed, the nurse should:
   1. try to distract his attention from his illness because he could not possibly be feeling pain in that foot
   2. ignore him, realizing that he probably has heard others speak of "ghost" pains after amputation
   3. realize that he may very well be experiencing these pains even though the foot has been removed
   4. tell him to report this to his surgeon because these pains often indicate that the surgery was not successful

Mrs. Johnson has been confined to bed for several weeks and refuses to change position or perform the exercises ordered by the doctor to maintain adequate circulation to the legs. One day she tells the doctor her leg hurts and he diagnoses her condition as thrombophlebitis.

102. Thrombophlebitis is:
   1. an inflammation of the vein caused by a blood clot in the blood vessel
   2. a traumatic inflammation of a blood vessel
   3. a ballooning of the wall of an artery
   4. an ulceration within the blood vessels

103. The most common symptom of thrombophlebitis is:
   1. cyanosis of the affected extremity
   2. pain in the calf of the leg
   3. severe swelling of the ankles
   4. bulging of the affected blood vessels

104. A nursing measure that is contraindicated in thrombophlebitis is:
   1. turning the patient from side to side
   2. elevating the head of the bed
   3. massaging the legs
   4. rubbing the back

105. Thrombophlebitis is a complication of a variety of illnesses and can best be avoided by:
   1. early ambulation and exercises to increase circulation
   2. administration of antibiotics

3. giving the patient daily doses of vitamin K
4. restricting physical activity of any kind after surgery

106. If you were called to a neighbor's house in an emergency and found that the father of the house, age 68, had apparently had a stroke, which of the following measures should you take until the ambulance arrives?

   a. turn the victim's head to the side to keep the airway open and free of mucus
   b. loosen tight clothing about the neck and waist
   c. help the victim to a sitting position to facilitate breathing
   d. massage the wrists to increase circulation
   e. try to arouse the victim and give him sips of brandy or whiskey

   1. all of these
   2. all but c
   3. a and b only
   4. c, d, and e

107. The medical term for stroke is:
   1. heart attack
   2. coronary occlusion
   3. subarachnoid hemorrhage
   4. cerebrovascular accident

108. The most common effects of a stroke are:
   1. mental deterioration
   2. paralysis of the lower extremities and deafness
   3. disturbances in speech and paralysis of one side of the body
   4. permanent paralysis of the upper extremities and blindness

109. Careful attention must be paid to positioning of the patient hospitalized after a stroke. The main objective in the nursing care of a stroke patient is to:
   1. prevent infection
   2. prevent complications that will make rehabilitation impossible
   3. provide adequate nutrition through tube feeding
   4. provide relief from pain and discomfort

110. To prevent foot drop in the stroke patient who has paralysis of a lower limb, it is most important to:
   1. provide adequate warmth
   2. use a foot board to keep the feet in a normal position
   3. massage the feet at least twice daily
   4. keep the feet clean and the toenails properly trimmed

111. When a stroke patient is turned on his side, it is important to:
   1. slightly elevate the head of the bed
   2. support the weak arm and leg with pillows
   3. use a trochanter roll to keep the back straight
   4. remove the pillow from under the patient's head

112. While a stroke patient is lying on his back, the lower arm and hand of the affected side should be placed:
   1. across his chest
   2. parallel with the body with the elbow extended
   3. either under his head pillow or supported on a pillow beside his chest and trunk
   4. under his hip to prevent contractures of the wrist and elbow

113. Use of a trochanter roll against the side of a lower limb, paralyzed by a stroke, will prevent:
   1. decubitus ulcers
   2. outward rotation of the hip
   3. inward rotation of the ankles
   4. foot drop

114. If a stroke victim expresses a desire to feed himself, the nurse should:
   1. discourage him because he will probably spill his food
   2. serve his tray just as she would to any other patient
   3. assist him with foods and liquids difficult to handle but encourage him to help himself as much as possible

   4. tell him it would be best to wait until he is completely well and able to feed himself
115. One of the best ways to encourage a convalescing stroke patient to exercise shoulder and arm muscles and at the same time make him less dependent on the nurse is by:
   1. sending him to physical therapy to exercise on special equipment
   2. instructing him to do several push-ups each day
   3. asking him to bathe himself and help make his bed each morning
   4. allowing him to comb his hair, wash his face, and brush his teeth even though he may be very slow while doing this at first
116. Which of the following is true in regard to the prognosis for stroke?
   1. All stroke victims are permanently paralyzed.
   2. Most stroke victims are partially paralyzed from the waist down.
   3. Stroke patients can usually regain most of the use of their affected limbs if they receive proper care.
   4. Most stroke victims become physically and mentally handicapped by their illness.

UNIT 9   DISEASES OF THE RESPIRATORY SYSTEM

I. Diagnostic Tests and Examinations
  A. Chest x-ray—film of the chest. No special preparation necessary.
  B. Bronchogram—x-ray film of the bronchial tree after a radiopaque dye has been introduced.
  C. Bronchoscopy—visualization of the inside of the trachea and bronchi, using a special instrument called the bronchoscope.
  D. Special nursing care
    1. Postural drainage may be ordered after a bronchogram for the purpose of facilitating the removal of the radiopaque oil from the bronchial tree.
    2. When patient's throat is anesthetized for bronchogram or bronchoscopy, food and fluids must be withheld until the gag reflex is present (usually at least 2 hours).

II. Common symptoms of respiratory diseases— cough, increased nasal and bronchial secretions, some elevation of temperature, varying degrees of respiratory difficulty

III. General Nursing Care
  A. Coughing—may or may not be beneficial, depending on type of cough and condition of patient.
    1. Types of cough
      a. Nonproductive—dry and harsh, no production of sputum; exhausting for patient and of no benefit in removing secretions in bronchial tree.
      b. Productive—deep and moist, produces varying amounts of sputum; may be beneficial.
    2. Cough mixtures
      a. Expectorant cough mixtures increase flow of secretions, making them easier to cough up. Example—SSKI
      b. Sedative cough mixtures depress the cough reflex and lessen the desire to cough. Example—those containing codeine.
      c. Cough mixtures are administered in small amounts and are NOT followed by water.
      d. May be left at bedside. Instruct patient to take small sips, and not to follow immediately with water.
  B. Increased secretions
    1. Care must be used in handling these because they are highly contagious.
    2. Patient is instructed to cough into a disposable tissue and discard the soiled tissue in a paper bag pinned to the bedside. Tissue is held so that it covers both nose and mouth during episodes of coughing or sneezing.
    3. Antispasmodics (bronchodilators) decrease the smooth-muscle tissue contractions of the bronchioles, thereby causing them to dilate and provide relief from respiratory distress. Examples include aminophylline, isoproterenol hydrochloride (Isuprel), and Adrenalin.
    4. Liquefying agents—administered by inhalation. Act to make bronchial secretions more liquid and easier to cough up and expectorate. Examples include sodium ethasulfate (Tergemist) and tyloxapol (Alevaire).
    5. Copious amounts of sputum should be expectorated into a waxed sputum cup.
    6. If sputum is foul-smelling, patient will need frequent mouth care, especially before meals.
  C. Respiratory distress
    1. Fowler's or semi-Fowler's position facilitates breathing.
    2. Air patient breathes is kept moist to prevent further irritation of the mucous membranes.
      a. Warm moist heat provided by vaporizer or steam kettle.
      b. Croupette provides a fine mist of cool, moist air.
  D. Rest
    1. Rest provided to avoid exertion which will place an added burden on the respiratory system.

2. Even minor infections require some rest in bed to prevent complications.

E. Diet
1. During acute stage the diet consists of high-calorie, high-vitamin liquids. Milk and milk products are especially important to provide the protein needed to build and repair tissue.
2. As patient progresses, his diet may be changed to a soft and then to a regular one.

F. Drugs
1. Antipyretics—to lower body temperature. Examples are aspirin and pyralgin.
2. Antihistamines—help dry up secretions of the nasal and bronchial mucosa. May produce undesirable side effects; e.g., extreme drowsiness. Examples are Benadryl and Chlor-Trimeton.
3. Antispasmodics—decrease the muscular contractions of the bronchioles and thereby relieve respiratory distress. Examples, aminophylline and Adrenalin.
4. Antibiotics—useful primarily in bacterial infections.

G. Intermittent positive-pressure breathing therapy.
1. Provides for increased inspiration of air into the lungs.
2. Helps overcome bronchial resistance to inward flow of air, aids in exchange of carbon dioxide and oxygen, makes coughing easier and more effective.
3. Machine may be used to deliver liquefying agents, bronchodilators, and antibiotics to respiratory tree.

H. Aerosol therapy
1. Used to apply medications directly onto the mucous membranes of the bronchial tree. Solutions may contain antibiotics, or bronchodilators such as Adrenalin.

I. Oxygen therapy
1. Administered for relief of oxygen lack in the blood and tissues.
2. Must be considered as a drug; to be given in specific doses of concentration and rate of flow.
3. If given in high concentrations over extended period of time, oxygen can have a toxic effect, producing depressed respirations and coma.
4. Modes of administration include mask, nasal prongs, nasal catheter and, less frequently, by tent (see Fig. 36).
   a. Mask. Mask should fit snugly so that there is no leakage of oxygen around the edges. Periodically the mask is removed and the face cleaned and powdered to avoid irritation.
   b. Nasal prongs. Most comfortable for patient. May cause drying of mucosa.

c. Nasal catheter. Should be changed at least every 8 hours and alternate nostrils used for insertion of catheter.
d. Tent. Must be free from holes and tears. Lower edge of tent is tucked under a sheet to prevent the escape of oxygen, which is heavier than air. Patient may need reassurance while adjusting to confinement of the tent.
5. Precautions
   a. Oxygen supports combustion, therefore fire is always a hazard. NO SMOKING signs are posted in the vicinity of the patient receiving oxygen therapy.
   b. All electrical equipment must be considered a potential source of sparks.

J. Irrigations
1. Helpful in eliminating thick tenacious mucus from the throat and nasal passages.
2. Force is never used in nasal irrigations because the solution may wash bacteria up into the sinuses and thereby spread the infection.

IV. **Diseases of the Respiratory System**
A. The common cold
1. Definition—an inflammation of the upper respiratory tract.
2. Cause—a viral infection.
3. Symptoms
   a. Starts with a mild sore throat or dry scratchy feeling in the nose and back of throat.
   b. Nasal congestion and watering eyes.
   c. Sneezing and nonproductive cough.
   d. Low-grade fever, if any.
4. Treatment and nursing care
   a. Primarily aimed at relief of symptoms.
   b. Patient should stay indoors and preferably in bed.
   c. Force fluids; citrus fruits good as source of vitamin C.
   d. Aspirin may help relieve aches and pains of a cold.
   e. Gargles and nose drops for relief of congestion and to help remove mucus.

B. Acute bronchitis
1. Definition—an acute inflammation of the bronchi.
2. Cause—may be viral or bacterial infection.
3. Symptoms
   a. Similar to those of the common cold.
   b. Cough is more persistent and soon becomes productive.
   c. Temperature elevated and may be so high as to cause febrile convulsions in children.
4. Treatment and nursing care

METHOD	MAX PER CENT OXYGEN	FLOW (L/min)	COMMENTS
A. *Nasal catheter*	30–40%	6–8	Comfortable. Higher flows provide up to 40% oxygen, but can cause respiratory depression and drying of mucosa.
B. *Nasal prongs*	30–40%	6–8	Comfortable. Higher flows provide up to 40% oxygen, but can cause respiratory depression and drying of mucosa.
C. *T-piece*	40–60%	4–12	Provides enriched oxygen mixtures and humidification. Used most often in weaning patients from ventilator assistance before endotracheal tube is removed.
D. *Face tent*	30–55%	4–8	Well tolerated. Good for supplying extra humidity.
E. *Venturi masks*	25–35%	4–8	Mask well tolerated. Accurate concentrations delivered.
F. *Mask without bag*	35–45% 45–55% 55–65%	6–8 10 10–12	Poorly tolerated. Significant CO_2 rebreathing possible at low flows. Highest percentage requires tight mask fit.
G. *Mask with bag*	40–55% 50–60% 90 + %	6 8 8–12	Poorly tolerated. Significant CO_2 rebreathing possible at low flows. Highest percentage requires tight mask fit and a large bag.
H. *Pressure-regulated ventilator*	40–100%	Direct from supply	Oxygen per cent unpredictable
I. *Volume-regulated ventilator*	20–100%	Direct from fupply	Bennett MA1, Ohio 560 can be set to any desired per cent.

FIGURE 36.   Methods of oxygen administration. (Sanderson, R. G.: *The Cardiac Patient,* Philadelphia, W. B. Saunders Co., 1972, pp. 310–312.)

a. Warm or cool moist air for patient to breathe.
b. Antibiotics for bacterial type of infection.
c. Postural drainage may help in removal of secretions in bronchial tree.

C. Pneumonia
1. Definition—an extensive inflammation of the lung tissue.
2. Two general types according to cause
   a. Bacterial—most often caused by the pneumococci.
   b. Primary atypical pneumonia or viral pneumonia—caused by virus or combination of organisms.
3. Symptoms
   a. Bacterial pneumonia has sudden onset with chills and fever.
   b. Viral pneumonia more gradual.
   c. Sharp, stabbing pain in chest or side, especially when coughing or taking a deep breath.
   d. Sputum becomes of characteristic rusty color.
   e. Fever blisters (herpes simplex) often occur with pneumonia.
4. Treatment and nursing care

a. Conservation of patient's strength—placed on absolute bed rest, treatments and nursing care scheduled so as to disturb the patient no more than necessary.
b. Relief of symptoms—fluids forced to combat dehydration; mouth care; protect patient from chilling and drafts. Abdominal distention relieved with low enemas or rectal tube.
c. Isolation of the patient and care taken with nasal secretions.
d. Observation of vital signs important.
e. Complications to be avoided by care during convalescent period include empyema and congestive heart failure.

D. Chronic obstructive lung disease (C.O.L.D.)
1. Definition—a term used to describe any condition in which the patient has constant respiratory distress due to a chronic pulmonary disease. Also called C.O.P.D. (chronic obstructive pulmonary disease). Chronic bronchitis, bronchial asthma and pulmonary emphysema are nearly always characterized by the symptoms of C.O.L.D.

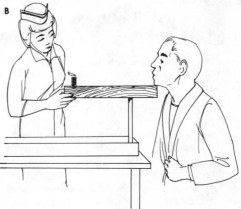

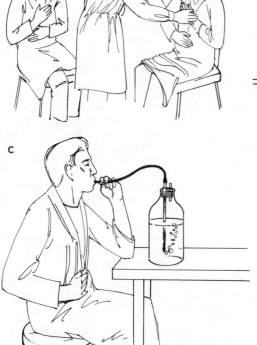

FIGURE 37.   Breathing exercises help to improve the patient's respiratory function. *A,* The physical therapist teaches patients abdominal breathing. Placing one hand on his chest and the other on his abdomen helps the patient to recognize when he is doing the exercise correctly. During abdominal breathing the movement of the abdomen is felt with each breath, whereas the chest remains quiet. *B,* Blowing out a candle at various distances. This exercise can be performed also without the chin rest by holding or placing the candle at various distances. *C,* A blow bottle like this one can be prepared easily for use at home or in the hospital. The long glass tube extends below the water and is connected to rubber tubing, through which the patient blows. By taking deep breaths and exhaling, the patient causes the water to bubble vigorously.

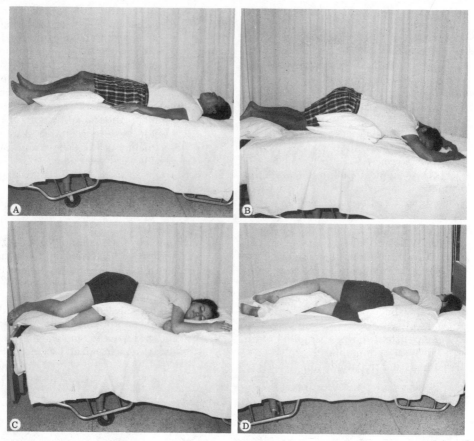

FIGURE 38.   Some postural drainage positions. (Krusen, F. H., et al.: *Handbook of Physical Medicine and Rehabilitation,* 2nd ed., Philadelphia, W. B. Saunders Company, 1971, p. 681.)

2. Symptoms—chronic, moist, wheezing type of cough, exertional dyspnea, barrel-shaped chest, anxious and strained facial expression, puffing out of the cheeks during expiration, and some degree of cyanosis.

3. Treatment—bronchodilator drugs and corticosteroid therapy, sometimes antibiotics are given to avoid serious respiratory infection. Exercises may be prescribed to increase lung capacity (see Fig. 37). IPPB therapy and postural drainage may be done to remove accumulated secretions and increase aeration of the lungs. Preventive measures such as good nutrition, avoidance of respiratory infections, and regulation of physical activity to avoid overexertion are very helpful.

E. Bronchiectasis
   1. Definition—a chronic disease of the respiratory system characterized by permanent dilatation of the bronchi.
   2. Cause—may be the result of a congenital defect in the alveoli or may be a complication of chronic respiratory infections.

3. Symptoms—most outstanding is cough with large amount of foul-smelling sputum. Coughing most noticeable in the morning. Fatigue and loss of weight also symptoms.

4. Treatment and nursing care
   a. There is no cure for bronchiectasis.
   b. Postural drainage used to remove stagnant sputum that has collected in the bronchial tree.
      1. Procedure should be done before meals.
      2. Special mouth care necessary after procedure to remove foul taste from the mouth.
      3. Various positions may be assumed but most important point is that thorax must be lower than rest of the trunk (Fig. 38).
   c. Drugs that relieve symptoms—bronchodilators, expectorants.
   d. Aerosol therapy.

F. Pleurisy
   1. Definition—an inflammation of the pleural membranes surrounding the lungs. With *effusion,* means an increase

in amount of serous fluid within pleural cavity.

2. Symptoms—sharp, stabbing pain in the chest.
3. Treatment and nursing care
   a. Bed rest and observation for signs of respiratory infection.
   b. Support of the chest wall by strapping with adhesive tape or Ace bandage may relieve pain.
   c. Thoracentesis—removal of fluid from pleural cavity when pleurisy with effusion is present.

G. Empyema
1. Definition—infection of the fluid within the pleural cavity.
2. Cause—may be staphylococcus, streptococcus, or pneumococcus.
3. Treatment and nursing care
   a. Antibiotics to remove infection.
   b. Thoracentesis.
   c. Rest and support of the chest wall.

H. Pulmonary emphysema
1. Definition—a chronic disease characterized by overdistention and permanent dilatation of the alveoli.
2. Cause—usually a result of repeated infections or inflammations of the respiratory tract and alveoli.
3. Symptoms—cyanosis and increased respirations. Barrel chest, clubbed fingers due to incomplete oxygenation of the extremities.
4. Treatment and nursing care
   a. Aerosol therapy.
   b. Periods of rest and avoidance of undue exertion.

I. Pulmonary tuberculosis
1. Definition—an infectious disease of the lung characterized by lesions within the lung tissue.
2. Cause—the tubercle bacillus.
3. Symptoms—cough, low-grade fever, loss of weight, night sweats, hemoptysis (spitting of blood).
4. Treatment and nursing care
   a. Rest, good nutrition, proper handling of nasal and bronchial secretions.
   b. Drugs used are usually given in combination; streptomycin, PAS, and INH.
   c. Surgery may be lobectomy or pneumonectomy. Thoracoplasty may be done to collapse and rest the affected lung.

V. Nursing Care of the Patient Undergoing Chest Surgery
A. Preoperative care
   1. Special exercises sometimes done to improve respiratory function.
   2. Diagnostic tests often done.
B. Postoperative care
   1. Close observation for signs of respiratory distress.
   2. Vital signs checked and recorded frequently.
   3. Position of patient depends on wishes of the physician; most often surgeon prefers having patient lie only on his back or on the operative side, to facilitate drainage from the operative area.
   4. Coughing and frequent changing of position necessary for adequate ventilation of good lung.
   5. Closed drainage apparatus often used. Drainage bottle must never be raised above the level of the patient's chest. Tubing must remain airtight and connected to the apparatus at all times so that pressure within the thoracic cavity will not be altered. Tubing must be kept open so that drainage can pass through.

VI. Nursing Care of the Patient with a Tracheotomy
A. Tracheotomy set consists of three parts, two hollow tubes and an obturator.
   1. Inner cannula which may be removed for cleansing.
   2. Outer cannula which should be removed only by the physician.
   3. Obturator which is used to insert the tubes and may later be used to obstruct the cannulae.
B. The nurse must remember that the patient with a new tracheotomy incision is always in danger of asphyxiation.
C. Tracheotomy tube must remain unobstructed because the patient must breathe through it as long as he has difficulty breathing normally.
D. The cotton tape that encircles the neck and ties at the back of the neck is used for the purpose of holding the tube in place, and must never be left untied.
E. When suctioning mucus from the inner cannula, care must be taken that the membranes of the throat are not damaged and that the opening of the tracheotomy is not obstructed with the catheter for long periods of time.
F. A small vaporizer at the bedside helps warm and moisten the air the patient breathes.
G. The inner cannula may be cleaned with hydrogen peroxide and pipe cleaners after it is removed.
H. Patient will be apprehensive until he adjusts to inability to talk. Nurse should give him a call bell and reassure him that someone is near at all times.

Questions

Joan Lester is a 15-year-old high school student who was seen at the hospital emergency clinic on a Sunday afternoon by the family physician. She had a high fever and persistent cough. Earlier in the week Joan's mother had kept her home from school because of a severe cold that Joan had caught from one of her classmates. On the following Friday evening Joan persuaded her mother to let her attend the football game. By Sunday morning Mrs. Lester realized that her daughter had more than a common cold.

1. The early symptoms of a common cold include:
   1. high fever and rash
   2. sneezing, nasal congestion, and mild sore throat
   3. low-grade fever and joint pain
   4. joint pain, headache, and visual disturbances
2. When one is suffering from a cold it is best to:
   1. restrict the diet to liquids only
   2. begin taking antibiotics immediately after symptoms begin
   3. get as much rest as possible, force fluids, and take aspirin to relieve mild discomfort
   4. get plenty of fresh air and exercise and restrict the fluid intake
3. Joan had complained of a "stuffy" nose. The mucous membranes of her nose and throat were inflamed. This area is best described as the:
   1. sinuses
   2. nasopharynx
   3. bronchi
   4. bronchioles
4. The cilia of the mucous membranes of the respiratory tract are:
   1. rugged folds on the surface
   2. tiny, hairlike projections
   3. small pockets or crypts
   4. glands that secrete mucus
5. The cilia:
   1. increase secretions during inflammation
   2. collect excess mucus
   3. prevent localization of an infection
   4. trap and help remove small foreign particles that are inhaled
6. A mild throat gargle is helpful in treating a cold because it:
   1. destroys bacteria in the respiratory tract
   2. removes nasal secretions and mucus from the bronchi
   3. reduces body temperature
   4. soothes the inflamed membranes of the throat
7. Antihistamines are sometimes used in the treatment of the common cold. The primary action of this group of drugs is:
   1. relief of aches and pains accompanying a cold
   2. drying up secretions of mucus
   3. production of sleep
   4. lowering of body temperature
8. A common side-effect of use of antihistamines is:
   1. loss of appetite
   2. diarrhea
   3. extreme drowsiness
   4. low-grade fever
9. An example of an antihistamine drug is:
   1. aspirin
   2. Chlor-Trimeton
   3. penicillin
   4. potassium iodide

10. Joan's physician decided that her cold had developed into acute bronchitis. He admitted her to the hospital for treatment and requested that a vaporizer be placed in her room as soon as she was admitted. His reason for using a vaporizer or steam kettle was to:
    1. provide additional oxygen for the patient
    2. prevent the spread of the disease to others
    3. provide warm moist air for the patient to breathe
    4. assist in the destruction of bacteria in the respiratory tract
11. At first Joan's cough was very dry and harsh. This type of cough is best described as:
    1. nonproductive
    2. productive
    3. persistent
    4. beneficial
12. The type of cough syrup given to Joan is classified as a sedative cough mixture. This medication:
    1. produces a large amount of sputum
    2. is irritating to the mucous membranes of the bronchi
    3. depresses the cough reflex and lessens the desire to cough
    4. makes the patient sleep by depressing the central nervous system
13. An example of a sedative cough mixture is:
    1. elixir of terpin hydrate
    2. elixir of terpin hydrate with codeine
    3. Robitussin
    4. SSKI — saturated solution of potassium iodide
14. Joan's mother asks why you have left the cough mixture at her bedside when the nurse on the evening shift would not leave Joan's "sleeping pill" there to be taken when she needed it. What would the best reply be?
    1. "Most nurses who work the evening shift are cranky and hard to get along with."
    2. "I really don't know why, but when she reports on duty today I will ask her about it."
    3. "It depends on the individual nurse as to whether or not she wants to leave a medication at a patient's bedside."
    4. "Cough mixtures can be left at a patient's bedside, but there must be a written order for the physician if any other medications are to be left there."
15. When administering a cough mixture, the nurse should be sure to:
    1. instruct the patient to drink a glass of milk with each dose
    2. remind the patient that all cough mixtures dry up secretions and keep one from coughing
    3. sign out for each dose on the narcotic record
    4. tell the patient to sip the medication and that it should not be followed immediately with water
16. To avoid contaminating others with the nasal and throat secretions which are highly contagious, Joan should be provided with:
    1. a supply of disposable tissues
    2. a mask to wear throughout the day
    3. a sputum cup
    4. a supply of clean cotton handkerchiefs
17. The proper method for disposing of used tissues is to place them in:
    1. an emesis basin
    2. a wastebasket under Joan's bed
    3. the bedpan in Joan's bedside cabinet
    4. a paper bag that has been cuffed so that it can be closed without touching the inside
18. When instructing Joan in the use of tissues it is most important for the nurse to:
    1. recommend a well-known brand
    2. give several demonstrations so Joan will know exactly what to do
    3. warn Joan that both the nose and the mouth must be covered during episodes of coughing and sneezing
    4. tell Joan that she will need to wear a mask if she refuses to do as she is told

19. Which of the following would be most beneficial to Joan as a bedtime snack?
    1. a carbonated beverage
    2. a chocolate milk shake
    3. tea and toast
    4. coffee and doughnuts

Mr. Cosby has been chronically ill with a respiratory disease for several years. He has lived on a farm all his life and has tried to cure his illness with patent medicines. Finally, his eldest son convinces Mr. Cosby that he should go to a large medical center near his home and be examined by a physician. With great reluctance Mr. Cosby agrees to admission for diagnostic tests.

20. The first test ordered for Mr. Cosby was a chest x-ray. For this examination:
    1. no special preparation is necessary other than dressing the patient in an x-ray gown
    2. the patient must have nothing by mouth for at least 8 hours
    3. the patient is given a cleansing enema the morning of the x-ray
    4. a special dye is injected into the trachea
21. The physician also scheduled an examination in which a special instrument is used to visualize the interior surface of the trachea and bronchi. This test is called:
    1. a bronchogram
    2. bronchoscopy
    3. cystoscopy
    4. laryngectomy
22. Mr. Cosby's throat was anesthetized for the diagnostic test. When he returns to his room it is most important for the nurse to:
    1. realize that Mr. Cosby will not be able to speak for several days
    2. suction his throat frequently for the next 24 hours
    3. give Mr. Cosby frequent throat irrigations to avoid hemorrhage
    4. withhold foods or liquids by mouth until his gag reflex has returned
23. Mr. Cosby was diagnosed as having C.O.L.D. (chronic obstructive lung disease). Postural drainage sometimes is used as a treatment for this condition. The purpose of this treatment is to:
    1. increase the blood supply to the lungs
    2. strengthen the muscles of respiration
    3. remove fluid from the pleural cavity
    4. help remove mucus that has accumulated in the bronchial tree and lungs
24. This procedure will be most effective and least disturbing to the patient if it is done:
    1. before breakfast and supper
    2. during visiting hours so he will be distracted from the treatment
    3. between the hours of 11 P.M. and 7 A.M.
    4. after breakfast and lunch
25. The primary aim of postural drainage is to provide for:
    1. an increase in the blood supply to the lungs
    2. strengthening the muscles of respiration
    3. removal of fluid from the pleural cavity
    4. removal of mucus that has collected in the lower bronchial tree
26. If Mr. Cosby refuses most of his meals once postural drainage has been done, the nurse can help eliminate the anorexia by giving him:
    1. a double dose of vitamins each day
    2. frequent mouth care, especially before each meal
    3. a liquid diet
    4. intravenous fluids containing minerals and vitamins
27. Patients with chronic obstructive lung disease frequently are given bronchodilators. These drugs:
    1. relax the diaphragm and the intercostal muscles, thereby increasing chest expansion
    2. decrease contraction of the smooth muscle tissue of the bronchi
    3. increase muscular contractions of the bronchi and alveoli, thereby aiding in the removal of secretions
    4. decrease the amount of secretions from the bronchial mucosa

28. Tergemist and Alevaire are administered by:
    1. mouth
    2. nasal spray
    3. inhalation
    4. injection
29. The above drugs are examples of:
    1. bronchodilators
    2. antibiotics
    3. antihistamines
    4. liquefying agents
30. The nurse can expect a patient with a chronic lung disorder such as emphysema to have sputum that is:
    1. thick and tenacious
    2. thin and watery
    3. blood-tinged
    4. highly contagious
31. Intermittent positive-pressure breathing is a type of therapy that often is ordered for patients with chronic lung disease. This therapy is used for patients of this type chiefly to:
    1. provide more aeration and expansion of the lungs than is possible without such assistance
    2. control the patient's respirations so that they are faster and more shallow
    3. administer cool moist air to the upper bronchi
    4. administer disinfectant solutions to the infected areas of the lungs
32. During postural drainage or use of the IPPB machine the nurse should provide the patient with:
    1. tissue wipes and an emesis basin or paper bag for disposal of used tissues
    2. adequate drinking water and a straw to facilitate drinking
    3. several towels to protect the bed linen and clothing
    4. extra pillows to elevate his lower extremities
33. Which of the following is *not* an exercise that could be used to improve a patient's respiratory function?
    1. blowing out candles at various distances
    2. using "blow bottles" and blowing bubbles into the water
    3. strengthening of the abdominal muscles
    4. lifting weights to strengthen the shoulder muscles
34. Before Mr. Cosby's discharge he was taught the purposes of postural drainage and the ways in which the treatment can be continued at home. This instruction was necessary primarily because:
    1. there is no cure for bronchiectasis and he will need to continue these treatments as long as he lives
    2. he may develop this condition again and will need to treat himself at home without seeking the advice of a physician
    3. bronchiectasis is highly contagious and other members of his family will probably have the disease and need to take the treatment
    4. all types of respiratory illness are treated with postural drainage and Mr. Cosby will have a tendency to develop a respiratory disease again
35. When Mr. Cosby left the hospital he was very appreciative of the help given him and was especially anxious to thank everyone individually for all they had done for him. Mr. Cosby's original reluctance to enter a hospital was probably based on:
    1. a very bad experience he had had in the past when dealing with doctors and nurses
    2. a fear of the unknown and anxiety about entering a strange environment
    3. his lack of respect for persons in the medical profession
    4. a feeling of superiority toward those who live and work in a big city

The following questions refer to various types of respiratory diseases.

36. The common symptom of asthma is:
    1. spitting of blood
    2. constant low-grade fever
    3. wheezing type of respiration
    4. decrease in the respiratory rate

37. The primary cause of asthma is thought to be:
    1. a bacterial infection
    2. a viral infection
    3. a congenital defect of the lungs
    4. an allergy to certain substances which is aggravated by emotional upsets
38. Epinephrine and aminophylline are used in the treatment of asthma because they:
    1. dilate the bronchi
    2. thin bronchial secretions
    3. are expectorants
    4. are antihistamines
39. An inflammation of the pleural membranes surrounding the lungs is called:
    1. pneumonia
    2. pleurisy
    3. bronchitis
    4. thoratitis
40. Pulmonary emphysema is a chronic disease which primarily affects the:
    1. bronchi
    2. alveoli of the lungs
    3. pleura
    4. trachea
41. The causative organism of tuberculosis is the tubercle:
    1. spirochete
    2. bacillus
    3. staphylococcus
    4. streptococcus
42. Hemoptysis is a medical term used to describe:
    1. spitting of blood
    2. secretion of profuse amounts of sputum
    3. emesis of blood
    4. thick tenacious mucus
43. The primary treatment of a patient with tuberculosis is:
    1. providing a warm environment
    2. a constant supply of cold fresh air
    3. high-carbohydrate, high-fat diet
    4. rest in bed

You are assigned to care for Miss Martha Jackson, who has pneumococcal pneumonia. She has been ill with pneumonia for 3 days.

44. Pneumonia is best defined as an inflammation of the:
    1. alveoli
    2. pleura
    3. tissues of the lung
    4. bronchi and bronchioles
45. When planning nursing care for Miss Jackson, you must remember that one of the most important aims in the treatment of pneumonia is:
    1. cleanliness of the patient and her environment
    2. frequent administration of oxygen to avoid dyspnea
    3. keeping the body temperature within normal range
    4. conservation of the patient's strength and energy
46. Miss Jackson developed "fever blisters" around her lips and nose. The medical term for these lesions is:
    1. herpes simplex
    2. hordoleum
    3. contact dermatitis
    4. decubitus ulcers
47. Care must be taken in handling Miss Jackson's nasal and bronchial secretions *primarily* because:
    1. they are unsightly and may upset the patient
    2. patients with pneumonia usually have bloody sputum
    3. suctioning is contraindicated in patients with pneumonia
    4. the secretions are highly contagious

48. Miss Jackson's fever was very high and the physician ordered a drug to lower her body temperature. Drugs of this kind are classified as:
    1. antibiotics
    2. antipyretics
    3. antiemetics
    4. antihistamines
49. An example of drugs which lower the temperature is:
    1. Benadryl
    2. streptomycin
    3. aspirin
    4. aminophylline

Mr. Kingsley, age 44, has just returned from the recovery room. His postoperative diagnosis is cancer of the lung. Right lobectomy was performed as a treatment.

50. Pneumonectomy is surgical removal of:
    1. a lobe of the lung
    2. an entire lung
    3. a growth located in the lung
    4. one or more of the alveoli of the lung
51. Lobectomy is:
    1. surgical removal of a lobe of the lung
    2. an incision into the pleural cavity for the purpose of drainage
    3. surgical removal of an entire lung
    4. an incision into the lung for the purpose of drainage
52. Mr. Kingsley's surgeon wrote an order for the patient to be allowed to lie on his operative side and back only. His reason for wanting the patient to lie on his operative side was to:
    1. prevent hemorrhage
    2. keep the operative area in view in case hemorrhage should occur
    3. make it easier to change the surgical dressings
    4. facilitate drainage from the operative area
53. During the surgical procedure, a thoracotomy tube was inserted and later it was attached to a closed drainage apparatus. A thoracotomy tube allows for drainage from the:
    1. trachea
    2. thoracic cavity
    3. thoracic artery
    4. remaining portion of the bronchi
54.. When transferring Mr. Kingsley from the recovery room bed to the bed in his room, it is most important that the:
    1. tube be disconnected from the drainage bottle
    2. physician be present in case hemorrhage occurs
    3. drainage bottle be placed on a standard above the patient's bed
    4. drainage bottle be kept below the level of the patient's chest
55. If at any time the closed drainage apparatus is opened or disconnected from the open thoracotomy tube:
    1. air will rush into the thoracic cavity and collapse the lung
    2. air will rush out of the thoracic cavity and allow the lung to expand
    3. water in the drainage bottle will flow into the lung and interfere with the patient's breathing
    4. hemorrhage will result because blood will drain through the tube
56. During the postoperative period of a patient who has had chest surgery, frequent turning, coughing, and deep breathing exercises are:
    1. prohibited because of the danger of hemorrhage
    2. supervised by the surgeon
    3. necessary to provide adequate ventilation of the unaffected lung
    4. encouraged only if they are not uncomfortable for the patient

Mrs. Hancock, age 33, was brought to the hospital emergency room following an automobile accident. In addition to a severe head injury, Mrs. Hancock was having extremely labored breathing. An emergency tracheotomy was performed and Mrs. Hancock was admitted to the intensive care unit.

57. A tracheotomy is best described as an incision into the:
    1. trachea for the purpose of removing a foreign body from the respiratory tract

2. bronchi to facilitate breathing
3. thorax to provide for drainage of mucus
4. trachea for the purpose of inserting a tube through which the patient breathes

58. Mrs. Hancock's tracheotomy tube was held in place by a cotton tape which encircled her neck and was tied at the back. This tape:
   1. is removed within a few hours after the tracheotomy is performed
   2. should not be taken off or left untied for any length of time
   3. is never replaced with a clean one
   4. must be kept sterile

59. Mrs. Hancock was comatose when admitted, but she soon regained consciousness. When she first awakened she appeared very apprehensive. A simple nursing measure that would be most helpful in relieving Mrs. Hancock's anxiety would be:
   1. explaining to her that she will soon learn to suction her own tracheotomy when it becomes obstructed with mucus
   2. to give her a hand bell to summon help when she needs it, and explain that she has temporarily lost her ability to make sounds
   3. leaving the light on in her room so she can tell when someone is there to help her
   4. showing Mrs. Hancock the location of the oxygen tank in case she needs to receive additional oxygen

60. When caring for a patient with a new tracheotomy incision, the nurse must be constantly alert for:
   1. symptoms of hemorrhage from the lungs
   2. loss of consciousness due to lack of oxygen
   3. respiratory difficulty caused by obstruction of the tube
   4. a drop in blood pressure as a symptom of shock

61. If the tracheotomy tube appears to be filling with mucus that is becoming dry and hard, the nurse can remove the:
   1. outer cannula and cleanse it with hot running water
   2. inner cannula and cleanse it with cotton tipped applicators dipped in alcohol
   3. outer cannula and suction the trachea thoroughly
   4. inner cannula and cleanse it with hydrogen peroxide and pipe cleaners

The following questions are concerned with the care of a patient receiving oxygen therapy.

62. When caring for a patient receiving oxygen by mask, the nurse should:
   1. leave the face mask in place at all times
   2. discontinue the oxygen and remove the mask when administering nursing care
   3. remove the mask and replace it with nasal prongs if the patient complains of discomfort
   4. remove the mask at least every 4 hours and wash and powder the patient's face

63. Whenever a patient is receiving oxygen, his environment should be kept free of all sources of sparks and flames because:
   1. oxygen is highly explosive
   2. oxygen supports combustion and a small fire spreads rapidly in its presence
   3. oxygen is lighter than air
   4. most hospitals include this precaution in their safety rules

64. The administration of oxygen should be considered to be the same as the administration of:
   1. a medication
   2. a harmless drug
   3. any other treatment that is the sole responsibility of the respiratory therapist
   4. any other measure that does not require a physician's written order

65. When given in high concentrations over an extended period of time, oxygen can:
   1. relieve severe cyanosis and dyspnea
   2. produce depressed respiration and coma
   3. prevent cardiac arrest
   4. prevent respiratory alkalosis

UNIT 10   THE URINARY SYSTEM

I. Special Diagnostic Tests and Examinations
  A. Urinalysis—one of the most common tests done to detect the presence of urinary disease. Abnormal constituents include blood, pus, bacteria, albumin.
    1. Collection of specimen
      a. Clean-voided specimen requires adequate cleansing of external genitalia before patient voids.
      b. Sterile specimen collected by catheterization.
    2. Specimen should be properly labeled and sent to the laboratory immediately.
  B. Urine culture—urine is examined for microorganisms causing an infection in the urinary tract.
    1. Patient is catheterized for specimen.
    2. Specimen is collected in culture tube and sent to laboratory. Care must be taken not to contaminate the inside of the tube while specimen is being obtained.
  C. X-ray examinations of urinary tract
    1. Intravenous pyelogram—dye is injected into the vein and excreted through the kidneys into the urine. Films are taken as radiopaque dye passes through kidneys, ureters, and bladder.
    2. Retrograde pyelogram—dye is injected directly into the ureters by way of a catheter passed through the bladder. This test is done at the time a cystoscopy is done.
    3. Cystogram—visualization of the bladder after sodium iodide has been instilled.
  D. Cystoscopy
    1. Visualization of the interior of the bladder through the use of a special instrument called a cystoscope.
    2. Useful in diagnosing tumors or local infections, strictures, etc.
    3. The physician can also remove small stones, obtain a biopsy from growths, and relieve strictures by using the cystoscope.
  E. Kidney function tests
    1. Used to determine the kidneys' ability to remove waste products from the blood, dilute the urine, or concentrate the urine.
    2. There are various types of kidney function tests. Nurse must be familiar with

hospital policies and wishes of the physician when preparing the patient and assisting with these tests.
  F. Blood urea nitrogen—determines amount of urea and wastes accumulating in the blood.

II. General Nursing Care of Patient with Urinary Disorder
  A. Measurement of intake and output
    1. Intelligent observation and accurate measurement of the intake and output of fluids are of primary importance in urological nursing.
    2. Measuring loss of body fluids
      a. Total urinary output requires measurement of all urine excreted by the kidneys. May be obtained by patient voiding or from urethral or ureteral catheters.
      b. Total output includes urine, emesis, watery stools, and an estimate of fluids lost through perspiration.
      c. Patients with edema are often weighed daily to estimate loss of body fluids. Weighed at same time each day, on same scales.
    3. Measurement of intake must include all fluids taken by mouth or administered by vein or through Levin tube or gastrostomy tube. Intake may be restricted in some cases.
    4. If catheter is irrigated and solution allowed to drain into drainage bottle, the amount of irrigating fluid must be subtracted from urinary output (Fig. 39).
  B. Care of the patient using a retention catheter—retention catheter has bulb on end to hold it in place; is left in bladder so that urine is constantly drained from bladder (Fig. 40).
    1. Drainage bottle must always be kept below the level of the bladder.
    2. Amount of drainage in bottle is measured at least every 8 hours. Drainage observed for color and content.
    3. Tubing and apparatus used for collecting urine must be sterile when connected to the catheter because the urinary system is considered to be sterile.

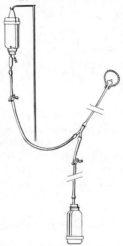

FIGURE 39.   Irrigation apparatus. (Sutton: *Bedside Nursing Techniques.* 2nd ed.)

4. Presence of bright red blood in catheter or tubing should be reported immediately.
5. External genitalia must be cleansed thoroughly with soap and water at least twice a day while the catheter is in place.
6. Irrigation of the bladder done according to physician's specific orders. (See Part V, "Basic Nursing," for further information.)
7. After catheter is removed, patient is checked frequently for retention of urine in the bladder. Bleeding, incontinence, or dribbling of urine should be reported.
C. Other means of establishing urinary flow
  1. Ureteral catheters—tubes of very small gauge. They are inserted directly into the ureters, usually by way of a cystoscope.

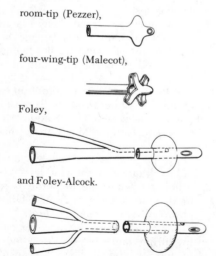

room-tip (Pezzer),

four-wing-tip (Malecot),

Foley,

and Foley-Alcock.

FIGURE 40.   Retention catheters. (Sutton: *Bedside Nursing Techniques.* 2nd ed.)

  2. Ureterostomy tube—inserted into a surgical incision made into the ureter by way of the abdominal wall.
  3. Nephrostomy and pyelostomy tubes—placed directly into the kidney pelvis.
  4. Care of these tubes requires special skills and should not be attempted without direct supervision by a urologist or a registered nurse.

III. **Inflammations of the Urinary Tract**
  A. Nephritis—a general inflammation of the kidneys with degeneration of the kidney cells. There is no bacterial invasion of the kidney and the disease is classified as noninfectious. There are two types of of nephritis—acute and chronic.
    1. Acute glomeruloneophritis—seen primarily in children and young adults. Often follows an episode of streptococcal infection.
      a. Symptoms include widespread edema, puffiness about the eyes, visual disturbances, and hypertension.
      b. Treatment and nursing care
        1. Rest is of primary importance.
        2. Low-sodium diet and restriction of fluid intake recommended when edema is severe.
    2. Chronic glomerulonephritis—may be considered as a stage of acute glomerulonephritis if the disease is not cured in its acute stage.
      a. Treatment is symptomatic.
      b. Prognosis is poor; however some patients live for years while others rapidly develop renal failure and uremia.
  B. Pyelonephritis
    1. Definition—an infection of the kidney. Caused by bacterial invasion of the urinary tract and kidneys.
    2. Symptoms
      a. In acute stages there is nausea, vomiting, fever, chills, and pain in the kidney region.
      b. In the chronic phase there is gradual scarring of the kidney tissues with loss of weight, low-grade fever, and weakness.
      c. In both acute and chronic pyelonephritis the urine contains pus, bacteria, and albumin.
    3. Treatment and nursing care
      a. Infections of the kidney are often associated with an obstruction in the urinary tract. Treatment of the infection begins with removal of the cause if it can be determined.
      b. Medications include antibiotics,

which will destroy the specific micro-organism causing the infection.

c. Rest and forcing of fluids are important as long as the infection is present.

C. Cystitis
1. Definition—an inflammation of the bladder. One of the most common disorders of the urinary tract. Occurs more often in females because of the proximity of the bladder to the genital area.
2. Symptoms
   a. Frequency and urgency of urination.
   b. Dysuria—pain on urination.
   c. Sitz baths and vaginal douches help relieve the pain associated with cystitis.

IV. Obstruction of the Urinary Tract
A. Nephroptosis
1. Definition—a "dropping" of the kidney from its normal position.
2. Symptoms
   a. Does not usually present symptoms until it causes kinking of the ureters, with interference in the flow of urine from the kidney.
   b. In some patients there is pain in the kidney region that is aggravated by standing and relieved by lying down and elevating his hips.
3. Treatment and nursing care
   a. Abdominal supports or braces may be worn to help support the kidney in its normal position.
   b. Nephropexy (surgical fixation of the kidney in its normal position) may be done.
B. Renal calculi (nephrolithiasis)
1. Definition—kidney stones. They may be found anywhere in the urinary tract and vary in size from very small crystals to stones the size of an orange.
2. Symptoms
   a. With large stones there is dull pain in the kidney region and an increased production of urine.
   b. Very small stones may try to pass down the ureters and in so doing they cause renal colic. The symptoms include sudden, severe pain beginning in the flank of the affected side and radiating down the ureter to the genitalia. Nausea, vomiting, and profuse perspiration may also be present.
3. Treatment and nursing care
   a. At first the urologist may choose to wait and see if the stone will pass through the urinary tract. The nurse is then responsible for straining all

urine passed by the patient. Gauze or cheesecloth squares are used for this.
   b. If the stone does not pass through, it must be removed by surgical means.

V. Care of the Patient Undergoing Surgery of the Kidney
A. Types of surgery
1. Nephrectomy—surgical removal of the kidney.
2. Nephrostomy—surgical incision into the kidney for the purpose of providing for drainage from the kidney.
B. Postoperative care
1. Patient must be checked carefully for tubes and catheters that may have been inserted during surgery. These may be attached to various types of drainage or irrigation equipment.
2. Hemorrhage is a common complication following surgery of the kidney.
   a. Dressings may be tinged with bright pink drainage, but the presence of blood should be reported.
   b. Some drains have a sterile safety pin attached to the end. These must never be left open or attached to the bed linen or the patient's clothing.
   c. Adequate drainage from the unaffected kidney is of concern to the surgeon, and the nurse is responsible for accurate measuring and recording of urinary output from the bladder.
   d. Fluids may be restricted during the immediate postoperative period in order to avoid overburdening the kidney.

VI. Renal Failure
A. Definition—a disturbance in the normal functioning of the kidneys. Waste products remain in the blood and the patient is said to have *uremia*.
B. Symptoms
1. Acute uremia—occurs suddenly and may be a result of poisoning caused by mercury, transfusion reaction, prolonged shock, or dehydration.
2. Chronic uremia—occurs gradually as more and more kidney cells are destroyed and cease to function. May follow prolonged inflammation of the renal cells.
3. Both types are characterized by loss of appetite, vomiting, visual disturbances, muscular twitching, convulsions, coma, and eventually death if the situation cannot be reversed.
C. Treatment and nursing care
1. Aimed at decreasing the workload of the kidneys and establishing a normal water and electrolyte balance.
2. In some acute cases an artificial kidney

may be used to remove waste products from the blood.

3. Nursing care may be very difficult, as the increase of waste products in the blood adds to the discomfort of the patient.

a. Mouth care must be done frequently to remove foul taste and odors from the mouth.

b. Deposits of urea salts on the skin cause itching. Mild vinegar solution will help remove these salts and relieve itching.

c. Quiet environment and safety precautions to keep the patient from injuring himself are necessary when uremia is severe. Increased pressure within the cranial cavity may cause delirium and convulsions.

Questions

Mrs. Fisher, a 52-year-old mother of two teenage daughters, has been ill with chronic glomerulonephritis for the past 15 years. She first noticed symptoms of nephritis several weeks after a severe sore throat, which she treated with home remedies. She has had flare-ups of symptoms periodically since that time. Her present admission notes state that Mrs. Fisher has recently experienced a gradual increase in edema, visual disturbances, and episodes of nausea and vomiting. On the day of her admission to the hospital she was preparing breakfast when she began having muscular twitching and complained of a severe headache. Her diagnosis was chronic glomerulonephritis, acute exacerbation.

1. As soon as he admitted Mrs. Fisher to the hospital, her physician ordered a stat blood urea nitrogen. This test is done to determine the:
    1. concentration of urine
    2. amount of urea and nitrogen wastes accumulating in the urine
    3. waste products being left in the blood because of failure of the kidneys to remove them
    4. amount of bacteria being left in the blood because of the failure of the kidneys to remove them

2. A urine culture was also ordered. For this test the nurse must:
    1. catheterize the patient to obtain a specimen
    2. cleanse the genitalia before obtaining a voided specimen
    3. have the patient void directly into the culture tube
    4. restrict fluids for 6 hours before obtaining a specimen

3. While collecting the specimen for a culture, it is most important for the nurse to:
    1. obtain at least 100 ml. of urine for the test
    2. use a sterile bedpan for collecting the specimen
    3. call the laboratory in advance so it can prepare for the test
    4. be careful not to contaminate the inside of the culture tube with microorganisms outside the patient's urinary tract

4. Mrs. Fisher's total intake and output were to be measured carefully. Total intake includes:
    1. water taken by mouth and fluids given by vein
    2. all liquids taken orally, including milk, tea, and coffee, and all liquids given by vein
    3. only the liquids given by vein, since Mrs. Fisher was having episodes of vomiting
    4. fluids taken by mouth only

5. Mrs. Fisher's total output would include:
    1. all fluids lost by vomiting, urination, or profuse perspiration
    2. recording the number of times she voided or had a bowel movement
    3. the amount of urine voided during the day
    4. only the urine obtained by catheter

6. Since Mrs. Fisher had the symptom of muscular twitching, the nurse should:

     a. restrain the patient's upper extremities to keep her from falling out of bed

     b. keep noise and other stimuli at a minimum to reduce the possibility of convulsions in the patient

     c. apply side rails and use other measures such as padding the head of the bed to prevent injury to the patient during involuntary muscular movements

     d. inform the physician that a sedative is needed to keep the patient quiet

     1. all of these
     2. a and b
     3. b and c
     4. c and d

7. A retention catheter was inserted into Mrs. Fisher's bladder by way of the urethra. A retention catheter is one that is:

     1. left in the kidney pelvis
     2. used when a patient has urinary retention
     3. used only when the patient cannot retain urine in the bladder
     4. designed so that it has a bulb on the end to keep it in the bladder for a period of time

8. In the female the urinary meatus is located:

     1. about ¼ inch (6 mm.) below the neck of the bladder
     2. between the vaginal orifice and rectum
     3. about 6 inches (15 cm.) below the neck of the bladder
     4. between the clitoris and vaginal orifice

9. When attaching the drainage tubing and bottle to the end of the catheter, the nurse must:

     1. avoid letting air into the catheter
     2. be sure the drainage apparatus is sterile and is not contaminated while it is being connected to the catheter
     3. irrigate the bladder immediately before the apparatus is connected to the catheter
     4. always keep the drainage bottle 18 inches (46 cm.) above the level of the bladder

10. As long as the retention catheter is in place, the patient will be more comfortable if the:

     1. tubing is pinned to the sheet so there is slight tension on the catheter
     2. genital area is powdered liberally with talcum powder to prevent irritation
     3. genital area around the catheter is gently cleansed with soap and water several times a day
     4. drainage tubing is looped over the abdomen to prevent pulling on the catheter

11. The physician requested that Mrs. Fisher's weight be taken and recorded daily. The reason for this is to determine the:

     1. amount of body fat lost
     2. amount of tissue fluid lost
     3. ability of the kidneys to concentrate urine
     4. amount of fluids taken by vein within a 24-hour period

12. When weighing Mrs. Fisher it is most important to:

     1. weigh her in the late afternoon
     2. force fluids several hours before she is weighed
     3. use a scale which measures weight in grams
     4. weigh her at the same time each day, using the same scale each time

13. Mrs. Fisher's illness did not respond well to treatment and she was soon critically ill with uremia due to renal failure. A nursing measure that will help relieve itching and discomfort from deposits of urea salts on the skin is:

     1. bathing the skin with alcohol
     2. applying lotion to the skin
     3. sponging the skin with a diluted vinegar solution
     4. rubbing the skin with mineral oil

14. As Mrs. Fisher's condition became worse she began to realize that she was gravely ill. One day she asked to have a minister come to see her. In this case the nurse should:
    1. realize that the patient is probably delirious and does not know what she is saying
    2. tell a member of the family that Mrs. Fisher is dying and needs a minister
    3. call the minister as requested by the patient
    4. wait until the next time the hospital chaplain makes rounds and ask him to call a minister
15. At 9:00 A.M. 1 week after her admission Mrs. Fisher died. Her family was with her at the time and were asked to leave the room momentarily while the physician pronounced her dead. Before the family is allowed to reenter the room the nurse should:
    1. place Mrs. Fisher's body in a natural sleeping position and close her eyes
    2. wrap Mrs. Fisher's body in a morgue sheet and tie an identifying tag on her foot
    3. remove all personal articles from the room and ask one of the family members to sign for them
    4. transfer the body from the bed to the stretcher in preparation for moving it to the morgue

Mr. Cole, age 37, was awakened at 2:00 A.M. with a severe pain in his right flank. The pain radiated down the inner aspect of his right leg. When he got up to urinate he noticed a small amount of blood in his urine. The pain continued and he began to vomit. His wife became alarmed and called a physician, who told her to bring Mr. Cole to the hospital emergency room immediately. Mr. Cole was then admitted to the hospital for treatment of kidney stones.

16. The medical term for kidney stones is:
    1. uremia
    2. renal calculi or nephrolithiasis
    3. nephroptosis
    4. hydronephrosis
17. Mr. Cole's urine was to be strained. The chief purpose of straining his urine was to:
    1. remove blood clots for examination
    2. remove bits of tissue that may have been excreted in the urine
    3. check to see if the stone is passed in the urine
    4. obtain a more accurate record of his urinary output
18. The type of material used for straining the urine is usually:
    1. wire mesh
    2. plastic
    3. unbleached muslin
    4. gauze or cheesecloth
19. Mr. Cole was scheduled for an intravenous pyelogram. In this test, x-ray films are taken after a radiopaque dye has been:
    1. instilled into the bladder
    2. injected into the ureters
    3. injected into a vein
    4. injected into the kidney pelvis
20. The stone was found to be lodged in Mr. Cole's right ureter. The ureters are:
    1. two small tubes leading from the kidneys to the bladder
    2. the small basins located just below each kidney
    3. the small tubes leading from the bladder to the outside
    4. two small tubes leading from the renal arteries to the kidneys
21. Mr. Cole was taken to surgery and the surgeon used a cystoscope to remove the stone from the ureter. A cystoscope is a special instrument used to:
    1. examine the kidney
    2. visualize the interior of the bladder and also to remove foreign bodies from the bladder or ureters
    3. enlarge the urethra so the stone can be washed out by the urine
    4. remove small stones from the ureter and large stones from the kidney

The following questions refer to various disorders of the urinary system.

22. Acute glomerulonephritis frequently follows infections elsewhere in the body. These infections are most often caused by:
    1. streptococci
    2. staphylococci
    3. influenza viruses
    4. tubercle bacilli

23. Pyelonephritis is caused by:
    1. accumulation of urine in the kidney
    2. a bacterial infection in the urinary tract
    3. formation of stones in the urinary tract
    4. a noninfectious inflammation of the kidney cells

24. In pyelonephritis the urine contains:
    1. bacteria and pus
    2. large amounts of blood
    3. necrotic tissue from disintegrating kidney cells
    4. large amounts of mucus

25. Cystitis is:
    a. one of the most common disorders of the urinary tract
    b. more common in males than in females
    c. characterized by chills and a high fever
    d. characterized by frequency and urgency of urination

    1. all of these
    2. b and c
    3. a and d
    4. b and d

26. The appearance of blood in the urine is referred to as:
    1. dysuria
    2. oliguria
    3. anuria
    4. hematuria

27. Painful urination is referred to as:
    1. dysuria
    2. oliguria
    3. anuria
    4. hematuria

28. Two nursing measures that are helpful in reducing the discomfort of cystitis are:
    1. low soapsuds enema and frequent catheterizations
    2. sitz bath and vaginal irrigations
    3. administration of antibiotics and analgesic drugs
    4. saline enema and bladder irrigations

29. A serious complication that must always be considered following surgery of the kidney is:
    1. hemorrhage
    2. excessive loss of body fluids
    3. edema
    4. dehydration

30. In the postoperative care of a patient who has had surgery of the kidney, the nurse must be especially careful to:
    1. measure and record urinary output from the unaffected kidney
    2. avoid turning the patient onto his operative side
    3. reinforce the dressings when bright red blood drains from the operative site
    4. firmly anchor all drains and catheters to the patient's clothing so they will not be misplaced

UNIT 11   THE ENDOCRINE SYSTEM

I. Introduction
A. Endocrine glands are ductless and empty their secretions directly into the blood. The substances secreted are called *hormones,* and they are chemical substances which excite activity in the various organs of the body.
B. The endocrine glands are interrelated; i.e., one gland may stimulate the activity of another gland.
C. Most diseases of the endocrine glands are concerned with overactivity or underactivity of the glands. The prefix *hypo* refers to underactivity; *hyper* refers to overactivity of the gland.

II. The Thyroid Gland
A. Special diagnostic tests and examinations
1. Protein-bound iodine—measures the amount of protein-bound iodine present in the blood. Normally there are 4 to 8 mcg. in the plasma. The amount is decreased in hypothyroidism and increased in hyperthyroidism.
2. Radioactive iodine (^{131}I) uptake. The thyroid gland readily absorbs and utilizes iodine in the production of its hormone, *thyroxin.* The overactive gland accumulates more radioactive iodine than the underactive gland. Amount of iodine absorbed is measured with a scintillation counter because the iodine has been made radioactive. Normal thyroid will remove as much as 15 to 50 per cent of the radioiodide. The enlarged and overactive thyroid may remove as much as 90 per cent.
3. Thyroid scanning. Patient swallows radioactive iodine and a scanner is passed back and forth across the throat. The pattern of scan shows concentration of iodine in the thyroid and other tissues.
4. Palpation of the thyroid gland may reveal an enlargement of the gland.
B. Disorders of the thyroid gland
1. Simple goiter—an enlargement of the thyroid gland. There is no increase in the secretion of thyroxin.
   a. Caused by a decrease in the intake of iodine.

b. Symptoms include enlargement of the neck, difficulty in swallowing, and dyspnea.
c. Treatment includes administration of iodine preparations and inclusion of iodine in the diet (iodized salt most common form).
d. Surgical removal of the gland may be necessary if it has enlarged to the point that it interferes with swallowing and breathing.
2. Hyperthyroidism—overactivity of the thyroid gland. Also known as Graves' disease, toxic goiter.
   a. Cause is unknown; related to emotional and physical stress.
   b. Symptoms include extreme nervousness, increase of appetite with loss of weight, emotional disorders, and a speed-up of all body processes.
   c. Treatment may be medical, surgical, or both.
      1. Iodine preparations and other drugs, particularly propylthiouracil, which block the release of thyroxin from the gland are given.
      2. Diet is high-calorie, high-vitamin to help maintain normal body weight.
      3. Surgical removal of the thyroid gland (thyroidectomy) is necessary if medical treatment is not successful.
   d. Postoperative nursing care includes
      1. Placing patient in Fowler's position as soon as he has reacted.
      2. Support of the head with sandbags to relieve tension on the sutures.
      3. Keep patient quiet and discourage talking.
      4. Observe carefully for bleeding, swelling, or tightness of bandage; difficulty in breathing, difficulty in swallowing.
      5. Tracheotomy set should be kept at bedside.
3. Hypothyroidism—underactivity of the thyroid gland. In children it is called *cretinism*; in adults it is *myxedema.*
   a. Symptoms include mental and physi-

cal retardation, in children. Older patients are very lethargic and tend to be slow mentally.

   b. Treated with thyroid extract, with gradual increase in dosage as patient adjusts to the drug.

III. The Parathyroids

A. The hormone *parathormone,* secreted by the parathyroids, helps maintain a constant calcium balance in the blood.

B. A disturbance in the secretion of parathormone may be due to a tumor of the gland or to injury to the gland during thyroidectomy.

C. Hyperparathyroidism — oversecretion of the hormone.

   1. Results in depletion of calcium from the bones. They become tender and painful and may break spontaneously. Other symptoms result from an excess of calcium in the blood and include the formation of kidney stones.

   2. Treatment consists of surgical removal of the tumor on the gland when one is present, or removal of all but one of the parathyroid glands.

D. Hypoparathyroidism — undersecretion of the hormone.

   1. Symptoms are the result of a deficiency of calcium in the blood. Outstanding symptom is *tetany* (muscular spasms). Tracheal spasms may produce dyspnea and cyanosis.

   2. Treatment is administration of calcium and of vitamin D, which increases the absorption of calcium.

IV. Disorders of Carbohydrate Metabolism

A. Special diagnostic tests and examinations

   1. Urinalysis — testing the urine for sugar. When the level of sugar in the blood is high some will spill over into the urine.

   2. Blood sugar — normal range of blood sugar is 80 to 120 mg. per 100 ml. of blood; an increase indicates improper utilization of sugar in the blood.

   3. Glucose tolerance — determines the individual's ability to utilize glucose in the blood.

B. Diabetes mellitus

   1. Definition — a disease resulting from an inability of the body to use and store carbohydrates in a normal manner. Primarily, this is due to an insufficient amount of insulin in the body.

   2. Cause is not definitely known. Heredity does play a part in development of the disease.

   3. Symptoms

     a. Elevation of blood sugar and presence of sugar in the urine.

     b. Polyuria (increased urination).

     c. Polydipsia (increased thirst).

     d. Polyphagia (increased appetite) with weight loss in some cases, weight gain in others.

     e. Fatigue and muscular weakness.

   4. Treatment and nursing care — aimed at control of the diabetes and prevention of complications. There is no cure for diabetes.

     a. Diet is calculated on an individual basis depending on amount of exercise taken, ability to utilize carbohydrates, and metabolic needs for building body tissues and producing energy. Usually is low in carbohydrate, high in protein content, and contains a moderate amount of fat.

       1. Patient is given a special diet with lists of foods to substitute for those restricted on his diet.

       2. Mild diabetics can control their disease with diet.

     b. Administration of insulin

       1. Insulin is given by injection to replace the deficiency in production. Its action is to lower the blood sugar by increasing the body's ability to utilize carbohydrates.

       2. Types of insulin are listed in Table 14.

       3. Insulin is measured in units. U40 insulin contains 40 units of insulin per ml. (cc.). U100 contains 100 units per ml.

       4. Patient is taught to administer his own insulin. Sites are rotated to increase absorption of insulin and

Table 14. Types of Insulin

TYPES OF INSULIN	APPEARANCE	ACTION BEGINS	PEAK OF ACTION	ACTION LASTS
Regular	Clear	30 minutes to 1 hour	2 to 3 hours	6 to 8 hours
Globin zinc	Amber	2 hours	8 hours	24 hours
Protamine zinc	Cloudy	4 to 6 hours	12 to 24 hours	48 hours
NPH	Cloudy	4 hours	8 to 12 hours	28 to 30 hours
Lente	Cloudy	1 to 2 hours	8 to 12 hours	28 to 30 hours

Table 15. Symptoms of Diabetic Coma and Insulin Reaction

DIABETIC COMA	INSULIN REACTION
Gradual onset, may be more rapid in active children.	Sudden onset, begins abruptly
Skin hot and dry, face may be flushed	Perspiration, skin pale, cold, and clammy
Deep, labored breathing	Shallow breathing
Nausea	Hunger
Drowsiness and lethargy	Mental confusion, strange behavior, nervousness
Fruity odor to breath	Double vision
Loss of consciousness	Loss of consciousness, convulsions (rarely)
Urine contains much sugar	There may be sugar in the urine, depending on the type of insulin and when it was taken
Blood sugar high	Blood sugar low

reduce irritation of the tissues. Sites include upper arms, thighs, and abdomen.
  c. Complications of insulin administration
    1. Diabetic coma and insulin reaction (Table 15).
    2. Diabetics are susceptible to disturbances arising from poor circulation of blood. They have a tendency to develop arteriosclerosis. Proper care of the feet very important (Fig. 41).

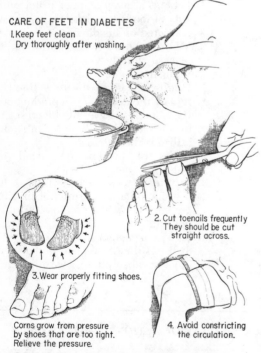

CARE OF FEET IN DIABETES
1. Keep feet clean
   Dry thoroughly after washing.

2. Cut toenails frequently
   They should be cut straight across.

3. Wear properly fitting shoes.

Corns grow from pressure by shoes that are too tight. Relieve the pressure.

4. Avoid constricting the circulation.

5. Avoid burning or freezing, bruising or cutting the feet.
6. Report any sore anywhere, but especially one on the foot that fails to heal.

FIGURE 41. The care of the feet in diabetes. (Dowling, H. F., and Jones, T.: *That the Patient May Know*, Philadelphia, W. B. Saunders Company, 1959.)

3. Diabetic also has poor resistance to infections. Meticulous skin care and prompt attention to breaks in the skin are imperative.
4. Changes in vision may result from retinitis, which is common in diabetics. Regular visits to opthalmologist necessary to prevent blindness and other visual defects.
  d. Oral agents—Orinase and Diabinase are *not* oral forms of insulin. They are now considered to have certain toxic effects, and their use is contraindicated except in a few special situations.

V. Diseases of the Adrenal Glands
  A. Addison's disease
    1. Definition—a disease resulting from underactivity of the adrenal cortex. May be caused by tumor, inflammation, or infection of the gland.
    2. Symptoms
      a. Early symptoms include fatigue, irritability, and loss of weight.
      b. Nausea and vomiting appear later, and patient may have severe dehydration and circulatory failure.
    3. Treatment and nursing care
      a. Replacement of the adrenal hormones lacking in the body. Cortisone and other steroids must be taken for the rest of the individual's life.
      b. Moderation in all activities and habits of good personal hygiene are essential.

VI. Cushing's Syndrome
  A. Definition—a disease resulting from an increased production of hormones from the adrenal cortex.
  B. Symptoms
    1. Typical "moon" face, muscular weakness.

2. Abnormal sexual development and some mental disturbances.
C. Treatment and nursing care
  1. Attempts are made to find the underlying cause.
  2. Patient will have disturbances in his water and electrolyte balance. Intake and output must be carefully measured and recorded.
  3. Low-sodium, high-potassium diet may be ordered.
  4. Severe mental depression is often present and patient must be prevented from injuring himself or taking his own life.

Questions

1. Mrs. Nelson is scheduled for a radioactive iodine uptake. Iodine is used in this test because the thyroid gland:
   1. rejects iodine that has been made radioactive
   2. absorbs and concentrates iodine in its tissues
   3. excretes the radioactive iodine through the sweat glands
   4. chemically removes the radioactivity from the iodine
2. If Mrs. Nelson's thyroid gland is hyperactive, you would expect the gland to:
   1. remove about 10 per cent of the radioactive iodine from the bloodstream
   2. remove about 80 to 90 per cent of the radioactive iodine from the bloodstream
   3. excrete most of the iodine within 24 hours
   4. absorb none of the radioactive iodine
3. Mrs. Nelson asks you about the thyroid scanning for which she is also scheduled. You should tell her that after she ingests the radioactive iodine:
   1. she will be isolated from others for about 2 days
   2. several blood samples will be drawn to determine the amount of iodine in her bloodstream
   3. a scanner will be passed back and forth across her throat and no discomfort will be involved
   4. the scanner will deliver radioactive beams to her thyroid in order to reduce its size
4. Mrs. Nelson was diagnosed as having an overactive thyroid gland. The medical term for this condition is:
   1. diabetes mellitus
   2. hyperthyroidism
   3. hypothyroidism
   4. simple goiter
5. The mineral that is most important for proper development and functioning of the thyroid gland is:
   1. iron
   2. sodium
   3. chlorine
   4. iodine
6. Mrs. Nelson was scheduled for surgical removal of the thyroid gland. This surgical procedure is called a:
   1. thyroidectomy
   2. thyroidostomy
   3. thyroid extract
   4. thyroidotomy
7. Upon her return from surgery, Mrs. Nelson should be watched closely, and the nurse must be especially alert for:
   1. local swelling and respiratory difficulty
   2. urinary retention
   3. abdominal distention
   4. severe headache which may indicate nerve damage

8. After she has reacted from the anesthesia, Mrs. Nelson would probably be most comfortable:
   1. in the Trendelenburg position
   2. in Fowler's position
   3. lying face down
   4. lying on her left side

9. To avoid strain on the suture line during the immediate postoperative period, the nurse should:
   1. support Mrs. Nelson's head with sandbags and advise her to talk as little as possible
   2. ask Mrs. Nelson to refrain from moving about in bed and restrain her if necessary
   3. place a pillow under Mrs. Nelson's head so that her chin is resting on her chest
   4. apply several layers of wide adhesive tape over the surgical dressing

10. Since respiratory difficulty may occur immediately after surgery, it is most advisable to:
    1. have a respiratory stimulant at the bedside
    2. place the patient in an oxygen tent for the first 72 hours
    3. keep a tracheotomy set at the bedside until all danger has passed
    4. apply continuous hot compresses to the surgical incision for the first 24 hours

Mrs. Snow is a 46-year-old mother of three children. She has recently complained of extreme fatigue, loss of weight, increased urination, and excessive thirst. A physical examination by her physician and a routine urinalysis in his office indicated that Mrs. Snow was a diabetic.

11. Mrs. Snow was sent to the hospital laboratory the following morning for a fasting blood sugar test. Her level of blood sugar was 210 mg. per 100 ml. of blood. This indicates that Mrs. Snow:
    1. had not refrained from eating before the test
    2. was suffering from a deficiency of glucose in the blood
    3. was not properly utilizing the glucose in her blood
    4. had an abnormal amount of insulin in her blood

12. After the diagnosis of diabetes was confirmed, Mrs. Snow was admitted to the hospital for administration of insulin and regulation of her diet. In regard to the treatment of diabetes, the practical nurse should know that this disease:
    1. can be cured by insulin
    2. can be controlled by diet and the administration of insulin
    3. is a hopeless disease that is eventually fatal in all cases
    4. has no specific treatment other than regular injections of insulin

13. Diabetes mellitus is a disease in which the body is unable to use and store:
    1. proteins
    2. fats
    3. carbohydrates
    4. minerals

14. Insulin is secreted by the:
    1. pituitary gland
    2. thyroid gland
    3. islets of Langerhans, which are situated on the pancreas
    4. adrenal glands

15. The action of insulin in the body is to:
    1. increase the metabolic rate and all other body processes
    2. lower the blood sugar by increasing the utilization of carbohydrates
    3. improve the body's resistance to infection by destroying bacteria
    4. decrease the blood sugar by chemically changing sugar to amino acids

16. In general, the diet of a diabetic should be:
    1. high in proteins, fats, and carbohydrates
    2. low in carbohydrates and high in fats and proteins
    3. high in fats and low in proteins and carbohydrates
    4. low in carbohydrates, high in proteins, and moderate in fat content

17. Mrs. Snow was taught to administer her own insulin. She was advised to rotate the site of injections primarily because:
1. there is danger of damage to the nerves near the surface of the skin after repeated injections
2. this plan reduces the danger of irritation to the tissues and increases absorption of insulin
3. it is less difficult to give your own injections if the sites are rotated
4. infection is less likely to occur if a different site is chosen for each injection

18. The type of insulin that provides the most rapid action is:
1. regular
2. lente
3. protamine zinc
4. globin zinc

19. Some types of insulin are cloudy and should be thoroughly mixed before the insulin is withdrawn from the vial. The best method for doing this is by:
1. vigorously shaking the vial
2. gently rolling the vial between the palms of the hands
3. heating the insulin to boiling point
4. withdrawing the insulin from the vial and then vigorously shaking the syringe

20. Mrs. Snow was informed of the symptoms of a mild insulin reaction. When she feels this reaction coming on it would be best for her to:
1. give herself an injection of 50 per cent glucose
2. drink a glass of sweetened orange juice or eat a few pieces of hard candy
3. give herself a small dose of insulin
4. change the type of insulin she is taking and notify her doctor that she is doing so

21. A patient in diabetic coma will have:
1. symptoms of shock and a high blood sugar
2. drowsiness, high blood sugar, hot dry skin
3. hunger, low blood sugar, and loss of consciousness
4. mental confusion, convulsions, and normal blood sugar

22. The term U100 in reference to strengths of insulin means that there are 100 units:
1. per 10-ml. vial
2. in each dose to be given the patient
3. per ml. or cc.
4. in each ounce

23. 3 cc. of U40 insulin would contain:
1. 40 units of insulin
2. 30 units of insulin
3. 20 units of regular insulin and 40 units of another type
4. 120 units of insulin

24. Mrs. Snow's urine was tested for sugar three times a day. The usual time for testing her urine would be:
1. 30 minutes before each meal
2. 30 minutes after each meal
3. between meals and at bedtime
4. 30 minutes after insulin is given

25. Mrs. Snow's physician ordered regular insulin on a sliding scale of 3 units for each plus of sugar in the urine. How much regular insulin whould be given if Mrs. Snow's sugar was 3 plus?
1. 12 units
2. 3 units
3. 9 units
4. 30 units

26. Mrs. Snow asked why she could not take insulin by mouth rather than by injection. What would the best answer to this question be?
    1. Insulin cannot be tolerated by mouth because it is very irritating to the mucous membranes of the mouth and stomach.
    2. There is not yet any form of oral insulin available. To be effective it must be taken by injection.
    3. Oral insulin is for diabetics who will not or cannot follow their diet as they should.
    4. Your physician does not believe in giving oral insulin to his patients.
27. Mrs. Snow was taught the proper care of her feet and advised of measures to improve circulation to her extremities primarily because:
    1. diabetics have a tendency to develop arteriosclerosis and circulatory disturbances
    2. she has varicose veins, which all diabetics have
    3. all diabetics eventually develop gangrene of one or both lower extremities
    4. she is overweight and has an abnormal amount of pressure on her feet and legs
28. Before she was dismissed from the hospital, Mrs. Snow was told that she might, at some time, develop an insulin reaction or diabetic coma. To avoid confusion and delay in getting medical attention when needed, Mrs. Snow was advised to:
    1. refrain from traveling alone
    2. inform all her associates of her condition
    3. keep her physician informed of her whereabouts at all times
    4. wear some form of identification stating that she is a diabetic
29. Mild cases of diabetes are best treated by:
    1. diet and exercise
    2. oral hypoglycemic drugs
    3. weekly injections of insulin
    4. oral doses of insulin

The following questions refer to various disorders of the endocrine glands.

30. Parathormone is secreted by the parathyroid glands. This hormone is important in maintaining a:
    1. constant level of insulin in the body
    2. normal acid-base balance in the body
    3. normal electrolyte balance in the body
    4. constant level of calcium in the blood
31. Any condition which produces a deficiency of parathormone in the body will result in:
    1. weakness of the bones
    2. an increase in the blood sugar level
    3. muscular twitching and spasms of the voluntary muscles
    4. deposits of calcium in the kidney
32. A decrease in the production of thyroxin in the early stages of life will result in:
    1. an increased metabolic rate and loss of weight
    2. retardation of mental and physical growth and development
    3. development of a goiter
    4. development of diabetes later in life
33. Addison's disease is the result of:
    1. an increased production of all the steroids
    2. a decrease in the production of hormones from the adrenal cortex
    3. an increase in production of thyroxin
    4. a decrease in production of parathormone

UNIT 12   THE FEMALE AND MALE REPRODUCTIVE SYSTEMS

I. Special Diagnostic Tests and Examinations
A. The pelvic examination
  1. Ideal time is between menstrual periods; however, if patient has abnormal bleeding the examination cannot be delayed until bleeding stops.
  2. Nurse should remain with the patient during the examination.
  3. Preparation includes the following
     a. Explaining the procedure to the patient if she does not know what to expect.
     b. Proper draping of the patient and providing privacy are necessary.
     c. Patient should void immediately before the examination so the bladder will be empty and the patient will be less uncomfortable and more relaxed.
     d. Equipment, such as vaginal speculum, gloves, lubricant, etc., is assembled before the physician is summoned to the examining room.
  4. Vaginal douches should not be taken immediately before the examination because they remove secretions and tissues that may help the physician in his diagnosis.
B. Smears and cultures—samplings of material from the reproductive tract are removed and examined in the laboratory.
  1. Papanicolaou smear useful in diagnosing cancer of the cervix.
  2. Cultures useful in determining causative microorganisms in an infection.
C. Dilatation and curettage—dilatation of the cervix and curettage (scraping) of the uterus to remove endometrial tissues or other material inside the uterus. May be used as diagnostic test or as treatment of certain disorders of the reproductive system.

II. Disorders of Menstruation
A. Amenorrhea—absence of menstruation.
B. Dysmenorrhea—painful or difficult menstruation.
  1. May be mild or severe depending on the cause.
  2. Mild discomforts of menstruation may be relieved by
     a. Moderate exercise and adequate rest.
     b. Warm baths.
     c. Removal of tight clothing.
     d. Well-balanced, nonconstipating diet.
C. Menorrhagia—excessive loss of blood during the menstrual period.
D. Metrorrhagia—uterine bleeding or spotting which occurs at times other than the menstrual period. Must always be reported to a gynecologist as it may be a symptom of malignancy or other serious disorder.

III. Infections of the Genital Tract
A. Gonorrhea—a venereal disease caused by the gonococcus.
  1. Symptoms—about 90 per cent of the women with gonorrhea have no symptoms or very mild symptoms of a pelvic inflammatory disease (see below).
  2. Diagnosis established by identification of the organism on a smear or culture.
  3. Treatment—large doses of penicillin or some other antibiotic.
  4. It is a highly infectious disease; no immunity is established.
  5. Extreme care must be taken when nursing these patients. Vaginal discharge is highly contagious.
B. Syphilis—also a venereal disease, but is not restricted to the genital tract. May involve any organ in the body.
  1. In the primary stage there are chancres (open sores) on the mouth or genital area. These may subside without treatment but the disease will still be present. During this stage secretions from the chancres and the patient's blood are both considered to be highly contagious.
  2. In the secondary and tertiary stages the disease may present symptoms of a number of serious diseases.
  3. Treatment includes use of antibiotics; most useful in the first stage. After the disease has progressed to the third stage little can be done for the patient.
C. Pelvic inflammatory disease—an infection of the pelvis, outside the uterus. Most

often involves the fallopian tubes and ovaries.

1. May be caused by any microorganisms capable of causing an infection.
2. Symptoms include profuse vaginal discharge, purulent in nature; severe pain in the lower abdomen; elevated temperature; nausea and vomiting.
3. Treatment most effective if begun in the early stages before the infection becomes widespread. Antibiotics used, heat is applied to the lower abdomen, rest and general hygienic measures used to help patient overcome the infection.

D. Trichomonas vaginitis — an inflammation of the vaginal mucosa, caused by the trichomonas parasite, *Trichomonas vaginalis.*

1. Symptoms include persistent leukorrhea (white discharge), inflammation, and swelling of the vaginal mucosa and external genitalia.
2. Difficult to control. Vinegar douches or other applications which change the chemical environment of the vagina are most helpful in relieving symptoms and reducing inflammation.
3. Metronidazole (Flagyl) is drug of choice.

E. Monilial vaginitis — caused by *Candida albicans*, a member of the yeast family.

1. Symptoms — watery discharge with cheese-like flakes, severe itching, and inflammation.
2. Treated with antifungal agent.

F. Genital herpes — caused by herpesvirus hominis, Type II.

1. Lesions on external genitalia similar to "fever blisters."
2. Usually is fatal in the newborn who contracts the infection during birth.
3. Difficult to treat and control.

IV. **Tumors of the Uterus**

A. Fibroids — benign tumors of the wall of the uterus.

1. May subside spontaneously after menopause or may require surgical removal.
2. Symptoms include bleeding, which is common to all types of tumors in the genital tract. As tumor enlarges it causes an increase in size and feeling of heaviness in the lower abdomen.

B. Malignant tumors — most commonly found originating in the cervix.

1. Symptoms are bleeding and pressure as tumor enlarges.
2. Treatment — surgical removal and some form of radiation therapy.

V. **Uterine Displacement**

A. Definition — an extreme tilting of the uterus from its normal position in the pelvis.

B. Types

1. Anteflexion — a bending forward of the uterus.
2. Retroflexion — a bending backward of the uterus.
3. Retroversion — a tilting backward of the uterus without bending.
4. Retrocession — a backward displacement of the uterus without bending.
5. Prolapse of the uterus — a falling or lowering of the uterus into the vaginal canal.

C. Symptoms include backache, feeling of heaviness in the pelvis, white vaginal discharge, and fatigue.

D. Treatment necessary when symptoms are severe. Surgical correction may be necessary, or the uterus may be held in its normal position with a pessary.

VI. **Nursing Care of the Patient Undergoing Vaginal Surgery**

A. Preoperative care

1. Pubic and perianal hair is shaved to reduce danger of infection.
2. Douches using a surgical detergent or disinfectant are often ordered the evening before and morning of surgery. These are done to cleanse the surgical area and reduce the danger of infection.

B. Postoperative care

1. Patient must be watched carefully for signs of hemorrhage.
2. Perineal irrigations may be ordered to cleanse the operative site and promote healing. If irrigations are not specifically ordered the area should be cleansed several times a day, using a clean wash cloth, soap, and water.
3. Perineal light may be used to reduce discomfort and promote healing of the suture line. Light should be at least 12 inches (30 cm.) from the perineum and a 50-watt bulb used to lessen the danger of burning the patient.
4. To avoid constipation and straining at stool which might open the surgical incision, mineral oil is sometimes administered every night.
5. Patient may experience anxiety about surgery of the genital tract. Will need explanation of the type of surgery and the effect it will have on her menstrual cycle, role as a wife, and feminine characteristics.
6. When a hysterectomy is performed, the surgeon usually leaves a part of an ovary so that female hormones will continue to be secreted.
7. Nurse should know that in order for menstruation to occur, two organs are essential: (1) the uterus, and (2) at least part of one ovary.

VII. **Nursing Care of Patient Undergoing Mastectomy**
  A. Introduction
    1. Simple mastectomy — removal of a breast.
    2. Radical mastectomy — removal of the entire breast and adjacent tissue, including the underlying pectoral muscles and axillary lymph nodes.
  B. Preoperative care
    1. Surgical preparation of the skin varies little from that of any major surgery.
    2. Emotional aspects must be considered; patient should be prepared for radical mastectomy so she will know what to expect. Plans are made for the wearing of a prosthesis after healing takes place.
  C. Postoperative care
    1. Pressure dressing over operative site is applied to reduce the danger of hemorrhage. Patient must be checked frequently and dressings observed for signs of bleeding. Dressings on back of chest must not be overlooked.
    2. Any numbness of the lower arm, inability to move the fingers, or severe swelling of the arm should be reported immediately as they may indicate impairment of circulation to the arm.
    3. Deep breathing and coughing are necessary even though they will be painful for the patient.
    4. When getting patient up out of bed the first few times she must be well supported as she will have a tendency to lose her balance after removal of the breast.
    5. Special exercises are begun when ordered by the physician. These exercises include brushing the hair, wall climbing with the hands, and other movements which will strengthen the arm and chest muscles.
    6. Selection of prosthesis and fitting of breast forms are done when physician feels that patient may safely wear them.

VIII. **Infections of the Male Genital Tract**
  A. Urethritis — an inflammation of the urethra; may be caused by streptococcus, staphylococcus, or gonococcus.
    1. Frequency, urgency, and burning on urination are the most common symptoms.
    2. Treatment consists of administration of antibiotics and local application of a mild antiseptic to control infection.
  B. Prostatitis — an inflammation of the prostate gland, may be caused by any pathogenic microorganism which finds its way into the genital tract.
    1. Dysuria and pain and tenderness in the perineal region are the most common symptoms.
    2. Treatment includes administration of antibiotics, bed rest, and local applications of heat to reduce discomfort.
  C. Epididymitis — inflammation of the epididymis.
    1. Symptoms include local pain in the scrotal area, elevated temperature, and extreme fatigue.
    2. Treatment includes administration of antibiotics and local applications of cold.
  D. Orchitis — inflammation of the testes. A common complication of mumps in the adult male.
    1. Symptoms similar to those of epididymitis.
    2. Treatment is similar to that of epididymitis. In addition, the individual may receive gamma globulin to reduce severity of mumps.

IX. **Tumors of the Prostate Gland**
  A. Types
    1. Benign prostatic hypertrophy — benign enlargement of the prostate gland.
    2. Cancer of the prostate — malignant growth of cells in the prostate gland.
  B. Symptoms include urinary difficulty because the enlarged prostate presses against the urethra and blocks the flow of urine from the bladder. Benign prostatic hypertrophy occurs most often in males over the age of 55.
  C. Treatment — surgical removal of all or part of the prostate gland.
    1. Types of surgical procedures
      a. Radical prostatectomy — removal of the entire prostate gland and its capsule. Incision is made through the perineum.
      b. Suprapubic prostatectomy — removal of the prostate through an incision directly over the bladder. The bladder is opened and the urethral mucosa is incised.
      c. Retropubic prostatectomy — prostate is removed through a low abdominal incision, but the bladder is not opened.
      d. Transurethral prostatic resection — removal of part of the prostate by way of the urethra. There is no surgical incision.
    2. Postoperative care varies according to type of surgical procedure.
      a. Postoperative hemorrhage is most common complication to be avoided.

1. Catheter must be kept open and draining.
2. Urine must be watched carefully for signs of excessive bleeding. Bits of tissue and small clots are to be expected.
3. Catheter is irrigated frequently to remove clots and other material that may obstruct the catheter. Severe pain in the bladder region may indicate an obstructed catheter.
4. Care must be used not to oversedate the patient, especially since he is most likely to be elderly.

Questions

Mrs. Heath, a 40-year-old mother of three, has experienced bleeding between her menstrual periods for several months. She made an appointment for an examination by a gynecologist.

1. If you were the office nurse confirming the appointment for Mrs. Heath, you should caution her against:
   1. choosing a date on which she expects to have vaginal bleeding
   2. taking a douche immediately before coming to the doctor's office
   3. taking a tub bath immediately before coming to the doctor's office
   4. taking any foods or fluids for 8 hours prior to the visit to the doctor's office
2. Prior to a pelvic examination in the gynecologist's office, it is most important for the nurse to:
   1. direct the patient to the bathroom to empty her bladder
   2. administer a low enema
   3. catheterize the patient for a specimen
   4. scrub the perineal area with pHisoHex for 5 minutes
3. The chief purpose for this nursing measure is to:
   1. obtain a stool specimen
   2. remove flatus and feces from the intestinal tract
   3. sterilize the skin around the vagina
   4. avoid discomfort for the patient and enable the physician to palpate the pelvic organs more easily
4. The patient will be more relaxed and cooperative during the gynecologic examination if the nurse will:
   1. leave the room during the examination
   2. assure the patient that all the instruments have been sterilized
   3. explain the procedure to the patient if she does not know what to expect
   4. remind the patient that modesty is not important during any type of physical examination
5. The physician explained to Mrs. Heath that he would do a Papanicolaou smear of the cervical secretions. The purpose of this test is to:
   1. determine the presence of microorganisms that may be the cause of a disease
   2. rule out or confirm pregnancy
   3. rule out the possibility of a venereal disease
   4. determine the presence of malignant cells in the cervical secretions
6. After the examination Mrs. Heath's gynecologist recommended that she be admitted to the hospital for further diagnostic tests. After her admission Mrs. Heath was scheduled for a dilatation and curettage. This procedure involves:
   1. dilation of the cervix and scraping of the uterus
   2. removal of several samples of cervical tissue
   3. x-ray examination of the reproductive tract
   4. visual examination of the interior of the uterus

7. Mrs. Heath's condition was diagnosed as carcinoma of the cervix in its early stages. She was immediately scheduled for a vaginal hysterectomy. This procedure involves surgical removal of the:
   1. uterus and vagina through an abdominal incision
   2. uterus by way of the vagina
   3. uterus, tubes, and ovaries through an abdominal incision
   4. cervix and tubes by way of the vagina

8. The evening before surgery Mrs. Heath received a Zephiran douche. The purpose of this procedure is to:
   1. help minimize vaginal bleeding
   2. cleanse the vaginal canal
   3. remove malignant cells from the vaginal canal
   4. sterilize the operative area

9. During the immediate postoperative period it is most important for the nurse to:
   1. observe Mrs. Heath carefully for hemorrhage, which is a common complication of vaginal surgery
   2. keep Mrs. Heath in the Trendelenburg position to avoid strain on the sutures
   3. irrigate the operative area with normal saline to prevent infection
   4. catheterize Mrs. Heath every 4 hours to prevent overexpansion of the bladder

10. Mrs. Heath is to receive perineal irrigations beginning the first postoperative day. Before administering the irrigations the nurse should:
    1. warm the solution to body temperature
    2. assist the patient onto the commode for the procedure
    3. position the patient on her abdomen
    4. remove any soiled pads or dressings and discard them in the patient's wastebasket

11. During the perineal irrigation the nurse must remember to:
    a. use one cotton ball for each stroke when cleansing the area
    b. hold the irrigating can at least 18 inches (46 cm.) above the patient
    c. wipe toward the rectal area so as to avoid contamination of the operative area
    d. instruct the patient to void as soon after the procedure as possible

    1. all of these
    2. a and c
    3. b and d
    4. all but b

12. Mrs. Heath is also to receive a perineal light after each irrigation. In order to prevent burning the patient, it is necessary to:
    1. use only a 100-watt bulb for the lamp
    2. place the bulb 6 inches (15 cm.) from the perineum
    3. check frequently for redness and discomfort
    4. always remove the lamp within 10 minutes of application

13. Sometimes a perineal irrigation is not ordered for a patient receiving a perineal light. When an irrigation is not specifically ordered the nurse should:
    1. refrain from cleansing the area because of the danger of infection
    2. cleanse the area with tap water only
    3. chart her reasons for not cleansing the patient
    4. wash the perineal area thoroughly, using soap and water and a clean washcloth

14. On the third postoperative day Mrs. Heath's retention catheter was removed. The retention catheter had been inserted before vaginal surgery was done because:
    a. there is danger of contamination of the sterile field during surgery if the bladder is full
    b. many patients having vaginal surgery have difficulty voiding after surgery

    1. all of these
    2. all but c
    3. c and d
    4. a and b

    c. most patients with disorders of the reproductive system are incontinent
    d. there is less danger of damaging the bladder during surgery if it is kept empty during the procedure

15. Mrs. Heath's physician ordered daily catheterization for residual urine after the retention catheter was removed. When checking for residual urine it is most important for the nurse to:
    1. catheterize the patient early in the morning before she arises
    2. force fluids for several hours before the procedure
    3. send the specimen to the laboratory immediately after it is obtained
    4. instruct the patient to void immediately before she is catheterized

16. Mrs. Heath seemed worried about the aftereffects of her surgery and asked you if she would continue to have menstrual periods. The practical nurse should know that in order for menstruation to take place the following organs must be present and functioning:
    1. uterus and uterine tubes
    2. uterus only
    3. uterus and at least part of one ovary
    4. uterine tubes and one or both ovaries

17. Mrs. Heath also told you that the surgeon had told her he had not removed her ovaries. His reason for leaving the ovaries intact was to:
    1. allow for future pregnancies
    2. provide for continuing secretion of the ovarian hormones
    3. make the surgical procedure less difficult and prolonged
    4. lessen the danger of hemorrhage in the postoperative period

The following questions (18 through 26) refer to various disorders of the female reproductive system.

18. The term used to designate painful menstruation is:
    1. amenorrhea
    2. dysmenorrhea
    3. metrorrhagia
    4. hypermenorrhea

19. Relief from minor discomforts accompanying menstruation can best be obtained by:
    1. eliminating the daily bath and taking a daily laxative
    2. taking a cold shower and applying an icebag to the abdomen
    3. avoiding exercise and remaining in bed as much as possible
    4. taking moderate exercise, avoiding tight clothing, and eating a well-balanced, nonconstipating diet

20. A definite diagnosis of gonorrhea is obtained by:
    1. discovering the gonococcus in a specimen of vaginal discharge
    2. the symptoms of profuse vaginal discharge and painful urination
    3. testing the blood of the patient for gonococci
    4. an x-ray examination of the pelvic organs

21. Gonorrhea is a venereal disease and:
    1. is incurable once it reaches the fallopian tubes
    2. can be treated successfully with penicillin or streptomycin
    3. can be caught only once, after which an individual becomes immune to the disease
    4. is not classified as an infectious disease

22. When caring for a patient with gonorrhea, the nurse must be especially careful to avoid:
    1. contact with the patient's nasal secretions
    2. contact with the vaginal discharge
    3. handling syringes and needles used for injections for the patient
    4. coming in contact with the skin lesions of the patient

23. Syphilis is also a venereal disease and can affect:
    1. only the reproductive organs
    2. males only
    3. the entire body as well as the genital organs
    4. females only

24. The outstanding symptom of monilial vaginitis is a vaginal discharge that is:
    1. purulent and foul-smelling
    2. watery, cheese-like, and accompanied by itching and inflammation of the vulva
    3. bloody, and occurs at the time of ovulation
    4. blood-tinged, and occurs at regular monthly intervals
25. Benign tumors of the uterus are commonly referred to as:
    1. lipomas
    2. fibroids
    3. carcinomas
    4. sarcomas
26. The most common symptom of all uterine tumors is:
    1. bleeding at times other than the menstrual period
    2. rapid enlargement of the uterus
    3. profuse vaginal discharge
    4. cessation of menstruation

You are assigned to care for Miss Bryant, who has just returned from surgery. She has had a radical mastectomy for treatment of a malignant tumor of the breast.

27. A radical mastectomy involves removal of:
    1. a tumor and its capsule
    2. the entire breast and adjacent lymph nodes under the arm
    3. both breasts
    4. the tumor and adjacent fatty tissue
28. Miss Bryant has a pressure dressing over the surgical area. When checking the dressing for hemorrhage it will be necessary for you to:
    1. remove the uppermost layers of the dressing
    2. turn the patient frequently in order to check the dressings
    3. remove the entire dressing to observe the operative site
    4. always keep the patient turned onto the side opposite the operative side so that bleeding can be observed readily
29. If, during the first 24 hours after surgery, Miss Bryant complains of numbness and swelling of the lower arm on the operative side, the nurse should know that:
    1. there may be swelling under the pressure dressing causing it to become tighter and blocking circulation of blood to the arm
    2. this is not unusual for patients who have had a radical mastectomy
    3. this is one of the first signs of hemorrhage from the operative area
    4. there has probably been some damage to the nerves in the arm and paralysis is inevitable
30. One of the simplest ways of performing necessary exercises after a mastectomy is:
    1. weight lifting
    2. brushing the hair
    3. mopping the floor
    4. dusting the room
31. There were times during the postoperative period when Miss Bryant became depressed and withdrawn. The practical nurse should realize that:
    1. Miss Bryant is probably showing the early symptoms of a psychosis
    2. this is a difficult time of adjustment for most patients who have a mastectomy
    3. Miss Bryant is a very vain creature and needs flattery to get her out of this mood
    4. it would be best to leave Miss Bryant alone at this time and let her solve her own personal problems
32. Miss Bryant asks you when she will be able to obtain a prosthesis and begin wearing it. What would the best answer to this question be?
    1. When you can afford one.
    2. This will depend on the amount of scar tissue you will have.
    3. The physician must decide when healing is sufficient and the prosthesis can be worn comfortably.
    4. Some people can never adjust to a prosthesis after mastectomy.

Mr. McGregor, age 72, has been experiencing difficulty in urinating for the past several months. He was examined by his family physician and found to have an enlarged prostate gland.

33. An enlarged prostate gland interferes with urination because this gland:
    1. is located near the kidneys and presses against them
    2. encircles the urethra just below the neck of the bladder
    3. secretes a substance important in the formation of urine
    4. controls the sphincter muscle at the end of the urethra

34. Mr. McGregor was admitted to the hospital and scheduled for a transurethral prostatic resection. In this procedure:
    1. an incision is made into the perineum and the entire prostate gland is removed
    2. the prostate gland is removed through an incision directly over the bladder
    3. a low abdominal incision is made and the prostate gland is removed
    4. part of the prostate gland is removed by way of the urethra

35. Which of the following symptoms should be reported promptly if noticed during Mr. McGregor's immediate postoperative period?
    1. pinkish drainage from the operative site
    2. bits of clots and tissue passing through the catheter and into the drainage bottle
    3. large amounts of urine passing through the catheter
    4. appearance of bright red blood in the catheter and drainage bottle

36. If Mr. McGregor complains of severe pain in the bladder region, the nurse's *first* action should be to:
    1. check to see if the catheter is open and draining freely
    2. administer another dose of an analgesic medication because elderly patients require large amount of sedation
    3. clamp the catheter and gently massage the bladder region
    4. summon the physician immediately

37. Frequent irrigations of the bladder are usually ordered following a prostatectomy. The chief purpose of these irrigations is to:
    1. prevent infection in the bladder by destroying all bacteria
    2. keep the urinary tract free from scar tissue
    3. control hemorrhage from the bladder
    4. remove blood clots and shreds of tissue which may obstruct the catheter

The following questions refer to various diseases of the male reproductive system.

38. Orchitis is a complication of mumps and sometimes occurs in the adult male. Orchitis is an inflammation of the:
    1. prostate gland
    2. testes
    3. epididymis
    4. glans penis

39. The surgical procedure in which part of the foreskin is removed from the penis is called a:
    1. circumcision
    2. orchidectomy
    3. penectomy
    4. epididymectomy

40. A condition in which the foreskin cannot be retracted over the glans penis is called:
    1. prostatitis
    2. phimosis
    3. cryptorchidism
    4. hydrocele

UNIT 13   DISEASES OF THE NERVOUS SYSTEM

I. Common Neurological Terms
A. Paraplegia—paralysis of the lower extremities or lower part of the body. Commonly associated with spinal injury.
B. Hemiplegia—paralysis of one side of the body. Commonly associated with cerebral damage.
C. Quadriplegia—paralysis of all four extremities.
D. Flaccid paralysis—paralysis in which the muscles are limp and flabby.
E. Spastic paralysis—paralysis in which the muscles are tense and rigid.
F. Amnesia—loss of memory.
G. Aphasia—loss of the ability to speak.

II. Special Examinations and Diagnostic Tests
A. Neurological examination—measures the ability of the body to perform certain motor and sensory functions.
1. Tests ability of the cranial nerves to control sensory and motor activities.
   a. Senses of taste, smell, sight, hearing.
   b. Facial expressions.
   c. Gag reflex.
   d. Ability to move the eyes.
2. Tests groups of large muscles
   a. Evaluates patient's gait while walking and running.
   b. Checks posture while standing.
   c. Tests strength of hand grip.
3. Reflexes—involuntary muscular contraction in response to a stimulus.
B. Lumbar puncture—insertion of a hollow needle into the arachnoid space between the third and fourth lumbar vertebrae.
1. Purposes
   a. To obtain a specimen of spinal fluid from the spinal cavity for chemical analysis.
   b. To obtain a specimen of spinal fluid for microscopic examination.
   c. To measure the pressure within the cerebrospinal cavities.
   d. To determine if there is a blocking of the flow of spinal fluid.
   e. To remove blood or pus from the arachnoid space.
   f. To reduce intracranial pressure.
   g. For spinal anesthesia.

h. To inject air for x-ray examination of the skull.
2. Nursing care—patient is usually kept flat in bed for at least 8 hours after a lumbar puncture to reduce headache.
C. Electroencephalogram—a test that records the activity of the brain tissues.

III. General Nursing Care of the Patient with a Neurological Disorder
A. Care of the skin
1. Patient must be turned frequently. With loss of motion of various parts of the body there is also loss of feeling. The patient does not complain of discomfort from lying in one position too long because he does not feel any discomfort.
2. Intramuscular injections *should not* be given in the areas of the body which have no feeling.
3. All points of pressure should be massaged frequently to increase circulation.
B. Providing for self-care
1. All patients with neurological disorders are not totally helpless. The patient should be encouraged to do as much for himself as possible.
2. The furniture in the room should be arranged conveniently for the patient.
3. Side rails should be applied to assist the nurse in turning the patient.
4. A trapeze bar may help the patient in lifting himself onto a bedpan.
5. Feeding himself may be slow or clumsy for the patient but he should be allowed to feed himself if possible.
6. Avoid pushing the patient into activities beyond his physical limitations.
7. Proper handling of extremities will help prevent involuntary spasms of the muscles (Fig. 42).
C. Prevention of complications
1. Proper positioning of the patient.
2. Passive exercises to prevent deformities.
D. Emotional aspects
1. Emotional disturbances and personality changes often accompany these disorders.
   a. Outbursts of anger or depression are not uncommon.

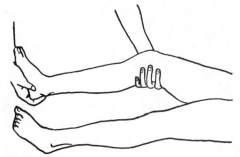

FIGURE 42. Proper method of handling a limb when muscle spasm is likely to result from stimulation. Note that the palms of the hands are used and the joints above and below the affected muscles are supported. (Wiebe: *Orthopedics in Nursing.*)

     b. Patient may lose the will to live.
  2. The nurse must help the patient to adjust to his handicaps.
 E. Rehabilitation
  1. In some cases, rehabilitation is limited to keeping the patient happily occupied as the disease progresses.
  2. If possible, rehabilitation should be planned so that the patient is able to be an active member of the community in spite of his handicap.

IV. Infections of the Brain and Spinal Cord
 A. Meningitis—an inflammation of the membranous lining of the brain and spinal cord; may be caused by many bacteria and viruses.
  1. Symptoms
    a. Severe and persistent headache.
    b. Pain and stiffness of the neck.
    c. Irritability.
    d. Photophobia (sensitivity to light).
    e. Hypersensitivity of the skin.
  2. Special treatment and nursing care
    a. Administer specific antibiotics.
    b. Maintain strict isolation.
    c. Keep room quiet and dimly lighted.
    d. Observe for signs of temperature elevation and convulsions.
    e. Cool compresses or an icebag to the head may help relieve delirium.
 B. Encephalitis—inflammation of the brain tissue; most frequently caused by a virus.
  1. Symptoms
    a. Headache.
    b. Fever.
    c. Lethargy.
    d. Muscular weakness.
    e. Mental confusion, visual disturbances, and disorientation may be present.
  2. Special treatment and nursing care
    a. Administer specific antibiotics.
    b. Isolation if it is the infectious type.

    c. Frequent checking of vital signs.
    d. Constant attendance to prevent injury to self during period of disorientation.
    e. Measures to lower temperature.
 C. Poliomyelitis—an acute inflammation of the anterior horn of the spinal cord; may be caused by three strains of viruses.
  1. Prevention—immunization now available.
    a. Salk vaccine.
    b. Sabin vaccine.
  2. Symptoms
    a. Upper respiratory infection.
    b. Fever.
    c. Severe headache.
    d. Stiffness of the neck.
  3. Special treatment and nursing care
    a. Application of heat to the muscles for relief of painful contractions.
    b. Observe carefully for respiratory difficulties.

V. Head Injuries
 A. Types
  1. Concussion—a head injury in which the brain is compressed by a portion of the skull and temporary anemia of the brain tissue results.
  2. Contusion—the brain tissue is bruised and swelling occurs, pressing the brain tissue against the skull.
 B. Symptoms—depend on severity of brain damage. Vomiting, headache, and loss of consciousness often occur.
 C. Special treatment and nursing care
  1. Bed linen may be arranged so that the patient's head will be at the foot of the bed, and dressings may be observed more easily.
  2. Observation one of the most important aspects of nursing care.
  3. Patient should be observed for the following
    a. Changes in blood pressure, pulse, or respirations.
    b. Extreme restlessness.
    c. Deepening stupor or loss of consciousness.
    d. Headache which increases in intensity.
    e. Vomiting, especially persistent projectile vomiting.
    f. Pupils that are unequal in size.
    g. Leakage of cerebrospinal fluid (clear, yellow, or pink tinged) from nose or ear.
    h. Inability to move one or more extremities.

VI. Injuries of the Spinal Cord

A. Symptoms and emergency treatment—An injured person should be treated as a case of spinal cord injury until a definite diagnosis is made if
   1. He complains of neck pain.
   2. He cannot move his legs.
   3. He has no feeling in his legs.

B. Immediate care
   1. Patient must be transported to hospital on a stretcher or board.
   2. The back *must* be kept straight.

C. The nurse is primarily concerned with prevention of
   1. Decubitus ulcers.
   2. Urinary complications.
   3. Orthopedic deformities.

VII. Ruptured Intervertebral Disc—a condition in which part of the fibrous cartilage disc prolapses and pinches the adjacent nerve root by pressing it against the bone

A. Symptoms
   1. Pain in lower back which radiates down the back of one leg to the foot.
   2. Walking is extremely painful.

B. Treatment and nursing care
   1. Medical
      a. Firm mattress with bed board.
      b. Bed rest.
      c. Hydrocollator pack or heating pad to reduce muscle spasm.
      d. Pelvic traction may be applied.
      e. Use of specially designed corsets or back braces to maintain proper alignment of the spine.
      f. When patient is turned, he should be "log-rolled":
         1. Patient folds his arms across his chest.
         2. He flexes the knee opposite the side on which he is to turn.
         3. The patient is rolled over as shown in Figure 43.
   2. Surgical—laminectomy (excision of the posterior arch of the vertebra).

VIII. Myasthenia Gravis—literally, grave muscle weakness

A. Symptoms
   1. Progressive muscular weakness of the skeletal muscles.
   2. The fatigue is relieved by rest, but soon returns.

B. Treatment—mainly drug therapy
   1. Neostigmine (Prostigmin).
   2. Pyridostigmine (Mestinon).

C. Myasthenic crisis—a period of severe weakness which may result in death owing to weakness of the throat muscles and respiratory failure.
   1. Nurse must be in constant attendance.
   2. Throat and mouth must be suctioned frequently.
   3. Nurse can reassure patient by her calm and competent manner.
   4. A tracheotomy and artificial respirator may be necessary to maintain life.

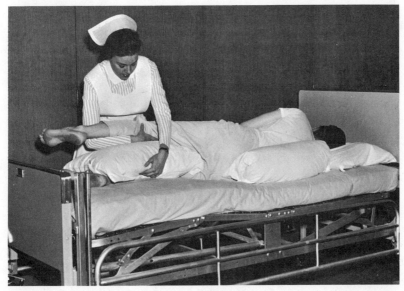

FIGURE 43.   Proper alignment and support with pillows when patient is "log-rolled" following surgery. This method of turning and support is used for patient who has had laminectomy or a spinal fusion. (Pasternak, S.: *American Journal of Nursing,* 62:77, 1962.)

IX. Parkinson's Disease — a degenerative disease of the nerve cells of the brain
  A. Symptoms
    1. Tremor — most marked in the fingers, causing the individual to constantly perform a "pill rolling" movement.
    2. Rigidity — of the skeletal muscles.
  B. Treatment
    1. Medications that produce mild sedation and muscular relaxation.
    2. Surgery — neurosurgical procedure that destroys certain areas of nerve cells and thereby eliminates the tremor and muscular rigidity.

X. Epilepsy — a term used to describe sudden and uncontrollable seizures, in which the individual has muscular twitching and a temporary loss of consciousness
  A. Causes
    1. Unknown.
    2. May be a symptom of brain damage.
  B. Types
    1. Petit mal — a brief lapse of consciousness; may pass unnoticed by a casual observer; may consist of only a vacant stare that lasts for a second or two.
    2. Grand mal — major convulsions in which the patient may lose consciousness for minutes.
      a. Seizure is often preceded by an *aura*, a specific warning which enables the patient to sense that an attack is coming; examples, flash of light, dimming of vision, peculiar odor.
      b. Sequence of events
        1. Usually heralded by a sharp cry.
        2. Muscles are held rigid and skin becomes cyanotic.
        3. After a few seconds, jerking movements begin.
        4. As the convulsion subsides, patient falls asleep and usually awakens hours later with headache and depression.
      c. Protection for patient
        1. If patient has warning, he should lie down.
        2. Head should be protected from injury.
        3. Insert mouth gag, if possible.
        4. Loosen all tight clothing.
      d. Drugs
        1. Dilantin — reduces convulsive seizures.

Questions

1. The word hemiplegia means:
   1. paralysis of one side of the body
   2. paralysis of all four extremities
   3. paralysis of the upper extremities
   4. paralysis of the lower extremities and lower half of the body
2. Flaccid paralysis is paralysis in which the muscles are:
   1. limp and flabby
   2. tense and rigid
   3. unable to function on one side of the body
   4. subject to continuous spasms
3. A reflex is best defined as:
   1. the response one gets from tapping the knee cap with a percussion hammer
   2. an involuntary muscular contraction in response to a stimulus
   3. a sign of meningeal irritation
   4. a voluntary movement of the skeletal muscles
4. The cerebrospinal fluid is located:
   1. inside the dura mater
   2. in the spaces of the arachnoid meninges
   3. in the brain
   4. in the brain and spinal cord tissues
5. A lumbar puncture or spinal tap is done for all but ONE of the following reasons:
   1. to measure the pressure within the cerebrospinal cavities
   2. to remove blood or pus from the arachnoid spaces
   3. for spinal anesthesia
   4. to inject a disinfectant

6. The diagnostic test that may be done to determine whether the *activities* of the brain tissues are normal is called:
    1. an electroencephalogram
    2. a pneumoencephalogram
    3. a ventriculogram
    4. a neurogram
7. Patients who have paralysis of certain parts of the body must be given skin care because:
    a. they have no feeling in these affected parts and have no warning that the skin is being damaged
    b. circulation to the affected parts is poor and the skin in the area breaks down quite readily
    c. injections are frequently given in the paralyzed area and thus provide openings for the entrance of bacteria
    d. these patients cannot move and change their positions when necessary

    1. all of these
    2. all but c
    3. c and d
    4. a and b
8. Mealtime can be made more pleasant for a partially paralyzed patient if:
    1. the nurse feeds him so that he will not have accidents and spill his food
    2. he is left to do everything for himself and thus is encouraged to help himself
    3. the nurse prepares his food by cutting meat, spreading butter, etc. and then allows him to feed himself as much as possible
    4. a member of his family feeds him each of his meals
9. In some neurological disorders in which there is irritation or damage to the spinal nerves, the patient may be subject to painful, involuntary spasms of the extremities. To avoid stimulating the muscles and bringing on these spasms when handling the extremities, the nurse should:
    1. firmly grasp the muscle in the center of the limb and lift the limb gently
    2. place the palms of her hands under the joint rather than on the affected muscles
    3. place her hands under the muscles and lift from below
    4. splint the limb with a pillow before lifting
10. Meningitis can be caused by:
    1. any bacteria capable of causing an infection
    2. many different viruses
    3. the meningococcus
    4. all of these
11. Patients with meningitis often suffer from photophobia and extreme irritability. These symptoms require special attention to the patient's environment, and it is most important for the nurse to:
    1. provide a quiet environment and avoid bright lights in the patient's room
    2. ventilate the room properly and provide sufficient sunlight for the patient
    3. eliminate strong odors or unpleasant sights which may provoke vomiting
    4. allow frequent visitors to keep the patient from feeling lonely and depressed
12. Delirium and high fever often accompany infectious diseases of the brain and meninges. A nursing measure that would be most helpful in relieving delirium would be:
    1. administration of phenobarbital every 4 hours
    2. application of a hot water bottle to the neck
    3. forcing fluids by mouth
    4. application of cool compresses or an icebag to the head
13. One of the most important aspects of nursing care of patients with head injuries is:
    1. restraining the patient to prevent self-injury
    2. administration of sedatives to avoid convulsions
    3. careful observation of the patient's vital signs
    4. prevention of paralysis by frequent turning

14. Nursing care of patients having brain surgery can be simplified if:
  1. the top bed linens are not tucked in at the sides
  2. the bed is made so that the patient's head is at the foot
  3. a cotton mattress is placed on the bed
  4. the patient is kept restrained at all times

15. Physicians usually do not wish to give sedatives to patients who have suffered head injuries because these drugs may:
  1. produce coma
  2. mask the patient's true symptoms
  3. depress the respirations
  4. lead to hemorrhage within the skull

16. Following any type of accident, an individual would most probably be suspected of having injury to the spinal cord if:
  a. he could not move his lower extremities
  b. he complained of severe pain in the neck
  c. he was unconscious
  d. he apparently had an open wound of the head

  1. a and b
  2. all but a
  3. all but b
  4. c only

17. When transporting an individual who is suspected of having an injury to the spinal cord, it is most important to:
  1. flex the victim's knees and keep his head bent down on the chest
  2. keep him in a sitting position
  3. have him walk if at all possible
  4. keep the neck and back straight and well supported

18. Which of the following is true of epilepsy?
  a. It is an inherited disease, and epileptics should never marry.
  b. It is always accompanied by mental retardation.
  c. It is sometimes a symptom of damage to some of the brain cells.
  d. It is characterized by convulsive seizures over which the victim has no control.

  1. all of these
  2. a and b
  3. b and c
  4. c and d

19. About half the known epileptics describe a feeling of warning that they are going to have a seizure. This warning occurs just before the attack and is called:
  1. a prodromal symptom
  2. a sequela
  3. an aura
  4. an obsession

20. The nurse can be most helpful to a person having an epileptic seizure if she will:
  a. help him to a sitting position so as to maintain an open airway
  b. place some kind of padding under his head
  c. place a tongue blade or other padded article between his upper and lower teeth to prevent involuntary biting of the tongue
  d. loosen all tight clothing

  1. all of these
  2. all but a
  3. c and d
  4. a and b

21. If a physician orders "log-rolling" for a patient with an injury of the spine, the nurse can accomplish this best by:
  a. folding the patient's arms across his chest
  b. flexing the knee opposite the side onto which he is to turn
  c. rolling the patient's entire body simultaneously
  d. raising the head of the bed slightly

  1. all of these
  2. all but d
  3. a and b
  4. c and d

22. After "log-rolling" the patient onto his side, it is most important for the nurse to:
  1. support the back with pillows and place a pillow lengthwise between the lower extremities to avoid strain on the back
  2. elevate the head of the bed slightly to prevent pressure on the shoulder
  3. raise the knee rest slightly to avoid pressure on the hips
  4. remove the pillow from under the patient's head and place it under his shoulders

UNIT 14   DISORDERS OF THE EYES, EARS, AND THROAT

SECTION 1   DISORDERS OF THE EYES

I. Introduction

A. Statistics show that about half the people in the United States have defective vision to some degree.

B. Basic facts of eye care
  1. Headache, burning, itching, and redness of the eyes are symptoms of a visual defect and should be investigated by an ophthalmologist.
  2. Adequate diet and good nutrition play an important role in the conservation of sight, but no single type of food will improve the eyesight. Vitamin deficiences can produce visual defects.
  3. Children do not outgrow crossed eyes. Neglect of *strabismus* (crossed eyes) can lead to a serious loss of vision.
  4. Visual defects should be corrected by prescription lenses, not by "reading glasses" purchased at the dime store.
  5. Terminology to be understood in regard to persons concerned with care of the eyes
     a. Ophthalmologist or oculist—a medical doctor who specializes in the diagnosis and treatment of visual defects and diseases of the eye.
     b. Optometrist—one who is trained only in scientific examination of the eyes for the purpose of prescribing glasses. He is not qualified to treat diseases of the eye.
     c. Optician—one who is trained to make glasses and optical instruments.

II. Diagnostic Tests and Examinations

A. Snellen's chart—most commonly used test. It is read at a distance of 20 feet (6.1 m.) and consists of rows of letters, each row smaller than the one above it. A normal reading is 20/20.

B. Jaeger's test types—test an individual's ability to see objects close at hand. Use different sizes of printer's types.

C. Refraction—individual reads Snellen's chart through various types of lenses. When he chooses the lenses through which he can best read the chart, these are prescribed in glasses for him.

D. Intraocular pressure—measurement of the pressure within the eyeball. This is done with a tonometer and is used in the diagnosis of glaucoma.

III. Common Visual Defects

A. Refraction errors are the most common types. This means that the light rays entering the eyeball are not bent so that they focus on the retina properly. These errors may be caused by a number of structural defects in the eyeball (Fig. 44).

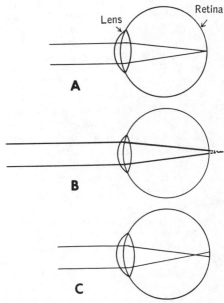

FIGURE 44. *A*, Normal vision. Lens bends light rays so that they focus directly on the retina. *B*, Hyperopia. Lens is too close to retina. Thus light rays converge at point beyond the retina. *C*, Myopia. Lens is too far away from retina, causing light rays to converge before they reach the retina. (Modified from Sackheim, G. I.: *Practical Physics for Nurses*, 2nd ed., Philadelphia, W. B. Saunders Co., 1962.)

1. Farsightedness—*hyperopia.*
2. Nearsightedness—*myopia.*
3. Astigmatism—difficulty in focusing the horizontal and vertical rays so that they strike the retina.
4. These conditions may be treated by wearing glasses in which the lenses have been shaped so that the light rays are brought into proper focus on the retina.

B. Injuries and infections of the eye
   1. Foreign bodies
      a. If not deeply imbedded in the tissues, they may be removed by touching the foreign object with the corner of a clean handkerchief.
      b. If object cannot be removed easily, the patient should consult an ophthalmologist immediately.
   2. Conjunctivitis—an inflammation of the mucous membrane lining the upper and lower lids and covering the front of the eyeball.
      a. May be caused by streptococcus, staphylococcus, and gonococcus.
      b. Pink-eye caused by Koch-Weeks bacillus. It is highly infectious.
      c. Symptoms include redness, swelling, and excessive tearing.
      d. Treated with antibiotics and steroids. May be given systemically or applied locally in the form of eye drops or ointments. In addition, the eyes may be treated with hot or cold moist compresses and irrigations.
   3. Sty (hordeolum)—an infection of the small lubricating gland around the edge of the eyelids.
      a. Redness, burning, and itching of the eyelids among the first symptoms. Later a small pustule forms on the lid.
      b. Treated with warm moist compresses to encourage rupture and drainage of the sty. Surgical incision and drainage may be necessary if the sty does not localize with this treatment.

C. Cataract
   1. Definition—an opacity of the lens resulting in impairment of vision. Most often occurs as a result of the aging process.
   2. Treatment
      a. Surgical removal of the affected lens is the only effective method of treatment.
      b. Preoperative care of the patient having a cataract extraction includes familiarizing the patient with his environment in the hospital so that he will not be frightened and confused after surgery when his eyes are bandaged.
   c. Postoperative care
      1. Most important that the patient avoid strain on the sutures. Coughing, sneezing, or sudden movements of the head must be avoided.
      2. Amount of physical activity allowed the patient depends on the desires of the surgeon.
      3. Eyelids may be cleaned with compresses and saline irrigations. Remember that only the lids are cleaned; the eyeball is not disturbed.

D. Glaucoma
   1. Definition—an increase in intraocular pressure. The cause is not known but it is primarily a disease of persons over the age of 40.
   2. Symptoms are very mild in the early stages and the individual does not realize that anything is wrong until permanent damage has been done to the eye and vision has been impaired. Danger signals of glaucoma include: blurred or hazy vision, difficulty in adjusting to darkened rooms, narrowing of vision at the sides of one or both eyes, and seeing rainbow-colored rings around lights.
   3. Treatment and nursing care
      a. Drugs include the *myotics* (those that constrict the pupil). Examples are pilocarpine, eserine, and neostigmine.
      b. Surgery may be performed in some cases. It is done to establish a means by which the aqueous humor may flow out of the eyeball when pressure builds up inside the eyeball.

IV. **General Principles in the Care of the Blind**
   A. Emotional aspects must always be considered. Depression and despair are to be expected until the individual adjusts to his loss of vision.
   B. Avoid shouting at those who are blind.
   C. Speak to the blind person as you enter the room and do not touch him until he is aware of your presence.
   D. Leave doors completely closed or completely open to avoid accidents. Be careful to keep the floor free from obstacles.
   E. Do not pity the blind. They wish to be treated as normal people and prefer to ask for help rather than have someone do everything for them.

SECTION 2   DISORDERS OF THE EARS

I. Introduction
A. Loss of hearing may be classified as sensorineural or conductive
   1. Sensorineural deafness (nerve deafness) is brought about by a disorder of the eighth cranial nerve.
   2. Conductive loss of hearing occurs when there is a barrier in the canal, eardrum, or middle ear and the sound waves are not conducted from the outside to the auditory nerve.
B. Loss of hearing affects one of ten persons in this country to some degree.

II. Special Diagnostic Tests and Examinations
A. Tuning fork tests used to determine individual's ability to detect sound waves produced by vibration of the fork.
B. Audiometry—use of special machine to determine and measure sound perception.

III. Infections of the Ear
A. Otitis media—an abscess or inflammation of the middle ear. Usually a complication of an acute infection of the throat or sinuses.
   1. Symptoms include pain in the ear, fever, and drainage from the ear.
   2. Treatment includes use of analgesics to relieve pain and antibiotics to inhibit the growth of the causative microorganism. *Myringotomy,* or incision and drainage of the eardrum, may be done to relieve pressure inside the ear and to allow for drainage of exudate.
B. Mastoiditis—a bacterial infection of the cells of the mastoid bone. Most often occurs when infection is spread from the middle ear.
   1. Symptoms include earache and tenderness over the mastoid bone.
   2. Antibiotics are used to treat the infection. Myringotomy is done to drain exudate and prevent spread of the infection. *Mastoidectomy* (removal of necrotic bone cells from the mastoid) is necessary in many cases when the infection has become extensive and does not respond to antibiotic therapy.
C. Otosclerosis
   1. Definition—destruction of the bones in the middle ear, with formation of sclerotic bone cells. Bones become fixed and do not transmit sound waves to the auditory nerve.
   2. Symptoms include a peculiar type of hearing loss in which the individual can hear his own voice very clearly, but cannot hear others speaking unless they raise their voices.
   3. Treatment—may be treated with a properly fitted hearing aid or by surgery. *Fenestration* is a surgical procedure in which a new "window" is made for the passage of sound. *Stapedectomy* is surgical removal of the stapes and insertion of a prosthesis.

IV. General Principles in the Care of the Deaf and Hard of Hearing
A. Nurse should always be alert to signs of hearing loss
   1. A listless expression.
   2. Frequent requests for repetition of a statement.
   3. Mispronunciation of words.
   4. Inattention or failure to respond when questioned.
   5. Tendency to avoid people.
B. Nurse must remember that speaking slowly and distinctly to one with a loss of hearing is preferred to shouting at him.
C. Always remember to face the person when you speak to him.
D. Phrase your questions so that the patient must answer with more than "yes" or "no."

SECTION 3   DISORDERS OF THE THROAT

I. Pharyngitis—Inflammation of the Pharynx
A. One of the most common afflictions of mankind. Frequently a symptom of various types of illness.
B. Symptoms include dry, scratchy feeling in the throat, slight fever, chills, and malaise.
C. Treated with hot saline gargles or throat irrigations. Antibiotics and sulfonamides

may help prevent secondary bacterial infections when the pharyngitis is severe.

II. Tonsillitis—inflammation of the tonsils, usually caused by streptococci or staphylococci

A. Symptoms may be similar to those of pharyngitis; however, the two are completely different disorders.

B. Acute tonsillitis produces symptoms of sore throat, fever, and chills. Treated with antibiotics, rest in bed, aspirin, and forcing fluids.

C. Chronic tonsillitis produces enlargement of the tonsils and adenoids. Individual has frequent colds, breathes through his mouth, and often snores in his sleep. Gives the general impression of being in poor physical health and may be considered to be mentally dull because of his facial expression and impairment in his hearing.

D. Care of patient undergoing tonsillectomy and adenoidectomy

1. This should not be considered a minor operation because there is always the danger of hemorrhage.

2. Patient is watched carefully for signs of external bleeding. Vital signs are recorded often; patient watched for frequent swallowing which may indicate bleeding from the operative site.

3. Ice collar applied to the neck will reduce swelling and discourage development of hemorrhage.

4. Diet usually consists of ice-cold liquids, ice cream, and chilled gelatins and custards.

5. During convalescent stage citrus fruits, hot liquids, and rough foods are restricted until healing is complete.

Questions

Mrs. Bond is a 50-year-old neighbor of yours whom you have known for several years. Within the past few months she has mentioned to you that she has frequent headaches and burning and itching of her eyes. Her eyes tire easily and become very red and watery whenever she reads or sews. She asks your advice about going to an optometrist to get some "reading glasses."

1. As a practical nurse you should know that an optometrist is:
   1. a medical doctor who specializes in the diagnosis and treatment of visual defects and diseases of the eye
   2. an individual who is trained to make glasses and optical instruments
   3. an individual who is trained only in scientific examination of the eyes for the purpose of prescribing glasses
   4. a physician who examines the eyes for visual defects and prescribes lenses for glasses

2. Mrs. Bond's symptoms are most likely indicative of:
   1. normal changes that occur in the eye as a result of the aging process
   2. mild conjunctivitis that can be treated with irrigations of the eye
   3. simple eyestrain resulting from fatigue of the muscles of the eye
   4. some visual defect that should be investigated by an ophthalmologist

3. When Mrs. Bond had her eyes tested the physician used Snellen's chart. A normal reading for this test would be:
   1. 20/20 vision
   2. 20/100 vision
   3. 100/20 vision
   4. 10/100 vision

4. Mrs. Bond also was tested for proper focusing of light rays on the retina. The physician applied various types of lenses and asked Mrs. Bond to read Snellen's chart through the lenses. This test is known as:
   1. a refraction
   2. an audiometry
   3. a tonometry
   4. an infraction

5. In another test the physician determined the amount of intraocular pressure in each of Mrs. Bond's eyes. This test is extremely important in diagnosing:
    1. myopia
    2. astigmatism
    3. hyperopia
    4. glaucoma
6. The lay term for myopia is:
    1. crossed eyes
    2. astigmatism
    3. farsightedness
    4. nearsightedness
7. Mrs. Bond was found to have astigmatism. This condition is treated by prescribing lenses which:
    1. strengthen the muscles which move the eyeball
    2. magnify objects being seen
    3. assist in focusing light rays on the retina
    4. strengthen the muscles which move the lenses of the eyes

The following questions refer to various disorders of the eye.

8. If a foreign body is not deeply imbedded in the tissue of the eye, it can be removed most easily by:
    1. rubbing the eye gently
    2. irrigating the eye with boric acid solution
    3. touching the foreign body with a corner of a clean handkerchief
    4. using a sterilized needle to lift the foreign body from the eye
9. Conjunctivitis is best defined as an inflammation of:
    1. the glands around the edge of the eyelids
    2. the mucous membrane lining the eyelids and covering the front of the eyeball
    3. tear ducts of the eyes
    4. fluid within the eyeball
10. Pink-eye is caused by a specific organism and is considered to be:
    1. highly contagious
    2. an infection of the inner part of the eye
    3. a mild type of staphylococcal infection
    4. quickly cured by frequent irrigations of the eye with normal saline
11. A cataract is best defined as:
    1. cloudiness of the fluid within the eyeball
    2. a condition in which the pressure within the eyeball is increased
    3. an infection of the conjunctiva
    4. a condition in which the lens of the eye becomes cloudy and opaque
12. A cataract extraction involves:
    1. incision and drainage of fluid from the eyeball
    2. surgical removal of the lens of the eye
    3. enlargement of the pupil of the eye
    4. removal of a growth from the retina
13. During the immediate postoperative period following a cataract extraction, it is most important that the nurse:
    1. encourage deep breathing and coughing to properly ventilate the lungs
    2. observe the patient for signs of hemorrhage, which is a common complication
    3. instruct the patient to avoid coughing, sneezing, or sudden movement of the head which will place a strain on the sutures
    4. encourage the patient to get out of bed as soon as possible to avoid circulatory complications
14. If compresses or irrigations are ordered following a cataract extraction, the nurse should know that the chief purpose of these treatments is to:
    1. remove exudate from the eyelids
    2. irrigate the eyeball and conjunctival sac
    3. apply sufficient heat to localize the infection present
    4. remove and destroy bacteria on or near the operative site

15. A disease of the eye which is characterized by increased pressure within the eyeball is:
    1. cataract
    2. glaucoma
    3. strabismus
    4. astigmatism
16. Pressure within the eyeball is measured by an instrument called:
    1. an audiometer
    2. an oculometer
    3. a tonometer
    4. an ophthalmoscope
17. Which of the following symptoms would be indicative of the early stages of glaucoma?
    1. redness and excessive tearing
    2. difficulty in adjusting to darkened rooms after being in the light, and a narrowing of vision at the sides of one or both eyes
    3. increasing loss of vision and severe headache
    4. increasing difficulty in distinguishing colors
18. Whenever the nurse enters the room of a patient who is blind she should:
    1. speak to him so that he will be aware of her presence
    2. gently shake him to be sure he is awake before she speaks to him
    3. knock on the door and wait for him to invite her in
    4. be sure to speak loudly and distinctly so the patient can hear her
19. Deafness that is brought about by a disorder of the auditory nerve is referred to as:
    1. conductive deafness
    2. sensorineural deafness
    3. traumatic deafness
    4. obstructive deafness
20. Otitis media is an inflammation of the:
    1. auditory canal
    2. eardrum
    3. middle ear
    4. inner ear
21. Otitis media may be treated by incision of the eardrum. This procedure is referred to as:
    1. a mastoidectomy
    2. an adenoidectomy
    3. spontaneous rupture
    4. a myringotomy
22. An infection of the mastoid bone often occurs as a complication of:
    1. streptococcal infection of the throat
    2. otitis media
    3. sinusitis
    4. encephalitis
23. Otosclerosis produces loss of hearing in the affected ear primarily because:
    1. the auditory nerve is permanently damaged
    2. there is an obstruction in the external canal of the ear
    3. the small bones of the inner ear have become sclerotic and cannot vibrate
    4. the auditory nerve is inflamed
24. The most serious and common complication following a tonsillectomy and adenoidectomy is:
    1. asphyxia
    2. hemorrhage
    3. deafness
    4. loss of speech

25. Aside from the obvious signs of external bleeding following a tonsillectomy, the nurse should also suspect hemorrhage when the patient:
    1. is unable to make sounds
    2. appears to be swallowing repeatedly
    3. complains of severe pain in the operative region
    4. does not react to the anesthetic in a normal manner

26. To reduce swelling and bleeding from the operative site, it would be best for the nurse to:
    1. apply a hot water bottle to the neck
    2. place the patient in the Trendelenburg position
    3. keep the patient lying face down
    4. apply an ice collar to the neck

27. During the convalescent period, when healing of the operative site is not yet complete, it would be best for the patient to:
    1. avoid eating very cold foods
    2. stay on a clear liquid diet
    3. avoid hot liquids, highly spiced foods, and those with a good bit of roughage
    4. eat as he normally would so as to prevent deficiences in the intake of vitamins and minerals

Part VIII

FIRST AID AND EMERGENCY NURSING

I. **Introduction**
   A. Definition—first aid is the immediate temporary care given to the victim at the scene of an accident before medical attention can be obtained.
   B. General directions for first aid
      1. Remember to do first things first. The first consideration is to restore breathing if necessary. Other emergencies needing immediate care include severe bleeding and poisoning.
      2. Keep victim lying down
         a. Avoid unnecessary or rough handling.
         b. Maintain normal body temperature; do not overheat the victim.
      3. Check for injuries
         a. Obtain information about what happened to the victim.
         b. Find the parts of the body that may be injured.
         c. When in doubt about injury to a part, immobilize it.
      4. Plan course of action
         a. Call a physician or ambulance.
         b. Instruct helpers with their duties.
         c. Carry out indicated first aid.

II. **Wounds**
   A. Definition—a wound is a break in the skin or mucous membrane.
   B. Types
      1. Abrasion—rubbing or scraping off the skin by friction.
      2. Incision—sharp cut that tends to bleed freely.
      3. Laceration—jagged or irregular wound; flesh is torn.
      4. Puncture—skin is deeply penetrated, wound may penetrate underlying tissues.
   C. Infection
      1. Definition—growth of pathogenic microorganisms in wound.
      2. Signs and symptoms of infection
         a. Evidence does not appear immediately; may take from 2 to 7 days.
         b. Wound is tender, red, and swollen, and pus often appears.
         c. Sometimes there are red streaks along the affected limb and swollen nodules in the armpit or groin.
      3. Treatment for minor wounds includes thorough cleansing with soap and running water. A clean or sterile dry dressing is applied.
      4. Wounds from which bleeding is severe
         a. Main objective is to stop bleeding at once, always with pressure applied directly over the wound. A clean cloth is used whenever possible.
         b. Pressure to the blood vessel will diminish the bleeding but will not stop it completely (See Fig. 45).
         c. Use of a tourniquet is justifiable only rarely. The decision to apply a tour-

niquet is actually a decision to risk sacrificing a limb in order to save a life.

5. Tetanus (lockjaw) must always be borne in mind, especially with puncture wounds. Tetanus antitoxin is given if no prior immunization to tetanus has been established.

D. Nosebleed often occurs spontaneously and usually is the result of injury to the nose. Treated by keeping the person quiet in a sitting position or lying down with head and shoulders raised. Pressure against the sides of the nostrils will stop the flow of blood. Cold wet compresses applied to the face may help stop the bleeding.

III. Animal Bites

A. Animal should be restrained or prevented from escaping. Animal should not be killed unless this is done to protect others from being bitten.

B. Police, physician, and veterinarian should be notified immediately.

C. Wound is thoroughly cleansed as in other types of wounds.

D. Rabies must always be considered a possibility when animal has not been inoculated. This disease is invariably fatal in man once it has developed.

IV. Shock

A. Definition—the word has many meanings. In first aid it refers to circulatory failure following serious injury.

B. Symptoms of shock
   1. Shallow and irregular breathing.
   2. Pulse weak or absent.
   3. Skin pale, cold, and clammy.
   4. Pupils dilated, eyes have a vacant, lackluster appearance.

C. Treatment
   1. Keep the patient lying down. Elevate feet except when these symptoms develop.
      a. Evidence of a head injury.
      b. Difficulty in breathing.
      c. Severe pain when head is lowered.
   2. Application of external heat may be harmful. Use only enough light covering to maintain normal body temperature and prevent loss of body heat.
   3. Fluids of any kind should not be given if the patient is partly conscious or unconscious, has an abdominal wound, or might require surgery within a few

hours. If fluids are given, it is best to give tap water.

V. Artificial Respiration

A. Definition—bringing about a flow of air into and out of the lungs by mechanical means when natural breathing ceases.

B. Uses—in nonbreathing victims of (1) shock, (2) drowning, (3) gas poisoning, (4) drug poisoning, or (5) foreign body in the respiratory tract.

C. Most practical and effective method of artificial respiration is generally considered to be mouth-to-mouth or mouth-to-nose (Fig. 46).
   1. First step is tilting the head backward to lift the tongue away from the back of the throat. This simple maneuver may be all that is necessary for victim to resume breathing spontaneously.
   2. If the head tilt is not effective, opening the air passage adequately may be accomplished by positioning the lower jaw forward (jaw thrust). Once the head is placed in a position for optimum breathing, this position is maintained throughout the procedure of artificial respiration.
   3. Blow into the mouth of the victim, being sure that the nose is pinched

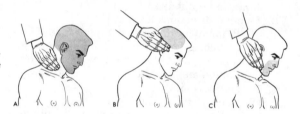

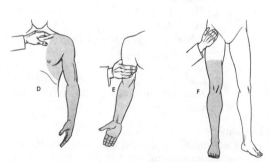

FIGURE 45. Pressure points. (Crawford, *Nursing Clinics of North America*, Vol. 2, No. 2, June 1967.)

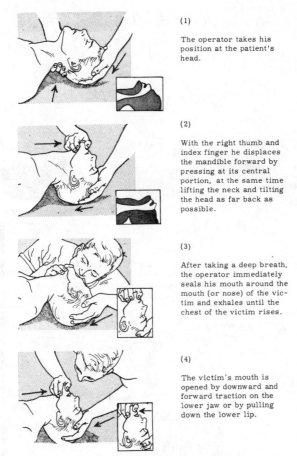

(1)

The operator takes his position at the patient's head.

(2)

With the right thumb and index finger he displaces the mandible forward by pressing at its central portion, at the same time lifting the neck and tilting the head as far back as possible.

(3)

After taking a deep breath, the operator immediately seals his mouth around the mouth (or nose) of the victim and exhales until the chest of the victim rises.

(4)

The victim's mouth is opened by downward and forward traction on the lower jaw or by pulling down the lower lip.

FIGURE 46. Technique of mouth-to-mouth resuscitation. (From Chatton, M. J., et al.: *Handbook of Medical Treatment.* 12th ed. Los Altos, Calif., Lange Medical Publishers, 1970.)

closed. In very small children the nose and mouth may be covered by the mouth of the person administering artificial respiration.

  4. For adults, one should blow vigorously 12 times per minute. For a child, relatively shallow breaths are blown into the lungs at the rate of about 20 per minute.

VI. Heart-Lung Resuscitation—indicated when heart has stopped beating and respirations have ceased.

  A. Symptoms of cardiac arrest are loss of consciousness, absence of pulse and heart sounds, and dilation of pupils.

  B. As soon as cardiac arrest is recognized initial treatment must be started. This consists of administering one or two sharp blows over the cardiac area.

  C. The lungs are then inflated rapidly 3 to 5 times;

  D. A firm support should be placed under the patient's chest if he is not lying on the floor or ground.

  E. External cardiac massage involves
    1. Depression of the lower third of the sternum to a depth of 1½ to 2 inches (38 to 51 mm.) using the heel of the hand,
    2. Holding the sternum down for ½ second,
    3. Rapid release of pressure without completely removing the hand from the sternum.

  F. Steps of heart-lung resuscitation (see Fig. 47).

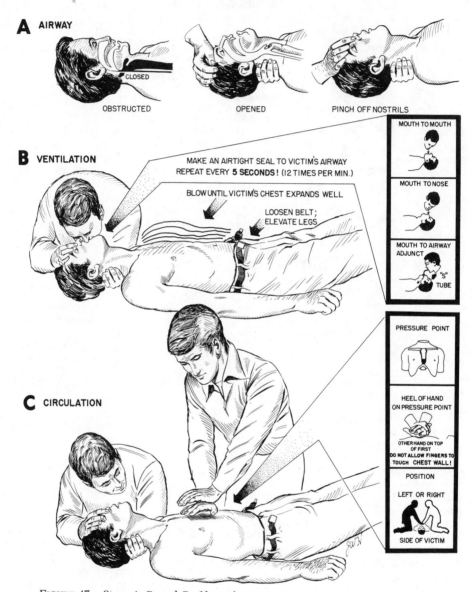

A AIRWAY

CLOSED

OBSTRUCTED   OPENED   PINCH OFF NOSTRILS

B VENTILATION

MAKE AN AIRTIGHT SEAL TO VICTIM'S AIRWAY
REPEAT EVERY **5 SECONDS**! (12 TIMES PER MIN.)

BLOW UNTIL VICTIM'S CHEST EXPANDS WELL

LOOSEN BELT;
ELEVATE LEGS

MOUTH TO MOUTH

MOUTH TO NOSE

MOUTH TO AIRWAY
ADJUNCT

"S" TUBE

C CIRCULATION

PRESSURE POINT

HEEL OF HAND
ON PRESSURE POINT

OTHER HAND ON TOP
OF FIRST
DO NOT ALLOW FINGERS TO
TOUCH CHEST WALL!

POSITION

LEFT OR RIGHT

SIDE OF VICTIM

FIGURE 47.   Steps A, B, and C of heart-lung resuscitation emergency treatment.

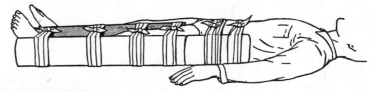

FIGURE 48. Splinted leg. (Miller and Miller: *Good Health: Personal and Community.*)

FOR BREAK IN UPPER LEG, OUTER BOARD SHOULD EXTEND TO WAIST; WRAP TOP PART OF BOARD SEPARATELY

VII. Poisoning by Mouth

A. Causes include attempts at suicide and accidental poisoning.

B. Prevention
1. Remember that most young children often cannot distinguish between what should be eaten and what should not be eaten.
2. Keep poisons, medicines, household disinfectants, etc. out of the reach of small children.
3. Educate older children regarding the danger of poisonous substances.
4. Do not keep remaining portions of partially used prescriptions in the home.

C. Signs and symptoms
1. Information from the victim or someone who saw the incident.
2. Sudden onset of pain or illness in a person previously well.
3. Finding the container where it does not belong.
4. Burns about the lips and mouth or a revealing odor to the breath.

D. First Aid
1. Not advisable to have victim drink large quantities of water or any other liquid
2. Induce vomiting except when
   a. Victim has swallowed a corrosive poison, a petroleum product, iodine, or strychnine.
   b. Victim is in a coma or has convulsions.
3. To induce vomiting give an emetic, usually syrup of ipecac. If none available place finger or spoon at back of throat.
4. Lavage may be done if vomiting should not or cannot be induced.
5. Give specific antidote for the poison. If not known, give activated charcoal in doses of 10 times the estimated ingested dose as a 25 per cent solution in water.
6. Keep victim calm and warm. Transfer to hospital or clinic immediately.
7. If at all possible, take container of poison to hospital.

VIII. Injuries to Bones, Muscles, and Joints

A. Signs and symptoms of fracture
1. Swelling, pain, tenderness, deformity, and pain on motion are the obvious signs.
2. Do not judge whether a fracture is present on the basis of loss of motion. Motion may be possible when a fracture is present.
3. X-ray examination is the most accurate form of diagnosis and should be done when there is any possibility of a fracture.

B. First aid for fractures
1. Immobilize the part immediately. "Splint them where they lie." (See Figures 48 and 49).
2. If fracture is compound and skin is broken, apply a sterile dressing over the wound.
3. Handle the affected part as little as possible.

C. Sprains
1. Definition—injury to the soft tissue around a joint.
2. Swelling, tenderness, and pain on motion are symptoms of a sprain.

D. First aid for sprains
1. Immobilize the part as you would for a fracture (Fig. 50).
2. Elevate the joint.
3. Apply cold wet compresses or an ice bag to affected joint.
4. Later the joint should be x-rayed for evidence of a small fracture.

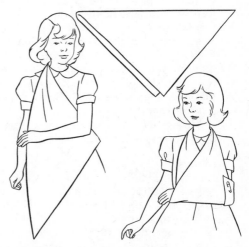

FIGURE 49. A triangular bandage or sling. (Culver: *Modern Bedside Nursing.* 8th ed.)

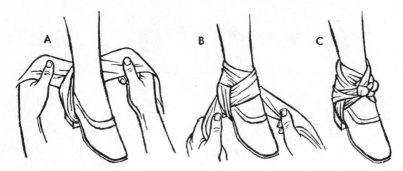

FIGURE 50. Temporary support for sprained ankle. (American Red Cross. 4th ed., © 1957.)

E. Dislocations
1. Definition—displacement of the bones of a joint.
2. Signs and symptoms
a. Similar to those of a fracture or sprain.
b. Abnormal shape to the joint.
3. First aid
a. Treat as a fracture and immobilize the joint.
b. Do not attempt to pull the bone into place.

IX. **Effects of Extreme Heat and Cold**
A. Burns—three general kinds
1. Thermal—heat.
2. Sunburn—ultraviolet rays.
3. Chemical—caustic substances; alkalis, acids, or other strong chemicals.
B. Classification
1. First degree—skin is reddened and hot to the touch.
2. Second degree—blisters form at site of burn.
3. Third degree—destruction of underlying structures as well as all layers of skin. Appears to be charred or may be dead white and lifeless in appearance.
C. Emergency treatment
1. Keep victim quiet and lying down.
2. Cover the burned area with sterile dressing, or, if they are not available, use clean sheets or towels. Dressings of this type keep out bacteria and air and reduce pain.
3. If burn is minor, cold compresses may be applied to reduce pain; a clean dressing is then applied. Do NOT rupture blisters.
4. Unless the burn is obviously not a second or third degree burn and is not extensive, NO ointment or salve should ever be applied.
5. In any type of *chemical* burn, the most important aspect of emergency treatment is to liberally apply water to dilute the chemical and reduce the amount of

damage done to the body tissues.
D. Frostbite
1. Definition—freezing of a part of the body. Parts more often affected are cheeks, nose, ears, fingers, and toes.
2. Signs and symptoms
a. Skin may be slightly flushed at first; later changes to a white or grayish-yellow color. Blisters may form.
b. There may be pain, and the affected part may feel intensely cold and numb.
3. Emergency treatment
a. Cover the frozen part and provide extra warmth to raise the body temperature to normal.
b. DO NOT RUB THE AREA. This increases damage to the tissues and increases the danger of gangrene.
c. Rewarm the affected part by placing it in water that is within the range of normal body temperature. DO NOT USE HOT WATER.
d. After rewarming the part, encourage the victim to exercise the affected part to increase circulation.

X. **Special Wounds**
A. Snake bites
1. Most snake bite fatalities in this country are caused by rattlesnakes. Other poisonous snakes in the United States include copperheads, cottonmouth moccasins, and the coral snake.
2. Emergency treatment
a. Keep the victim quiet. Muscular activity increases circulation of the venom throughout the body. Keep injured part lower than the rest of the body.
b. Apply a tourniquet above the bite if it is on an extremity. Tourniquet should be loose enough to allow for slight oozing of blood through the wound.
c. Apply cold compress to area to decrease circulation.

d. Cross-cuts over fang marks are *not* recommended by most experts because the cuts usually are not deep enough to do any good.

B. Scorpion stings
1. Most species of scorpions in this country do not inject a highly poisonous type of venom.
2. If sting is on an extremity, a constricting band is placed above the sting and left in place for 5 minutes.
3. The site of the sting should be packed in ice and medical attention should be obtained immediately.

C. Black widow spider bites
1. Almost all victims recover without serious complications. Small children and very old persons are likely to be most seriously affected.
2. First aid treatment is the same as for scorpion stings.

D. Insect bites and stings
1. Application of ice or ice water should be done immediately.
2. A paste made from baking soda, or compresses of ammonia water, relieve stinging and itching.

E. Tick bites
1. Some types of ticks transmit Rocky Mountain spotted fever.
2. Removal of entire body and head of tick is very important in the prevention of infection.
   a. Best method for removing the tick is to cover it with some type of heavy oil to close its breathing pores and then wait for it to remove its head. After 30 minutes, if head is still in the flesh, tweezers may be used to remove the tick.
   b. Lighted cigarettes, applications of heat, or use of tweezers to remove the tick as soon as it is found may damage the skin or leave parts of tick imbedded in the tissues.

F. Plant poisoning
1. Most common types are poison ivy, poison oak, and poison sumac.
2. Learning to identify the plants and avoiding contact with them is the best method of preventing poisoning.
   a. Poison ivy and oak have three leaflets.
   b. Leaves are usually glossy and dark green. Color may change to red or orange in the fall.
3. Signs and symptoms
   a. Itching, formation of small blisters at point of contact.
   b. Swelling of the part and fever may occur.
4. First aid
   a. Wash the part with soap and running water and then cleanse with alcohol.
   b. Calamine lotion may help relieve the itching.
   c. Serious reactions or extensive involvement should receive medical attention.

XI. **Emergency Childbirth**—steps to be taken when a physician or more experienced individual is not available.
A. Place mother on her back.
B. Keep vaginal area as clean and free from contamination as possible.
C. Do not attempt to push or pull infant through birth canal.
D. Wipe the infant's nose and mouth with a clean cloth to remove mucus and to clear air passages.
E. Leave infant between mother's knees and cover with a blanket or clean cloth. If it is apparent that medical help will not be available within an hour, some authorities recommend putting the infant to breast to stimulate uterine contractions and reduce bleeding.
F. The cord will not require attention unless a physician cannot be available within an hour. If the cord is to be cut, it must be tied securely about two inches (51 mm.) from the navel and again at about six inches (15 cm.). The cord is cut between the two ties, using a knife or scissors that has been sterilized.
G. The placenta should be saved for the physician's inspection.
H. The fundus should be massaged after the placenta is expelled to stimulate contraction of the uterus.

Questions

1. If a nurse came upon the scene of an accident and found that several persons had been injured, which of the following victims would require her *immediate* attention? The person having:
   1. a fracture of the lower leg
   2. severe bleeding

      3. multiple abrasions

      4. burns of the upper extremities

2. An abrasion is a wound made by:

      1. rubbing or scraping of the skin

      2. cutting deeply into the skin

      3. puncturing the skin

      4. jagged or irregular cutting of the skin

3. Penetrating the skin with a sharp instrument, such as a nail, causes which of the following types of wounds?

      1. laceration

      2. incision

      3. contusion

      4. puncture

4. If a wound is infected, the symptoms of infection are most likely to appear:

      1. immediately

      2. within 24 hours after injury

      3. from 2 to 7 days after injury

      4. several weeks after injury

5. The symptoms of a wound infection most often include:

      1. tenderness, swelling, redness, warm to touch, sometimes appearance of pus

      2. bloody and purulent drainage

      3. red streaks extending upward from wound, pain, swelling

      4. loss of motion, increased white blood cells, redness, sloughing of the tissues

6. The danger of tetanus should be considered in:

      1. puncture wounds only

      2. all lacerations

      3. severe burns

      4. all wounds

7. The lay term for tetanus is:

      1. gangrene

      2. lockjaw

      3. rabies

      4. blood poisoning

8. If a patient has not been immunized against tetanus prior to the injury, the doctor will most likely give:

      1. tetanus toxoid

      2. tetanus antitoxin

      3. tetanus serum

      4. tetanus gamma globulin

9. The most acceptable method for controlling severe bleeding is:

      1. application of a tourniquet for not more than 1 hour

      2. applying pressure directly over the wound

      3. elevation of the part

      4. application of a tourniquet until the victim is seen by a physician

10. If a person is bitten by a stray dog, it is most important to:

      1. prevent the animal from escaping

      2. kill the animal immediately

      3. attempt to locate the owner

      4. rush the victim to a veterinarian

11. Rabies is considered to be especially dangerous because it is:

      1. likely to cause mental deterioration

      2. invariably fatal once it develops

      3. caused by a virus

      4. widespread among domestic animals

12. The signs and symptoms of shock include:
    1. rapid pulse, cold moist skin
    2. slow pulse, flushed face, rapid respirations
    3. rapid respirations, rapid pulse, hot dry skin
    4. dyspnea, nausea, bounding pulse
13. When shock is present the immediate treatment usually includes:
    1. application of hot water bottles and blankets to elevate the body temperature
    2. elevation of the lower extremities and prevention of loss of body heat
    3. elevation of the head and application of hot water bottles to the lower extremities
    4. rubbing the wrists and applying cold cloths to the forehead
14. What is the best rule to follow in regard to administering fluids to a shock victim?
    1. If the victim has difficulty swallowing give only small sips of water.
    2. Alcoholic beverages are permissible in small amounts.
    3. Always administer salt and soda solutions to replace necessary electrolytes.
    4. Do not give anything by mouth if medical assistance will be available within a reasonable length of time.
15. According to the American National Red Cross, the most practical and effective method of artificial respiration is:
    1. back pressure-arm lift
    2. abdominal pressure
    3. mouth-to-mouth
    4. chest pressure-arm lift
16. The first step in resuscitation of a person who is not breathing is to:
    1. tilt the head backward and extend the neck
    2. place the victim in prone position
    3. blow vigorously into the victim's mouth three or four times
    4. grasp the victim's tongue and pull it forward
17. The ABC's of cardiopulmonary resuscitation are:
    1. always be careful
    2. artificial breathing and compression
    3. airway, breathing, circulation
    4. airway, breathing, consciousness
18. When administering mouth-to-mouth resuscitation, one should blow vigorously into the mouth of an adult victim and blow short puffs into the mouth of a child. The correct rate per minute for this blowing effort is:
    1. 20 for adults, 5 for children
    2. 12 for adults, 40 for children
    3. 20 for adults, 12 for children
    4. 12 for adults, 20 for children
19. Accidental poisoning in children is most often due to:
    1. the child's inability to distinguish between what should and should not be eaten
    2. the pleasant or sweet taste of most poisonous substances
    3. improper storage or preparation of foods
    4. improper labeling of poisonous substances
20. An emetic recommended to induce vomiting in cases of swallowed poison is:
    1. castor oil
    2. syrup of ipecac
    3. vinegar
    4. tincture of opium
21. One incidence of accidental poisoning in which vomiting should not be induced is the ingestion of:
    1. aspirin
    2. kerosene
    3. laxatives
    4. sleeping pills

22. When a victim is taken to an emergency clinic or doctor's office following ingestion of a poison it is most important to bring the:
    1. container for identification of the poison
    2. antidote used
    3. victim's hospitalization insurance policy
    4. vomitus obtained during first aid treatment
23. The substance that is given after vomiting has been induced in cases of swallowed poisons is:
    1. activated charcoal
    2. milk of magnesia
    3. syrup of ipecac
    4. acetic acid
24. A fracture in which a jagged edge of bone can be seen protruding through a break in the skin is called a:
    1. simple or closed fracture
    2. compound or open fracture
    3. greenstick fracture
    4. comminuted fracture
25. The most important point to remember in the emergency treatment of a fracture is to:
    1. use only splints from a standard first aid kit
    2. always elevate the part before splinting it
    3. apply ice bags to the part to reduce swelling before the splint is applied
    4. apply the splint before moving the victim
26. The safest and most accurate means of diagnosing a closed fracture is by:
    1. asking the victim if he can move the injured limb
    2. determining whether the victim can bear weight on the injured limb
    3. x-ray of the injured part
    4. examining the injured part for signs of a break in the skin

A practical nurse has volunteered to accompany a group of girl scouts on an overnight camping trip. In anticipation of the minor accidents that often occur on such an excursion, she brought along her first-aid kit. During the hike to the campsite Margie, a 13-year-old girl, slipped and hurt her ankle.

27. Margie sustained a minor sprain of the ankle. A sprain is:
    1. a dislocation of the bones of a joint
    2. a fracture in which the bone is slightly chipped
    3. a stretching of the ligaments around the joint
    4. an injury to a muscle due to overexertion
28. When applying a bandage to Margie's ankle the nurse should:
    1. pad the ankle with an article of clothing before applying the bandage
    2. have someone exert a steady pull on the foot while the bandage is applied
    3. remove Margie's shoe before applying the bandage
    4. leave the shoe on to give added support to the bandage
29. As soon as Margie arrived at the girl scout camp the nurse should have treated the sprain by taking the following measures:
    a. elevating the affected ankle
    b. applying cold compresses or an ice bag
    c. soaking the foot in hot Epsom salts solution
    d. massaging the ankle with liniment

    1. all but c
    2. b and d
    3. a and c
    4. a and b
30. Mrs. Thomas was severely burned when she fell asleep while smoking a cigarette, and ignited her clothing. If a nurse had been at the scene of the accident she should have:
    a. applied sterile petroleum jelly to the burned areas
    b. wrapped Mrs. Thomas in a clean sheet and made arrangements to take her to the hospital
    c. kept the patient calm and lying down
    d. applied a tourniquet to prevent hemorrhage

    1. all but b
    2. a, b, and c
    3. b and c
    4. c and d

31. A second degree burn can be recognized by the presence of:
    1. charring of the skin and underlying tissues
    2. a white and lifeless appearance to the skin
    3. blistering of the burned area
    4. redness of the burned area
32. A third degree burn:
    1. involves both layers of the skin and damage to the underlying tissues
    2. is accompanied by a severe and lasting pain until regeneration of the skin occurs
    3. heals without scarring
    4. involves only the epidermis
33. The most essential first aid treatment for a chemical burn of the skin is to:
    1. wash the area in baking soda solution
    2. wash with large quantities of water
    3. apply petroleum jelly to the area immediately
    4. wash the area with vinegar solution
34. In cases of minor burns, pain can be relieved and swelling reduced if:
    1. warm compresses are applied to the area
    2. the blisters are ruptured and the fluid allowed to drain
    3. cold compresses are applied to the area immediately
    4. butter or some other type of grease is applied immediately
35. When frostbite occurs, the affected part:
    1. appears to be white or yellowish-gray in color and feels intensely cold and numb
    2. becomes very red and has no sensation of heat or cold
    3. appears to be swollen and feels warm and comfortable
    4. remains normal in color but feels intensely hot
36. First aid treatment of frostbite involves:
    1. vigorously rubbing the area to increase circulation
    2. immersing the part in hot water
    3. elevating the part to reduce circulation
    4. covering the part to provide extra warmth, and then encouraging exercise of the part
37. To place a triangular bandage on the arm for use as a sling, the apex of the triangle is located at the:
    1. elbow
    2. wrist
    3. shoulder
    4. waist
38. When the two ends of a triangular bandage are tied at the back the knot should *never* be located:
    1. at the shoulder of the affected arm
    2. at the shoulder of the unaffected arm
    3. directly over the spine at the back of the neck
    4. over the jugular vein
39. A poisonous snake bite is treated by first applying a constricting band *above* the bite. The band should be applied so that it is tight enough to:
    1. prevent all circulation to the affected part
    2. allow for circulation in the surface vessels only
    3. allow for circulation in the deeper vessels and the surface vessels
    4. prevent circulation in the surface vessels but not shut off deep-lying vessels
40. The victim of a poisonous snake bite will have less venom circulating in his body if he is:
    1. given a mild stimulant such as coffee or some alcoholic drink
    2. kept quiet and the injured part is elevated above the level of the heart
    3. placed in an upright position and given sips of soda solution to drink
    4. kept lying down with the affected part lower than the rest of the body

41. First aid treatment of scorpion stings or black widow spider bites is aimed at preventing the spread of the venom through the body. One of the best ways of accomplishing this is by applying:
    1. hot compresses to the bite
    2. a tourniquet for at least 2 hours
    3. direct pressure over the bite
    4. ice or ice water to the bite

42. The safest and most effective means for removing a tick from the body is by:
    1. pulling it out with tweezers
    2. applying heat with a lighted cigarette
    3. covering the tick with a heavy oil, such as mineral oil or salad oil
    4. removing the head of the tick with a needle just as a splinter is removed

43. Poison ivy and poison oak are most easily recognized by:
    a. their three leaflets   1. all but d
    b. the glossy appearance   2. a and b
    c. their five leaflets   3. b and c
    d. their red stems   4. c and d

44. If a person realizes that he has been exposed to poisonous plants such as poison ivy or poison oak he should:
    1. receive injections of the plant serum
    2. wash the exposed area in warm, soapy water and rinse well
    3. avoid opening the blisters and spreading disease to other parts of the body
    4. rub the exposed area vigorously and apply some type of oil

45. Which of the following is *not* a sign of cardiac arrest?
    1. loss of consciousness
    2. absence of pulse
    3. dilatation of pupils
    4. hot, dry skin

46. When cardiac arrest is recognized, what is the first step to be taken?
    1. loosen constricting clothing
    2. administer one or two sharp blows to the chest
    3. inflate the lungs
    4. place the victim on his abdomen and clear airway

47. When only one operator is carrying out heart-lung resuscitation, what is the ratio of inflation of the lungs to compression of the sternum?
    1. 4 to 20
    2. 2 to 10
    3. 5 to 10
    4. 2 to 15

48. When two operators are carrying out heart-lung resuscitation, the person inflating the lungs should:
    1. ask the person giving cardiac massage to stop every tenth compression so he can inflate the lungs
    2. interpose one inflation after every fifth compression, working in rhythm with the other operator
    3. interpose one inflation during every fifth compression.
    4. ask the person giving cardiac massage to stop after 15 compressions and then rapidly inflate the lungs five times, repeating this cycle as long as necessary

49. If you were assisting a mother during an emergency childbirth, when would you cut the umbilical cord?
    1. just before the expulsion of the placenta
    2. immediately after expulsion of the placenta
    3. within 15 minutes after expulsion of the placenta
    4. not at all if a physician will be available within an hour after the birth

50. If you cut the cord where would you cut it?
    1. six inches (15 cm.) above the navel
    2. between the two places where the cord has been tied
    3. above the second tie and about seven inches (18 cm.) from the navel
    4. above and below the second tie

51. Why would it be advisable to put a baby to the breast immediately after birth if medical help will not be available for several hours?
    1. to avoid loss of the infant's body heat
    2. to prevent dehydration of the infant
    3. to prevent excessive uterine bleeding
    4. to keep the mother calm and her attention diverted from the emergency situation

Part IX
NURSING THE PATIENT WITH A COMMUNICABLE DISEASE

I. **Definitions of General Terms**
   A. Communicable disease—one that is spread by direct contact with the INFECTIOUS AGENTS causing the disease.
   B. Contamination—the presence of living pathogenic microorganisms in or on an article, person, or matter.
   C. Contact—any person or animal known to have been in association with an infected person and likely to develop a specific illness as a result.
   D. Carrier—a person who is without symptoms of an infectious disease but still harbors and spreads the living microorganisms to others.
   E. Disinfection—killing of pathogenic microorganisms by chemical or mechanical means.
      1. Concurrent disinfection—immediate destruction of microorganisms as they leave the body, or after they have contaminated linen, eating utensils, etc. in the patient's environment.
      2. Terminal disinfection—destruction of pathogenic microorganisms from the patient's environment after he is no longer considered to be a source of infection.
   F. Isolation—separating the patient from others and confining him to his unit until he is no longer a source of infection.

II. **General Principles of Nursing Care**
   A. Pathogenic microorganisms enter and leave the human body in a number of ways; for example, through the respiratory tract, intestinal tract, skin, and mucous membranes. All persons concerned with the care of a patient with a communicable disease should be thoroughly familiar with the ways in which that specific disease may be spread. Modes of transmission of infectious diseases include
      1. Direct contact with the body excreta or drainage from an ulcer, open sore, etc.
      2. Indirect contact with inanimate objects such as drinking glasses, toys, bed clothing, etc.
      3. Vectors—flies, fleas, mosquitoes, or other insects which are capable of spreading disease.
   B. The more prolonged the contact with an infected person and his surroundings, the more likely the chance for contamination.
   C. The single factor that is most important in preventing the spread of disease is proper handwashing. The hands are used for many nursing tasks, and are therefore most likely to be excellent sources of infections if they are not washed after each contact with a patient.

III. **Nursing Care of the Patient in Strict Isolation**
   A. General principles
      1. All unnecessary equipment and upholstered furniture should be removed from the patient's unit before he is admitted to the room.
      2. Once the patient has entered his room everything in the room must be considered contaminated.
      3. The door to the patient's room should be kept closed at all times.
      4. Visitors are restricted to members of the family and all persons entering the isolation unit should follow the isolation procedure required by the hospital.
      5. The spread of microorganisms can be kept at a minimum if it is always borne in mind that we touch only "clean to clean" and "contaminated to contaminated." Once a clean article has come in contact with a contaminated article, both must be considered to be contaminated.
   B. Special techniques

1. Hand washing is necessary each time the patient receives care or the nurse realizes that her hands are grossly contaminated.
   a. Use of running water is much preferred to the use of a basin of disinfectant solution.
   b. Friction between the hands during hand washing is very important in the removal of microorganisms from the lines and crevices in the skin.
   c. In medical asepsis the nurse is considered *un*contaminated and her hands are kept below the level of the elbows during the hand washing procedure.
   d. If bar soap is used, it is kept in the hands throughout the entire hand washing procedure until the hands are rinsed for the last time.
   e. The hands should be washed for at least 1 full minute.
   f. When foot pedals are not used to control the flow of water, the faucet handles are considered to be contaminated and a paper towel must be used to turn off the water after the hands have been cleaned.
2. The nurse wears a gown whenever she enters the patient's isolation unit and removes it when she leaves.
   a. If the gown has been worn previously, it must be considered contaminated on the outside, even though it may not be soiled. The gown is donned so that only the inside, back, and belt are touched by the nurse's hands.
3. Use of the face mask
   a. The mask is worn to protect the nurse from contamination by droplet infection. (Sneezing or coughing by the patient may release microorganisms from his respiratory tract. These microorganisms may then enter the nurse's respiratory tract.)
   b. A mask should fit the face snugly and cover both the nose and the mouth.
   c. A mask should not be worn for more than 1 hour. If it is necessary to stay in the patient's room for a longer period of time, the mask is discarded and replaced by a fresh one.
4. Dishes, trays, and eating utensils are kept in the patient's room. The food is transferred from the clean tray to the dishes kept in the patient's room. If paper plates and cups are used they are transferred in the same manner and then discarded after use.
5. Linen from the patient's room must be placed in a laundry bag marked "contaminated." The outside of the bag must be kept clean while transferring linen from the patient's room into the bag.
6. Feces and other body excretions can usually be disposed of in the hopper. If a hopper is not available, the excreta must be disinfected with chlorinated lime before it is discarded.
7. Papers, magazines, food wastes, and used tissues are wrapped in paper bags and burned in the incinerator.

IV. **Other Types of Isolation and Precautions**
   A. Strict isolation is not always necessary. For some types of infectious diseases handwashing before entering and after leaving the patient's room and observance of certain precautions are all that is needed.
   B. Enteric precautions—used for infectious diseases of the intestinal tract, transmitted through direct or indirect contact with feces.
      1. Gowns are worn by all persons having direct contact with patient.
      2. Gloves are worn by all persons having direct contact with patient or with articles contaminated with fecal material.
      3. Contaminated articles must be discarded or disinfected.
   C. Respiratory isolation—requires special care of all articles contaminated by respiratory secretions. Masks should be worn by all persons entering room if susceptible to the disease.
   D. Wound and skin precautions—special care must be taken with all dressings, linens, or other articles contaminated by drainage.
      1. Gowns and gloves must be worn by all persons having direct contact with patient.
      2. Masks are necessary only during dressing changes.
   E. Blood precautions—care must be used in handling all contaminated needles and syringes. Nurses must be especially careful to avoid contaminating themselves by smearing blood in open cuts or putting their hands around nose and mouth before hands are washed.
   F. Secretion precautions—used when transmission by direct contact with wounds and secretion or contaminated articles is a possibility. Only necessary if there is drainage or discharge from a lesion.
      1. Basically the use of a "no touch" technique and proper handwashing procedure will prevent transmission of the disease.
      2. Contaminated articles must be discarded or disinfected.

V. **Protective Isolation or Reverse Isolation**
   A. Purpose is to protect patient from infectious

agents that might be brought in from outside his environment.

B. Conditions in which this type of isolation is used (see Table 16) include:
1. Agranulocytosis
2. Lymphomas and leukemia
3. Certain patients receiving immunosuppressive therapy
4. Severe dermatitis
5. Extensive burns

C. For reverse isolation the patient must be in a private room with door closed. Gowns, masks, and gloves are worn. Under some circumstances caps and booties may also be worn.

D. Articles such as linen and bed clothes usually are sterilized prior to use in patient care. Mattresses and pillows are covered with impervious plastic and are cleaned thoroughly with a germicidal detergent immediately before patient is admitted to the room.

VI. **Specific Communicable Diseases**
See Part XII, "Pediatric Nursing," and Part VII, "Nursing the Adult Patient."

Table 16. More Common Infectious Diseases Requiring Isolation or Special Precautions °

DISEASE	ISOLATION OR PRECAUTION	DURATION
Chickenpox (varicella)	Respiratory isolation	For 7 days after eruption appears
Cholera	Enteric precautions	DI°°
Conjunctivitis, acute bacterial infection (sore eye, pink eye)	Secretion precautions	U°°
Diphtheria	Strict isolation	Until two cultures taken from the nose and throat at least 24 hours apart after cessation of antibiotic therapy are negative
Eczema vaccinatum	Strict isolation	DI
E. coli gastroenteritis	Enteric precautions	DI
Gas gangrene	Wound and skin precautions	DI
German measles (rubella)	Respiratory isolation	For 5 days after onset of rash
Gonorrhea, gonorrheal conjunctivitis	Secretion precautions	U
Hepatitis, infectious	Enteric precautions	DH°°
Hepatitis, serum	Enteric precautions, blood precautions	DH
Herpes simplex	Secretions precautions	DI
Herpes zoster, eruptive	Respiratory isolation	DI
Impetigo	Wound & skin precautions	DI
Malaria	Blood precautions	DH
Measles (rubeola) including encephalitis	Respiratory isolation	For 7 days after rash disappears
Meningitis, aseptic	Excretion precautions	DH
Meningitis, meningococcal	Respiratory isolation	U
Mumps (infectious parotitis)	Respiratory isolation	For 9 days after onset of swelling
Neonatal vesicular disease (herpes simplex)	Strict isolation	DI
Pertussis (whooping cough)	Respiratory isolation	DH
Scarlet fever	Secretion precautions	U
Smallpox (variola)	Strict isolation	Until all crusts are shed
Staphylococcal and streptococcal disease; burns, extensive	Strict isolation	DI
Dermatitis	Wound and skin precautions	DI
Enterocolitis	Strict isolation	DI
Pneumonia and draining lung abscess	Strict isolation	DI
Wounds	Wound and skin precautions	DI
Syphilis, mucocutaneous	Secretion precautions	U
Tuberculosis		
pulmonary sputum positive or suspect	Respiratory isolation	Until effective therapy begins and there is clinical improvement
extrapulmonary (open)	Secretion precautions	DI
Typhoid fever	Enteric precautions	Until three consecutive negative cultures of feces

°Modified from "Isolation Techniques for Use in Hospitals," U.S. Dept of Health, Education and Welfare. Public Health Service.

°°Code: DH—duration of hospitalization; DI—duration of illness (with wounds or lesions, DI means until they stop draining), U—until 24 hours after initiation of effective therapy.

Questions

Mrs. Kraft, age 22, was admitted to the hospital with a diagnosis of staphylococcal pneumonia and was placed on isolation.

1. Mrs. Kraft's physician wrote an order specifically stating that she was to be placed on isolation. This means that:
    1. Mrs. Kraft is to be confined to a unit separate from that of the other patients until she is no longer considered a source of infection
    2. only physicians and nurses are allowed to be near Mrs. Kraft
    3. Mrs. Kraft will be placed in a ward with medical patients only until her symptoms have subsided
    4. Mrs. Kraft will have a private duty nurse and the hospital personnel will not be allowed to care for her
2. Before Mrs. Kraft is taken to her room it is most important to:
    1. autoclave all equipment that will be needed to care for her during her hospitalization
    2. remove all unnecessary equipment and upholstered furniture in her room
    3. obtain a special mattress that can be autoclaved after she is dismissed
    4. seal all windows in her room so microorganisms cannot escape to the outside
3. Once Mrs. Kraft has been admitted to her room, everything in the room must be considered to be contaminated. The word contaminated refers to the presence of:
    1. dirt or dust on an object
    2. living pathogenic microorganisms in or on an object or person
    3. body secretions in or on an object
    4. harmless bacteria in or on an object
4. Mrs. Kraft's eating utensils, dishes, bedpan, thermometer, and so forth must remain in the unit or be sterilized before they are taken from the unit, primarily because:
    1. her illness can be spread to others by indirect contact
    2. her illness cannot be spread except by direct contact with the patient
    3. these articles are the ones that are most likely to be soiled
    4. it will be easier to clean these articles after they are sterilized
5. Hand washing is considered to be of primary importance when caring for a patient with a communicable disease chiefly because:
    1. most patients with a communicable disease have copious drainage of body fluids
    2. gloves are not effective barriers against bacteria
    3. the hands are used for many nursing tasks and therefore are capable of spreading infection very easily
    4. it is the quickest and most effective method for destroying bacteria
6. When the hands are being washed, it is best to use:
    1. very hot water to destroy the bacteria
    2. running water throughout the procedure
    3. a basin of disinfectant solution
    4. a very strong soap
7. In order to remove as many bacteria from the hands as possible, it is most effective to:
    1. soak them in a disinfectant solution for 15 minutes
    2. hold them under a very forceful stream of water
    3. fill the washbowl with water and completely immerse the hands
    4. rub the hands together and lather the skin between the fingers
8. In medical asepsis the nurse's arms are not considered to be contaminated. Her hands are contaminated before they are washed. If this is true then it is most important for her to:
    1. wash only her hands and avoid touching her wrists and arms
    2. hold her hands higher than her elbows while washing her hands to prevent the flow of contaminated water onto her hands
    3. hold her hands lower than her elbows throughout the washing procedure until she has dried her hands completely
    4. wash her upper and lower arms as well as her hands each time she leaves a patient's room

9. When a bar of soap is used to wash the hands it may serve as a source of contamination for the hands unless it is:
    1. kept in the hands during the entire washing procedure
    2. rinsed off with running water before it is used
    3. dipped into an antiseptic solution each time the hands are rinsed
    4. kept in an airtight container when it is not in use
10. Mrs. Kraft's room had an adjoining bath which was not equipped with foot pedals to control the flow of water into the lavatory. In this situation it is most important for the nurse to:
    1. use a clean paper towel to turn on the water before washing her hands
    2. use a clean paper towel to turn off the water after her hands are washed
    3. fill the basin with water and turn off the water before she finishes washing her hands
    4. have someone pour water from a pitcher onto her hands while she is washing them
11. Hand washing for medical asepsis is generally considered to be most effective if the hands are washed for at least:
    1. 5 minutes
    2. 10 minutes
    3. 30 seconds
    4. 1 full minute
12. Some hospitals do not require the nurse to don a fresh gown each time she enters an isolation unit. If a nurse is donning a previously worn gown she must remember that:
    1. only the outside is "clean"
    2. the entire gown is contaminated
    3. the entire gown is considered to be "clean"
    4. only the inside of the gown is considered "clean"
13. When a nurse is donning an isolation gown, the last item she touches is the:
    1. collar
    2. cuff of the sleeves
    3. hem of the gown
    4. belt that ties at the back of the gown
14. When removing a gown that is contaminated, but will be worn again, the nurse's first step is to:
    1. push up the sleeves beyond her elbow
    2. remove her arms from the sleeves
    3. untie the belt at the back
    4. wash her hands
15. The second step in removing the gown is to:
    1. wash the hands
    2. "shrug" the gown over the shoulders and turn it wrong side out
    3. reach up and pull the collar away from the neck
    4. push the sleeves away from the wrists
16. In medical asepsis a mask is worn by the nurse for the purpose of protecting the:
    1. patient from reinfection
    2. patient from cross infection from other patients
    3. nurse from droplet infection
    4. nurse from direct contact with microorganisms on the inanimate objects in the patient's room
17. When a mask is worn it should:
    1. fit loosely to avoid rebreathing of stale air
    2. fit snugly and cover the mouth
    3. fit snugly and cover both the nose and the mouth
    4. fit loosely so it can be removed quickly as soon as the nurse leaves the isolation unit
18. It is recommended that a mask should be worn for not more than:
    1. 8 hours
    2. 4 hours
    3. 2 hours
    4. 1 hour

19. At the end of each 8-hour shift, the contaminated linen was removed from Mrs. Kraft's unit and sterilized. All papers, tissues, and other wastes of this type were also removed and burned. These steps were carried out as part of a procedure referred to as:
    1. terminal disinfection
    2. concurrent disinfection
    3. surgical asepsis
    4. sterile technique
20. When removing the linen from Mrs. Kraft's room, it is most important to:
    1. place it in a special laundry bag kept in her room and then carry it directly to the laundry
    2. transfer the linen to a bag kept in a "clean" area and marked "contaminated," being careful to avoid contaminating the outside of the bag
    3. place it in a vat of disinfectant solution before taking it to the laundry
    4. wrap it in a clean sheet and put it down the laundry chute immediately
21. The papers, used tissues, and paper towels taken from Mrs. Kraft's room should be:
    1. enclosed in paper bags and burned
    2. taken to the utility room and discarded in the trash can
    3. flushed down the hopper in the work room
    4. given to the hospital housekeeper for disposal
22. A friend of Mrs. Kraft's asked you what type of flowers would be best to send to Mrs. Kraft. The best answer to this question would be:
    1. a permanent arrangement of artificial flowers that she can take home when she is discharged
    2. a potted plant that she can enjoy caring for while in the hospital and at home
    3. cut flowers in a disposable vase
    4. cut flowers in a vase that has been brought from Mrs. Kraft's home
23. One of the most important points to remember when caring for a patient with a communicable disease is:
    1. always avoid direct contact with the patient
    2. remember to touch "clean to clean" and "contaminated to contaminated"
    3. the length of time spent in contact with the patient and his environment has no relation to the degree of contamination
    4. most patients with a communicable disease are thoroughly familiar with the ways in which infection is spread
24. If a patient has a disease that can be spread by droplet infection, what type of isolation or precaution would be used to avoid infection of others?
    1. enteric precautions
    2. blood precautions
    3. respiratory isolation
    4. protective isolation
25. Some communicable diseases are spread by carriers. A carrier is best defined as:
    1. an inanimate object that is contaminated with pathogens
    2. an insect that harbors the causative organism of a disease
    3. a human who is ill with a communicable disease
    4. a human who is without symptoms but harbors the microorganisms of a communicable disease
26. A child with German measles (rubella) should be kept under:
    1. strict isolation
    2. respiratory isolation
    3. enteric precautions
    4. secretion precautions
27. The period of isolation for the child with measles would be for:
    1. 5 days after onset of rash
    2. 5 days after disappearance of rash
    3. 7 days after fever subsides
    4. 7 days after rash disappears

28. Which of the following diseases does not require respiratory isolation?
    1. mumps
    2. chickenpox
    3. whooping cough
    4. impetigo
29. Which of the following would be most important in the care of a patient with gonorrhea?
    1. use protective isolation technique
    2. be very careful with secretions, especially avoiding contamination of the nurse's eyes
    3. wear gown and mask each time direct contact with the patient is necessary
    4. soak all linens in disinfectant before sending them to laundry
30. When caring for a patient with syphilitic lesions of the mucous membrane, the nurse must use:
    1. strict isolation until the patient is discharged
    2. secretion precautions until 24 hours after effective therapy is begun
    3. respiratory precautions during entire course of illness
    4. enteric precautions until culture returns negative

Part X
NURSING THE EMOTIONALLY DISTURBED AND THE MENTALLY ILL

I. Introduction
A. Mental illness is the major health problem in the U. S. today.
B. In the past 10 or 15 years there has been almost a 76 per cent increase in the number of patients admitted to public mental hospitals but the number of discharges have increased by about 127 per cent. This is a result of improved methods of treatment that have drastically reduced the average length of stay in a mental institution.
C. Mental illness is a relative term and cannot be defined precisely. A person who is mentally healthy is one who (1) knows himself and is able to accept himself as he is, (2) has a sincere concern for others and the ability to love, (3) is directed more by inner values than by outer, (4) can be independent without hurting others in the process, and (5) is flexible enough to tolerate stress and frustration reasonably well.

II. General Terms to Be Understood
A. Autistic thinking—extreme daydreaming. A complete turning in on oneself.
B. Delusion—a false impression or idea. No amount of reasoning can change the idea.
C. Hallucination—a sensory impression without justifiable stimulus. Example: seeing, hearing, or feeling something that is not actually present.
D. Illusion—mistaken impression resulting from an actual stimulus. Example: lines on the wall are seen as snakes; wind blowing in the trees is interpreted as a baby crying.
E. Depression—an unremitting feeling of sadness.
F. Phobia—an unrealistic fear.
G. Obsession—an idea that persists in spite of one's efforts to avoid or ignore it.
H. Compulsion—an act that is carried out repeatedly, despite the person's wish to refrain from doing it or his realization that the act is irrational.
I. Euphoria—a feeling of elation and joy.

III. Causes of Psychogenic Mental Disorders
A. The individual fails to adapt to his environment because of a complicated interaction between himself as he is and the reality of his environment.
B. The individual may lack flexibility and develop rigid patterns of defense (adjustment patterns) which reduce his capacity for adjustment.
C. The individual may not have the temperament (energy) to face all the physical and emotional challenges of life.

IV. Personality and Behavior
A. Personality—the total of all distinguishing traits that are unique to a particular individual.
   1. Behavior can be symptomatic of a personality disorder.
   2. The major motivating forces behind behavior are biological and social factors.
      a. The goal of biological drives is satisfaction derived from release of tension of smooth muscles.
      b. The goal of social forces is the security derived from acceptance in the society of others.
   3. Personality develops according to one's physical, mental, and emotional make-up, all of which are influenced by heredity and environment.
B. Patterns of adjustment—mental mechanisms or behavioral patterns of adjustment that are used to resolve conflicts and provide relief from the stress and tension of everyday life. They become dangerous when one uses them habitually to escape reality.
   1. Regression—reverting to childish behavior that was successful in one's past.
   2. Projection—attributing to someone or something else one's own shortcomings (often called the blaming mechanism). Prevents one from reaching maturity because he refuses to admit his own weakness or to work to overcome them.

3. Identification—assuming the mannerisms, attitudes, and achievements of someone else as his own. Prevents one from accomplishing goals of his own and enjoying the rewards of his own achievements.
4. Rationalization—one seeks to explain his behavior by using half-truths or other false reasons for his actions. Often confused with reasoning and is probably the most frequently used of all defense mechanisms.
5. Repression—pushing into the subconscious mind thoughts or feelings that are painful. Unless they are released in an acceptable manner they can serve as powerful motivation for behavior later in life.
6. Sublimation—directing strong impulses into acceptable channels so that behavior is condoned by society.
7. Displacement—transfer of hostility or other strong feelings from original cause of feelings to another person or object.
8. Compensation—striving to make amends for some lack of or loss in personal characteristics. Overcompensation is directing one's energies too strenuously toward one aspect of his personality to the point of neglecting his total personality. Usually if the individual fails in one direction he will *overcompensate* by going the opposite direction—for example, from aggressiveness to withdrawal.

C. Exaggerated responses and deviations from normal behavior
1. The patient with a mental illness exhibits behavior that differs in degree but not in kind from that of a so-called normal individual.
2. An understanding of why he behaves abnormally can guide us toward helping him return to reality.
3. There are two broad categories of mental illness—*psychosis* and *psychoneurosis.* These are to be taken only as guides to an understanding of the patient's illness and *not* as a definite diagnosis of mental illness.
   a. Psychosis—a serious mental breakdown. The individual's entire personality may be affected. He has difficulty distinguishing between what is happening in the real world and what goes on in his mind. Psychotic individuals often fail to show appropriate emotions or feelings. They can lose physical as well as emotional control under normal everyday stress.
      1. Schizophrenia is a form of psychosis. Its exact cause is not known. Chemical changes in the brain and psychological conflict are considered as possible causes. It is characterized by a variety of symptoms, not all of which are necessarily severe and are not present in every schizophrenic. A typical symptom is an inability to think in a logical manner and to listen to reason.
      2. Paranoid schizophrenia is a type of schizophrenia in which the individual has delusions of persecution and feels that others are "against" him, or he may have delusions of grandeur in which he thinks he is deserving of great honor and respect.
   b. Psychoneurosis is a less serious form of mental breakdown in which the individual may suffer from phobia, compulsions, obsessions, and conversions.

D. Withdrawal patterns—the patient who is seriously withdrawn isolates himself from others because he feels they will not accept him. He often has a profound sense of unworthiness and a loss of self-respect, yet he desperately craves affection and companionship.
1. In passive withdrawal the patient makes no attempt to communicate with others and is unable to attach any enduring emotions to another. He has extreme apathy toward others and is very difficult to work with.
2. In active withdrawal his attempt at communications may be in the form of bizarre and inappropriate behavior. He may have delusions and hallucinations that motivate his erratic behavior.
3. Nursing care includes attitudes of acceptance, objectivity, active friendliness, kind firmness to avoid condoning his unacceptable actions, consistent interest in him.

E. Aggressive patterns—patient displays hostility openly by overt actions.
1. Patient may have greatly exaggerated mood changes—agitated depression, retarded depression, explosive excitement.
2. Patient may have a high "nuisance value" but he usually is easier to communicate with and has a better prognosis than the withdrawn patient.
3. Nursing care of patient involves providing a quiet, nonstimulating environment.
   a. Physical needs include adequate rest and prevention of self-injury.
   b. Patient must be allowed to express his hostility openly; his questions are answered simply and directly. His inappropriate actions are not condoned but neither are they criticized by the nurse.

F. Overactivity—frantic physical activity, usually without direction.
  1. The stimulus causing this is not always obvious.
  2. The patient should be handled in a calm, quiet manner.
  3. Most helpful to divert the patient's attention and activity into more reasonable channels, e.g., outdoor activity, sports, dancing, or pursuing a hobby or developing a talent.
  4. Mechanical restraints increase fear, tension, and anger and should be used only as a last resort to prevent the patient from injuring himself.
G. Underactivity—extreme apathy, depression, and lack of response to any stimulus.
  1. The amount of activity varies with individual patients. Some may be slightly withdrawn; others may be completely uncommunicative, and nothing seems to reach them.
  2. Special attention must be given to the patient's personal hygiene. Regular skin care with some type of exercise or activity is important in the prevention of circulatory complications and musculo-skeletal disorders. Some patients will sit or stand in one position for hours on end, day and night.
  3. Care must be used in what is said within the hearing of patients. They may not seem to see or hear, but most of them are aware of what is going on around them; they simply cannot make any type of response.

V. General Principles of Nursing Care
A. The patient must be accepted as he is. His behavior is recognized as a symptom of his illness and he is treated with kindness and respect.
B. Understanding of the patient is of primary importance.
C. The nurse must be objective in all of her dealings with the patient. She must not read her own thoughts and attitudes into the actions of the patient. She will need to remain calm and in control of herself, helping the patient find an outlet for his pent-up emotions.
D. It is important to be a good listener. Verbal communication with others often is very difficult or impossible for mentally ill patients. When the patient is inclined to talk about his problems or himself, he needs a sympathetic and attentive listener.
E. Communication with another on a verbal level involves four basic steps:
  1. Listening to the words the person is using.

  2. Repeating to him what you think he said.
  3. Questioning him to be sure you understand exactly what he is saying.
  4. Acting according to the information the person has given to you.
F. A person's physical actions are also a means of communicating with others. Refusing to eat, frantically pacing the floor, or slamming furniture about are all examples of ways in which the individual may be seeking help and relief from mental anxiety and tension.
G. The nurse must be familiar with the type of therapy to be used for each individual patient and must work with the psychiatrist and other members of the mental health team. She should be aware that her own actions and ways of dealing with the patient can be helpful or harmful. Her attitude and behavior become a form of therapy when properly used as a therapeutic tool.

VI. Organic Behavior Disorders
A. Organic behavior disorders are traumatic in origin and result from some injury to the cells of the brain or nervous system.
B. Acute organic disorders can be described as delirium. They usually appear suddenly and are caused by a toxin in the body.
  1. Treatment is aimed at removal of the toxin when possible and prevention of complications.
  2. Nursing care depends on the type of toxin present. The patient must be kept quiet and unstimulated.
C. Chronic behavior disorders can be described as *dementia*. Types include senile dementia, dementia paralytica of syphilitic origin, and arteriosclerotic dementia.
  1. Treatment is aimed at helping these patients live out their lives as comfortably and as fully as possible within the limitations of their abilities.
  2. Nursing care is concerned with helping the patient live in dignity and with self-respect. He needs social acceptance, companionship, and a feeling of worthiness.

VII. Forms of Treatment for Mentally Ill
A. Psychotherapy—communication between a trained person and a mental patient. The communication may be through speech or actions and allows the individual patient a means of taking a long, honest look at himself and his relations with others.
  1. Individual therapy involves one patient.
  2. Group therapy includes several patients under the guidance of a psychologist, psychiatrist, or other trained person.
  3. Mental patients who cannot talk about problems are seriously ill. An ability to talk about and discuss his feelings with

others indicates an improvement in the patient's condition.

B. Ataraxic drugs (tranquilizers)
1. These drugs relieve the symptoms; they do not cure the illness.
2. The chief action of the drugs is to produce emotional tranquility so that the patient is more cooperative and more easily reached by the psychotherapist.
C. Antidepressants—reduce feeling of depression
D. Electric shock therapy
1. Used to reduce physical and emotional tension and make the patient easier to approach for psychotherapy.
2. There is no pain associated with the treatment, but many patients fear the procedure and should receive some explanation of the procedure and reassurance before it is begun.
E. Insulin shock therapy
1. Similar in principle to electric shock therapy.
2. Patients' meals and amount of physical exercise should be observed carefully while this treatment is used.
3. Group therapy for patients getting insulin shock treatment is often quite successful. Most patients do not fear insulin shock as they do electric shock therapy.
F. Occupational therapy
1. Provides useful, constructive, or artistic activities for the patient. May include work done in the occupational therapy department and work done outside the department.
2. A form of occupational therapy in which the patient performs various chores in and around the institution is called industrial therapy. It must be borne in mind that this type of therapy must be done for the benefit of the patient and NOT for the benefit of the institution. In some mental hospitals the patient may receive a salary for the work he does until he is dismissed from the hospital.
G. Recreational therapy
1. Provides indoor and outdoor recreation programs for the mentally ill.
2. Hospital personnel and patients participate in this type of therapy.
3. Recreational therapy seems to be closer to normal community and home life and helps the patient adjust to living with others again and becoming socially acceptable.

VIII. **The Alcoholic Patient**
A. There is no one specific cause of alcoholism. The person uses alcohol as a crutch to help overcome emotional problems.
B. The person develops a compulsion to drink and experiences some kind of physical reaction to alcohol that is not experienced by normal persons.
C. It is not known why alcoholics choose alcohol rather than some other means of escaping reality, or why they develop psychological dependency on alcohol.
D. Alcoholism is *not* due to lack of will power.
E. Treatment requires some form of psychotherapy to help the alcoholic gain insight into his problem. He must admit that he cannot control his drinking.
F. Alcoholics Anonymous—one of the most successful organizations offering help to the alcoholic. Its greatest advantage is in giving the alcoholic an opportunity to see himself as useful and acceptable to others who have a similar problem.
G. Physical effects of alcoholism are a result of toxicity. Alcohol is a poison that is detoxified by the liver. It has a definite depressant effect on the brain and nervous system and can cause impairment of mental processes and disturbances in motor activity and coordination.
1. Delirium tremens—an acute toxic reaction to alcohol. Occurs in those who have been drinking heavily for at least 5 to 10 years. When alcohol is abruptly withdrawn the individual begins to experience typical reaction.
a. Symptoms include delusions, hallucinations, and a highly agitated state of mind.
b. Patient must be watched closely to avoid injury to himself or others.
c. Physical strain may lead to cardiac strain and hypertension.
d. Treatment includes tranquilizing drugs, improvement of patient's nutritional status, prevention of respiratory infections and other complications, and a calm, uncritical atmosphere.

IX. **The Drug Addict**
A. An individual who depends on the drug to help him adjust to conflict.
B. Opiates, cocaine, Demerol, sodium methadone, and the barbiturates are the more commonly misused drugs. The hallucinogenic drugs such as lysergic acid diethylamide (L.S.D.), mescaline, and peyote are not truly addictive, but are dangerous in that

they can precipitate a severe psychotic state in certain individuals.

C. Withdrawal symptoms—occur when drug is withheld from the addict. Less severe symptoms include weakness, anorexia, and insomnia; more severe signs include muscle cramps, high blood pressure, nausea, diarrhea, and prostration.

D. Treatment of drug addiction must be on a long-term basis. Rehabilitation is necessary because a personality defect is the basis of the addiction. Rehabilitation of the personality is often difficult because it involves helping the patient recognize the source of his problems and finding new ways to solve his emotional difficulties so that he no longer uses drugs to control his anxieties or cope with stress and tension.

X. The Suicidal Patient

A. These patients have profound feelings of unworthiness.

B. Such a person usually tries to give some warning that he is contemplating suicide. He may use such expressions as "I don't want to live any longer" or he may indirectly hint at his desire to end his life.

C. Depression, disorientations, defiance, and dissatisfaction with dependency on others are all states of mind or mood that can lead to suicide.

D. The nurse has a definite role in suicide prevention. She must listen to what her patients are trying to tell her and she must show by her actions that she considers them worthy of respect and attention.

Questions

1. Which of the following statements is true regarding mental illness?
   1. All mentally ill persons are dangerous and destructive.
   2. A person who is mentally ill is mentally retarded.
   3. Mental illness is the major health problem in the United States.
   4. There has been a gradual decrease in the occurrence of mental illness in this country.
2. One of the most important requirements for those who care for the mentally ill is:
   1. a knowledge of psychiatric terminology
   2. recognition of the mentally ill as persons who are sick and in need of help
   3. realization that mental illness is nearly always incurable
   4. ability to control and prevent emotional outbursts in others
3. In the past decade mental institutions in the country have:
   1. had a 50 per cent increase in the number of admissions and 10 per cent increase in the number of discharges
   2. admitted fewer patients but discharged 75 per cent more than in the previous decade
   3. admitted 76 per cent more patients than in previous years and dismissed 127 per cent more
   4. maintained an equal percentage in admission and discharges
4. The above statistics in regard to admissions and discharges from mental institutions are primarily a result of:
   1. increased facilities available for the mentally ill
   2. elimination of large central state hospitals and establishment of local clinics
   3. an increase in the number of psychiatrists practicing in this country
   4. improved methods of treatment that have reduced the average length of stay in a mental institution
5. A person who is mentally healthy has all of the following characteristics except:
   1. being independent without offending others
   2. having a sincere concern for others
   3. placing his values on material things rather than inner worth
   4. being able to accept himself as he knows himself to be

6. An autistic individual is most concerned with:
    1. himself
    2. his fellow beings
    3. material wealth
    4. the attitudes of others

7. Hearing voices that are not really present is an example of:
    1. a phobia
    2. an illusion
    3. an hallucination
    4. a delusion

8. Repeatedly carrying out an act such as washing one's hands in spite of a desire not to do so is an example of:
    1. a compulsion
    2. a phobia
    3. an hallucination
    4. an obsession

9. Some drugs, such as heroin, can produce a feeling of great elation and joy, especially when one first begins taking the drug. This feeling can best be called:
    1. mania
    2. phobia
    3. delusion
    4. euphoria

10. Human beings behave in certain ways primarily because they are seeking:
    1. a better life for themselves and those around them
    2. a means of escape from the realities of life and the responsibilities of being involved with others
    3. release from physical tension, and security in being accepted by others
    4. the true meaning of their existence and their role in society

11. When a psychotic patient is extremely uncooperative or repulsive in his speech or actions it is most important for the nurse to:
    1. let him know immediately that his behavior is not acceptable
    2. remain calm and accept his behavior as a symptom of his illness
    3. react as she would with any normal person and ignore him until he becomes more cooperative
    4. talk with him and frankly tell him that his actions are extremely repulsive to others

Match the following terms with their definitions:

12. Extreme daydreaming_____   1. Euphoria
13. The opposite of reality_____   2. Fantasy
14. Exaggerated feeling of elation_____   3. Depression
15. Unremitting feeling of sadness_____   4. Autistic thinking

16. Many reactions of the mentally ill are similar to normal reactions. The chief difference is that the mentally ill:
    a. react more strongly and to a much greater degree   1. all of these
    b. do not want to control their emotions   2. a and b
    c. cannot distinguish between fantasy and reality   3. c and d
    d. are deliberately trying to deceive others   4. a and c

17. Avoiding unpleasant past experiences by completely "forgetting" about them and trying to pretend that they never happened is an example of:
    1. regression
    2. rationalization
    3. repression
    4. projection

18. Mrs. Lackey insists that she is Queen Victoria and frequently refers to the psychiatric aides as her ladies-in-waiting. Mrs. Lackey's behavior is an example of carrying to extreme the defense mechanism of:
    1. rationalization
    2. regression
    3. identification
    4. compensation

19. Bob Thomas is a 19-year-old who is emotionally disturbed. His chief difficulty in getting along with others is his superior attitude and "bossy" manner. Bob actually feels very inferior to other people and his behavior is an example of extreme:
    1. compensation
    2. rationalization
    3. regression
    4. identification

20. Rationalization is one of the most frequently used defense mechanisms. It is dangerous when used to extreme primarily because:
    1. it leads to childish and immature behavior in times of stress
    2. it is a form of lying in which the individual justifies his behavior with false-hoods or half-truths and does not face his conflicts honestly
    3. the person who rationalizes is copying the behavior of others rather than developing his own personality
    4. rationalization leads to suppression of feelings that should be brought to the surface and handled through acceptable behavior

21. The nurse who becomes angry with her supervisor and "takes it out" on the nurse's aide with whom she works is using which of the following defense mechanisms?
    1. rationalization
    2. regression
    3. displacement
    4. compensation

22. The behavior pattern by which one avoids accepting full responsibility for his own actions and shortcomings by blaming someone or something else is called:
    1. projection
    2. identification
    3. rationalization
    4. compensation

23. If a patient who has been very loud and demanding and discourteous toward the staff suddenly becomes sullen and withdrawn, we might say that he is:
    1. rationalizing his behavior
    2. overcompensating for his aggressive behavior
    3. identifying with other patients in the hospital
    4. repressing his unpleasant thoughts and feelings

24. A schizophrenic individual:
    1. has difficulty distinguishing between reality and what goes on in his mind
    2. always has delusions of persecution and is easily offended
    3. usually can function well in society with a minimum of therapy
    4. responds well to reasoning and can easily be made aware of his failure to think logically

25. The patient who withdraws from the society of others is frequently suffering from:
    1. a deep sense of unworthiness and a loss of self respect
    2. an overwhelming sense of superiority which makes him feel above the need for the company of others
    3. a strong feeling of persecution with hostility toward other members of society
    4. an inability to communicate his feelings in any way other than verbally

26. Mrs. Bond has the reputation of being the "nuisance" of the ward. She finds numerous ways to gain the attention of the nursing staff, criticizes everything that is done for her, questions every action of the physicians and nurses, and often bangs around the furniture and threatens to leave if she doesn't receive better care. Her behavior can best be described as:
    1. deceptive
    2. withdrawn
    3. suicidal
    4. aggressive

27. The nurse should understand that Mrs. Bond's behavior is most likely an expression of:
    1. overdepression
    2. hostility
    3. overstimulation
    4. understimulation
28. In dealing with Mrs. Bond's behavior it would be best if the nurse would:
    1. isolate her from other patients who may be aggravating her anxiety
    2. ignore Mrs. Bond's demands so she will know that her behavior is not acceptable to others
    3. criticize her behavior at every opportunity so she will change her way of acting
    4. allow her to express her hostility openly but do not give the impression that her behavior is being condoned
29. When Mrs. Bond states that "all nurses are sweet to your face but they really don't care about their patients," the first thing the nurse should do is:
    1. ask Mrs. Bond if she would rather have another nurse assigned to care for her
    2. tell Mrs. Bond that she is wrong and that she has no real reason for feeling that way
    3. repeat Mrs. Bond's statement and ask her if that is what she has said
    4. ask Mrs. Bond if she feels the same way about the physicians and other members of the health team
30. Which of the following would be the best means of helping an overactive patient?
    1. isolating the patient so he will not be stimulated by other patients
    2. restricting his activities by mechanical restraint so he will not exhaust himself
    3. providing some reasonable activity, such as playing softball or basketball
    4. assigning him to the task of stripping all the beds in the ward and remaking them so he can work off some of his excess energy
31. Overactivity in a mentally ill person most often is characterized by:
    1. frantic activity that is apparently unreasonable and without purpose
    2. activity that is planned by the patient so that it will be most irritating to others
    3. spasmodic physical exertion followed by periods of inertia
    4. brief periods of extreme activity which quickly exhaust the patient and produce normal sleep
32. Mrs. Fisher is an extremely quiet patient who sits in a corner of the ward for hours on end. In order to help Mrs. Fisher it would be best for the nurse to:
    1. ignore her until she shows some sign of wanting help
    2. encourage Mrs. Fisher to play ping-pong or checkers with another patient
    3. take a few minutes during the day to sit with Mrs. Fisher and listen to her when she wants to talk
    4. warn the other patients not to talk with Mrs. Fisher because she obviously wants to be left alone
33. A very important aspect of nursing care of the extremely underactive patient is:
    1. providing a quiet atmosphere for the patient
    2. regular skin care and physical exercise to avoid circulatory and musculoskeletal complications
    3. directing the patient's activities into more useful channels
    4. providing a variety of interests for the patient so he will not become bored
34. A neurotic individual is best described as one who:
    1. has an incurable mental illness
    2. cannot control his emotions in a normal manner
    3. has a complete and profound change in his personality
    4. is unable to distinguish between fantasy and reality
35. A very serious mental breakdown with severe personality changes is best described as:
    1. a neurosis
    2. an emotional disturbance
    3. a hypochondria
    4. a psychosis

36. Organic behavior disorders differ from functional types of mental illness in that organic disorders are:
    1. always directly related to the individual's environment
    2. found only in elderly persons
    3. a result of injury to the brain cells or nervous system
    4. a result of inherited defective genes
37. Delirium is characterized by:
    1. a sudden onset with a toxin being the cause
    2. a chronic physical condition that has brought about damage to the brain cells
    3. a sudden onset with mild symptoms of anxiety and disorientation
    4. a gradual onset with increased loss of physical as well as mental capabilities
38. Psychotherapy is primarily a form of treatment in which the patient.
    1. is given a series of lectures by the psychiatrist
    2. receives various drugs which produce sleep and relaxation
    3. is given specific tasks to perform to keep him occupied
    4. is encouraged to face reality by talking about himself and his problems
39. Psychotherapy is possible only when the patient is:
    1. able to communicate with others through words or actions and express his true feelings
    2. quiet and willing to listen to advice from others
    3. heavily sedated or physically restrained so he will be more cooperative
    4. admitted to a mental institution where a psychiatrist is available
40. The newer ataraxic drugs being used in the treatment of mental illness are successful chiefly because they:
    1. stimulate underactive patients
    2. help relieve mental depression by producing forgetfulness
    3. make the patient more talkative and physically more active
    4. produce serenity and reduce emotional tension
41. Mrs. Little has been scheduled for electric shock therapy in the morning, but she has heard other patients discuss the treatment and is extremely apprehensive. In order to help Mrs. Little accept this treatment it would be best to:
    1. tell her that the treatment is for her own good and she must go through with it
    2. ignore Mrs. Little's attitude because it is typical of a mentally ill person
    3. take time to discuss the treatment with Mrs. Little and give her a brief explanation of the procedure
    4. tell Mrs. Little that there is nothing to the treatment and she has nothing to worry about
42. In many mental institutions some of the patients are permitted to work in the laundry, greenhouse, or other departments in and around the institution. When this type of privilege is allowed the patient for his own benefit it is referred to as:
    1. industrial therapy
    2. recreational therapy
    3. group therapy
    4. psychotherapy
43. Recreational therapy is especially helpful in the treatment of mental illness chiefly because it:
    1. gives the patient physical exercise
    2. relieves the workload of the hospital personnel
    3. helps pass the time
    4. puts the patient in a more normal situation that is similar to his home and community life
44. Which of the following is *not* true of alcoholism?
    1. the victim has a compulsion to drink alcohol
    2. the alcoholic apparently suffers from some kind of unique physical reaction to the alcohol itself
    3. the condition is caused by a lack of will power
    4. the alcoholic has become psychologically dependent on alcohol

45. Symptoms of delirium tremens include all but:
    1. delusions
    2. hallucinations
    3. extreme agitation
    4. hypotension

46. Delerium tremens usually is produced by:
    1. sudden withdrawal of alcohol from a person who has been drinking heavily for a number of years
    2. excessive drinking by a person who rarely drinks alcohol
    3. prolonged intake of alcohol over a period of several days
    4. rapid consumption of a large amount of alcohol by a person unused to drinking

47. Which of the following would be most important when caring for a patient with delirium tremens?
    1. taking the opportunity of his hospitalization to discuss Alcoholics Anonymous with him
    2. restricting fluid and food intake until he can tolerate alcohol
    3. providing a calm and uncritical atmosphere
    4. checking the patient's vital signs at least every 15 minutes

48. The hallucinogenic drugs such as L.S.D., mescaline, and peyote are dangerous chiefly because they:
    1. are strongly addictive
    2. lead to organic brain disorders
    3. can bring on a severe psychotic state
    4. are all related to the opiates

49. The suicidal person:
    1. usually experiences a sudden and severe psychic shock immediately before he attempts suicide
    2. rarely gives any warning that he may take his own life
    3. is likely to consider himself superior to others
    4. has a profound feeling of unworthiness

50. Which of the following states of mood is least likely to lead to suicide?
    1. depression
    2. defiance
    3. elation
    4. disorientation

Part XI

NURSING THE MOTHER AND HER NEWBORN INFANT

Revised by Verna Jane Muhl

UNIT 1   HUMAN REPRODUCTION AND PREGNANCY

I. Introduction
A. Terms and definitions
1. Abortion—the termination of pregnancy before viability, i.e., before the twentieth week of gestation.
2. Afterpains—uterine cramps caused by contraction of uterus following delivery. Last from 3 to 4 days; more commonly seen in women who have had previous pregnancies.
3. Areola—the dark pigmented ring about the female nipple.
4. Asphyxia neonatorum—the failure of a newborn baby to breathe.
5. Atelectasis neonatorum—imperfect expansion of the lungs of the newborn infant.
6. Braxton-Hicks contractions—irregular contractions of the uterus after the third month of pregnancy.
7. Breech birth—delivery in which feet or buttocks are presenting part.
8. Chloasma—darkening pigmentation of skin, especially of face; the mask of pregnancy.
9. Crowning—visibility of the fetal head in the birth canal just before delivery.
10. Dilatation—expansion of an opening, as the cervix prior to delivery.
11. Embryo—the fetus in its early stage of development, before the end of the third month.
12. Fetus—the product of conception after the third month of gestation.
13. Fontanel—the space formed when two or more sutures of the infant's skull come together.
14. Gestation—period of intrauterine fetal development.
15. Gravid—pregnant.
16. Icterus neonatorum—jaundice of newborn; referring to normal physiological jaundice.
17. Induction of labor—labor brought on by artificial means.
18. In utero—within the uterus.
19. Involution—the return of the uterus to its normal size after childbirth.
20. Lactation—milk production.
21. Lanugo—the fine hair covering the body of the fetus.
22. Lightening—the descent of the presenting part into the pelvis prior to labor.
23. Lochia—the vaginal discharge following delivery, lasting from 3 to 5 weeks.
24. Meconium—the first greenish stools of the newborn infant.
25. Milia—plugged sebaceous glands on face of newborn.
26. Miscarriage—the expulsion of the product of conception before the period of viability; same as abortion.
27. Multigravida—a woman during her second and subsequent pregnancies.
28. Multipara—a woman who has delivered two or more babies after the period of viability, regardless of whether they were alive or stillborn.

29. Neonate—newborn.
30. Obstetrics—the science and art of human reproduction.
31. Ophthalmia neonatorum—gonorrheal infection of the conjunctiva of the newborn.
32. Parturition—childbirth.
33. Precipitate delivery—a sudden delivery under unsterile conditions.
34. Presenting part—that part of the fetus which enters the pelvis first.
35. Primipara—a woman who has delivered her first child.
36. Puerperium—the period from delivery to completion of involution.
37. Quickening—the first movements of the fetus within the uterus, usually occurs between 4½ and 5 months of gestation; the feeling of life.
38. Stillbirth—the birth of a dead baby.
39. Vernix caseosa—a cheese-like material coating the fetus in utero.
40. Vertex birth—delivery in which top of head is presenting part.

B. Significant events that have influenced obstetrical care
   1. History of obstetrics
      a. Civilization's oldest branch of practicing medicine.
      b. First midwives were women of the family who cared for the mother and child.
      c. Puerperal fever took many lives.
      d. Semmelweis initiated aseptic care in Europe in the middle 1800's.
      e. Oliver Wendell Holmes advocated the same care in the United States.
   2. Recent trends
      a. The move toward more effective and better mother and child care is recent throughout the entire world.
      b. There has been increased emphasis on more and better care of mother and baby since the turn of the century.
      c. Local, state, and federal governments began to sponsor maternal and child care programs.
         1. Created Children's Bureau in 1912.
         2. Established prenatal and well-baby clinics.
         3. Established visiting nurse services.
         4. Established school health programs.
         5. Began to train midwives.
         6. Initiated immunization programs for prevention of infectious diseases.
      d. Public is being educated to the need for early and adequate medical supervision during pregnancy.
      e. Great advances have been made through research.
         1. Pasteurized milk.
         2. Antibiotics.
         3. Blood banks.
         4. Poliomyelitis vaccination.
         5. Rubella vaccination.
         6. Rubeola vaccination.
         7. Mumps vaccination.

II. Human Reproduction
A. Anatomy of reproductive systems (see Part III, Basic Sciences; Unit 1, Anatomy).
B. Physiology of reproduction
   1. Ovum—female sex cell.
   2. Sperm—male sex cell.
   3. Ovulation—expelling of mature ovum by ovaries; normally occurs 14 days prior to menstruation.
   4. Graafian follicle—sac containing the ovum.
   5. Estrogen—female hormone which stimulates the lining of the uterus (endometrium) to prepare a bed for the fertilized egg, produced by the graafian follicle.
   6. Menstruation—the shedding of the lining of the uterus by way of the vagina. Normally occurs once a month.
   7. Conception or fertilization—uniting of the ovum and sperm. Normally occurs in the fallopian tube.
   8. Corpus luteum—"yellow body" formed by the graafian follicle which produces progesterone.
   9. Progesterone—female hormone which stabilizes pregnancy.
   10. Placenta or afterbirth—a flattened, rounded organ which attaches to the inner surface of the uterine wall, from which arises the umbilical cord through which the fetus derives its food and oxygen from the maternal circulation via a large umbilical vein, and passes waste products to the maternal circulation for disposal via two umbilical arteries.
   11. Amniotic fluid—clear liquid within the amniotic sac (membrane) which surrounds the fetus. It helps to maintain the body temperature of the fetus and serves as a cushion against injury.
   12. Heredity and sex determination
      a. Chromosomes containing genes determine physical characteristics of growing embryo.
      b. Special chromosomes called the X or sex chromosomes determine the sex of the child.
   13. Multiple pregnancy—condition in which there is more than one fetus existing in the pregnant uterus at the same time.
      a. Identical twins—both fetuses develop from a single fertilized ovum and share the same placenta. Resemble one another very closely.

b. Fraternal twins—develop from two separate fertilized ova.

14. Duration of pregnancy—280 days; 38–40 weeks; 10 lunar months; 9 calendar months.

15. Calculation of expected date confinement (E.D.C.)—subtract 3 months from the first day of the last menstrual period and add 7 days (Nägele's rule).

C. Fetal development

1. First month—cell mass has developed into a minute embryo, but this body form has little resemblance to the body of the newborn infant, even though there is early evidence of eyes, ears, and extremities.

2. Second month—body form is becoming human. Eyes and ears are beginning to show definite positions; the face is forming, and so are the extremities.

3. Third month—the head, though still large, is erect; nasal bones are forming and so is the palate. Is able to swallow. Fingers and toes show beginning nail formation, and external genitalia reveal the sex. The embryo is now called a fetus.

4. Fourth month—heartbeat can be heard with a stethoscope, hair is present on the scalp and body, and the face begins to look human. Fetal movements are active.

5. Fifth month—skin is transparent; nails, eyebrows, and eyelashes are evident. Vernix caseosa covers the body.

6. Sixth month—the fetus is long and has a wrinkled red skin. The nostrils are open, but the eyes are shut.

7. Seventh month—movements are strong, and fine hair covers the thin red body. If delivered, the fetus could make a weak cry, but rarely survives at this stage of development.

8. Eighth month—the fetus usually doubles its weight during this month, but the skin is still wrinkled because of little fatty padding. May survive if delivered.

9. Ninth month—weighs from $5\frac{1}{2}$ to $7\frac{1}{2}$ pounds (2.5 to 3.4 kg.). Skin loses its wrinkled appearance as subcutaneous fat appears, and is pink in color. Fine body hair has disappeared, but hair growth tends to be heavy.

III. Pregnancy and Prenatal Care

A. Physiological changes in pregnancy

1. Uterus—increases in size and weight owing to muscle enlargement and increased blood supply.

2. Cervix—becomes more succulent and softer until its consistency is similar to that of the lips. The cervical canal is filled with a plug of mucus that acts as a barrier to bacteria.

3. Vagina—takes on a bluish color due to increased blood supply.

4. Abdomen—becomes stretched owing to enlargement of uterus; skin may break, causing markings, or scars, known as "striae of pregnancy."

5. Breasts—become enlarged and are sometimes painful. The nipples become more deeply pigmented and quite sensitive. A thin watery fluid called colostrum may be expressed after a few months' gestation.

6. Heart and circulatory system—owing to added work during pregnancy, the heart becomes somewhat enlarged and during the latter weeks of pregnancy is displaced by pressure from the pregnant uterus. The blood volume is increased but blood pressure and pulse should remain within normal limits. Varicosities may appear in the legs and about the vulva and anus (hemorrhoids).

7. Respiration—additional oxygen required causes the chest to expand to give increased capacity for inspired air. The respiratory rate is increased slightly during the last weeks of pregnancy.

8. Urinary tract—no marked changes in the kidneys, but they must perform more work. During the first 3 months and last month of pregnancy, pressure of the uterus on the urinary bladder causes frequency of urination.

9. Digestive tract—during early months of pregnancy, there is a slowing of peristalsis, resulting in a tendency to nausea and constipation.

10. Skin—in addition to striae of pregnancy and pigmentation of nipples, there is usually a darkened line extending from the navel to the pubic bone. Some patients develop the "mask of pregnancy" across the bridge of the nose and extending up around the hairline. This is thought to be due to hormonal changes.

11. Weight gain—from 10 to 15 pounds (4.5 to 6.8 kg.) of weight gain during pregnancy is thought to be due to the growing fetus, placenta, membranes, amniotic fluid, and enlarged uterine muscle. Care should be exercised to prevent a weight gain of over 18 to 25 pounds (8.2 to 11.3 kg.) during entire pregnancy.

B. Psychological adjustment in pregnancy—background, economic and social stability influence adjustment to pregnancy.

1. First trimester—initial happiness may be dampened by physiological discomforts.

2. Second trimester—physically and emotionally a pleasant and happy time.
3. Third trimester—becoming discouraged with waiting; may be physically uncomfortable. About two weeks prior to delivery, emotional well-being and a "surge of energy" are felt.

C. Diagnosis of pregnancy
  1. Presumptive signs
    a. Cessation of menses
    b. Morning sickness
    c. Frequency of urination
    d. Breast changes
    e. Quickening
  2. Probable signs
    a. Abdominal changes
    b. Uterine changes
    c. Changes in cervix
    d. Positive biologic test for pregnancy
  3. Positive signs
    a. Hearing and counting fetal heart sounds
    b. Fetal movements
    c. Outline of fetus on x-ray
    d. Palpation of fetus

D. Prenatal care
  1. First medical examination—about 3 weeks after first menstrual period is missed.
    a. Medical history regarding previous illnesses, menstrual history, previous pregnancies, and hereditary traits.
    b. Complete physical examination, including pelvic examination and measurements, to determine patient's general state of health.
    c. Laboratory tests—blood samples taken for serologic test, red cell count, hemoglobin, typing, and Rh determination. Complete urinalysis is done.
  2. Return visits—every 3 to 4 weeks during first 7 months of pregnancy, every 2 weeks during eighth month, and every week of the last 4 weeks.
  3. Danger signals to be reported
    a. Vaginal bleeding.
    b. Marked swelling of the legs or hands.
    c. Persistent vomiting.
    d. Uncontrollable leakage of water from the vagina.
    e. Persistent headaches or dizziness.
    f. Failure to feel fetal movement.
    g. Persistent abdominal cramping or pain.
    h. Elevated temperature with or without chills.
  4. Physical needs
    a. Nutrition
      1. Diet should be well balanced and the daily caloric intake determined according to the patient's size and amount of activity.
      2. Vitamin supplements will be prescribed by the physician.
    b. Oral hygiene
      1. Regular dental checkups.
      2. Brushing at least twice a day.
    c. Sleep and rest
      1. Avoid fatigue.
      2. Afternoon nap or rest with feet elevated.
      3. Adequate sleep each night.
    d. Exercise
      1. Walking best form of exercise.
      2. Moderate forms of exercise are allowed; avoid more strenuous forms such as tennis or horseback riding.
    e. Skin care
      1. Daily bath is essential—physician may recommend shower or sponge bath during latter weeks of pregnancy.
      2. Skin creams or lotions may be used as usual.
      3. Hair may appear oily due to increased activity of oil glands. Wash as needed.
    f. Breast care
      1. Good supporting brassiere is essential; may wear at night if more comfortable.
      2. Wash with warm water and mild soap during daily bath.
      3. Gentle massage of nipples with cocoa butter will help keep them soft for nursing.
    g. Elimination
      1. Daily elimination can be insured with proper diet and adequate amount of fluids.
      2. Physician should be consulted before taking a strong laxative or enema.
    h. Marital relations—seek physician's advice; in normal pregnancy, relations may occur to full term.
    i. Douches—should be avoided except on advice of physician.
    j. Employment—allowed as long as patient is comfortable and shows no signs of developing complications.
    k. Clothing
      1. Should be comfortable, attractive, and suited to the occasion.
      2. Should be without constricting bands at the waist.
      3. Garter belt or maternity girdle worn to support stockings, never garters.
      4. Shoes should be well fitted and low-heeled.
    l. Travel
      1. Optimal time to travel is in second trimester.
      2. Seek physician's advice for plans for travel in first and third trimester.

5. Emotional needs
   a. Great need for love and security and knowledge of husband's support.
   b. Acceptance of pregnancy by both parents and other members of the family.
   c. Couple should plan for financial needs to provide feeling of security.
   d. Sometimes unplanned pregnancy interferes with career and causes resentment by one or both parents.
   e. Guilt feelings may be encountered when resentment is felt.
   f. Fear of responsibility is seen sometimes in immature parents.
   g. Both husband and wife should have opportunity to discuss problems with some responsible person who can offer sound advice.
6. Educational needs
   a. Increased emphasis to prepare expectant parents for pregnancy, parturition, and parenthood.
   b. Childbirth education classes prepare expectant parents for more active participation in labor and childbirth.
      1. Dick-Read method emphasizes education, exercises, and relaxation techniques.
      2. Lamaze method emphasizes psychoprophylactic concepts of concentration and neuromuscular control, along with the use of massage, to promote a satisfying, dignified parturition in which both husband and wife are actively participating.

E. Discomforts of pregnancy
1. Morning sickness—may be relieved by taking small amounts of starches, such as dry cereal or crackers, before arising in the morning.
2. Frequency of urination—caused by pressure on the urinary bladder by the growing uterus. Usually present in the first and third trimester of pregnancy.
3. Varicose veins—usually due to pressure in the pelvis from the enlarged uterus. May be relieved by avoiding long periods of standing and by elevating the feet several times a day. Physician may suggest wearing elastic stockings or bandages during the day.
4. Hemorrhoids—also caused by pressure on the pelvis due to enlarged uterus. Constipation should be avoided or relieved on physician's advice. Cold compresses or witch hazel packs may help relieve discomfort. Physician may prescribe hemorrhoidal suppositories.

5. Vaginal discharge—normal secretions usually increase and may cause itching. If caused by yeast infection, physician will prescribe proper treatment.
6. Dyspnea—results from pressure on the diaphragm by the enlarged uterus. Cannot be wholly relieved until after lightening occurs.
7. Edema of extremities—usually seen during latter part of pregnancy. May be relieved by elevating the feet. Physician should be consulted if condition persists.
8. Heartburn—usually more common in later part of pregnancy. Thought to be due to decreased peristalsis. Frequent small feedings may relieve condition.
9. Muscle cramps—may be relieved by straightening leg and pushing ball of foot backward toward knee. If persists, contact physician.

F. Complications of pregnancy
1. Vaginal bleeding caused by
   a. Abortion—if abortion is threatened, physician may successfully prevent it by adequate and early treatment. Therapeutic abortion is legal termination of pregnancy when its continuation will endanger the mother's life.
   b. Ectopic pregnancy—a pregnancy which settles outside the uterus. After the diagnosis is made, the treatment is always surgical.
   c. Placenta previa—occurs when the placenta lies over the neck of the cervix instead of high up in the uterus.
   d. Abruptio placentae—occurs when the placenta prematurely separates from the uterine wall.
2. Hyperemesis gravidarum—excessive vomiting during pregnancy. Usually responds favorably to intravenous therapy. In rare instances, therapeutic abortion is necessary.
3. Toxemia of pregnancy—exact cause not known but it can be prevented with early and adequate medical care. It is characterized by edema, high blood pressure, and presence of albumin in the urine (albuminuria).
   a. Preeclampsia—toxemia without convulsions.
   b. Eclampsia—toxemia with accompanying convulsions and coma.
4. Infections
   a. Syphilis
      1. Detected early in pregnancy if serology is done.
      2. If treated early will not be transmitted to fetus.
      3. If untreated can be transmitted

to fetus. The mother may abort, or fetus may be deformed or show other signs of disease at birth.
b. Gonorrhea
  1. May be detected in pregnancy if vaginal discharge is prominent.
  2. Infection of eyes in newborn is possibility if mother is untreated.
  3. Prophylactic treatment of newborn's eyes is legal requirement in most states.
c. German measles
  1. If contracted during first trimester of pregnancy, baby may have congenital deformities, the most common ones being congenital cataracts, heart disease, mental retardation, and deafness.
d. Tuberculosis
  1. Mothers should be under treatment.
  2. Is not transmitted to the fetus in utero, but newborn will contact disease if left with untreated infected mother.
e. Mothers of high risk
  a. Diabetics—require special care to meet metabolic requirements.
  b. Heart disease—require special evaluation and supervision during pregnancy.
  c. ABO and Rh blood factor incompatibilities—require close monitoring throughout pregnancy.
G. Practical nurse's role in prenatal care
  1. Know and teach the value of early and adequate prenatal care.
  2. Offer emotional support to prospective mother.
  3. Instruct expectant parents in the care of the newborn baby.
  4. Be able to recognize and report signs of complications of pregnancy.

Questions

1. Obstetrics is that branch of medicine which deals with:
   1. disorders of the reproductive system
   2. the science and art of human reproduction
   3. the science and art of the care of children
   4. control of venereal disease
2. Advances in maternal and infant care include:
   a. health education programs for the public
   b. prenatal and well-baby clinics
   c. immunization programs
   d. development of special field of neonatology
   1. all of these
   2. all but a
   3. b and c
   4. a and d
3. The female sex glands are known as:
   1. ova
   2. sperm
   3. ovaries
   4. testes
4. The male sex cells are known as:
   1. ova
   2. sperm
   3. ovaries
   4. testes
5. The hormone secreted by the pituitary gland which causes maturation of graafian follicles is called the:
   1. corpus luteum
   2. progesterone
   3. follicle-stimulating hormone
   4. estrogen
6. Expulsion of a mature ovum by the ovary is known as:
   1. coitus
   2. conception
   3. menstruation
   4. ovulation

7. The organ into which sperm are deposited is the:
    1. uterus
    2. vagina
    3. fundus
    4. ovary
8. Union of a sperm and ovum is known as:
    1. ovulation
    2. conception
    3. implantation
    4. menstruation
9. Fertilization of the ovum by the sperm usually takes place in the:
    1. uterus
    2. vagina
    3. fallopian tube
    4. ovary
10. The hollow, pear-shaped muscular organ into which the fertilized egg embeds is the:
    1. ovary
    2. uterus
    3. vagina
    4. fundus
11. The walls of the uterus are made of strong, smooth muscle called:
    1. perimetrium
    2. endometrium
    3. menstruation
    4. myometrium
12. The uterine lining is called the:
    1. endometrium
    2. menstrual tissue
    3. myometrium
    4. perimetrium
13. The organ responsible for nourishing the fetus until birth is the:
    1. ovary
    2. uterus
    3. vagina
    4. placenta
14. Another name for the birth canal is the:
    1. cervix
    2. vagina
    3. uterus
    4. fallopian tube
15. Failure of conception will result in a periodic discharge of bloody fluids called:
    1. menstruation
    2. ovulation
    3. implantation
    4. fertilization
16. In a 28-day cycle, ovulation takes place:
    1. the first day of the menstrual period
    2. the last day of the menstrual period
    3. half way between menstrual periods
    4. the week preceding menstruation
17. The approximate duration of a normal pregnancy is:
    1. 38–40 weeks
    2. 42–45 weeks
    3. 20–22 weeks
    4. 30–32 weeks
18. The hormone secreted by the corpus luteum and placenta which inhibits uterine contractions is:
    1. progesterone
    2. estrogen
    3. follicle-stimulating hormone
    4. lactogenic hormone

19. Until the end of the third month, the product of conception is known as the:
    1. fetus
    2. embryo
    3. lanugo
    4. placenta
20. After the end of the third month, the product of conception is known as the:
    1. fetus
    2. embryo
    3. infant
    4. zygote
21. The fetus receives its blood supply and gets rid of its waste products through:
    1. the amniotic fluid
    2. two umbilical arteries and one umbilical vein
    3. the membranes surrounding the placenta
    4. the membranes surrounding the fetus
22. The first movements of the fetus within the uterus are known as:
    1. lightening
    2. quickening
    3. involution
    4. abortion
23. The first movements of the fetus in utero are normally felt:
    1. at the end of the third month
    2. just before term
    3. within the first 72 hours after conception
    4. between 4½ and 5 months gestation
24. The liquid surrounding the fetus in utero is known as:
    1. vernix caseosa
    2. colostrum
    3. meconium
    4. amniotic fluid
25. The fluid surrounding the fetus acts as a:
    a. cushion against injury to the unborn infant
    b. barrier to bacteria in the mother's bloodstream
    c. insulator to help maintain the body temperature of the fetus
    d. source of nourishment to the fetus

    1. all of these
    2. a and c
    3. b and c
    4. c and d
26. The fine downy hair covering the skin of the fetus in utero, most of which disappears by birth, is called:
    1. vernix caseosa
    2. meconium
    3. lanugo
    4. caput
27. The chief function of the vernix caseosa is to:
    1. serve as a cushion against injury to the fetus
    2. protect the skin from maceration in utero
    3. feed the growing fetus
    4. prevent absorption of waste products through the skin
28. Normal physiological changes of pregnancy that one may anticipate include:
    a. enlargement of breasts
    b. increased pigmentation of areola
    c. tendency to nausea
    d. abdominal cramping
    e. vaginal bleeding

    1. all of these
    2. all but b
    3. a, c, and e
    4. a, b, and c
29. The thin watery fluid secreted by the breast during pregnancy and before lactation begins is called:
    1. colostrum
    2. amniotic fluid
    3. progesterone
    4. meconium
30. Presumptive signs of pregnancy include:
    a. cessation of menstruation
    b. fetal movements
    c. morning sickness
    d. changes in cervix

    1. all of these
    2. all but b
    3. a and c
    4. c and d

31. Probable signs of pregnancy include:
   1. hearing fetal heart sounds
   2. outline of fetus on x-ray
   3. positive biological test for pregnancy
   4. cessation of menstruation
32. Positive signs of pregnancy include:
   a. hearing fetal heart sounds   1. all of these
   b. breast changes   2. all but b
   c. cessation of menstruation   3. all but c
   d. outline of fetus on x-ray   4. a and d
33. A woman who suspects that she is pregnant should consult her physician:
   1. as soon as she misses a menstrual period
   2. shortly after missing the second menstrual period
   3. as soon as morning sickness starts
   4. as soon as she feels the baby moving
34. The blood tests usually done on the expectant mother's first visit to the physician are:
   a. serology   1. all but c
   b. blood count and hemoglobin   2. all of these
   c. prothrombin time   3. a and c
   d. blood typing, including Rh factor   4. b and d
35. Diagnostic tests usually done on the first prenatal visit are:
   a. prothrombin time   1. all of these
   b. urinalysis for sugar and albumin   2. a and b
   c. blood pressure   3. b and c
   d. chest x-ray   4. c and d
36. A woman pregnant for the first time is known as a:
   a. primipara
   2. primigravida
   3. premarital
   4. multipara
37. In the fifth month of pregnancy, the expectant mother might expect which of the following procedures done in her regular office visit?
   a. urinalysis   1. all of these
   b. weight   2. all but c
   c. blood pressure   3. all but d
   d. listening for fetal heart sounds   4. a and b
38. When excess weight is gained in pregnancy:
   a. it is lost with difficulty after delivery   1. all of these
   b. it is lost immediately after delivery   2. all but d
   f. it may be associated with complications   3. a and c
   d. it means a large baby is developing   4. b and d
39. During the third trimester, the pregnant woman may have which of these?
   a. morning sickness   1. all of these
   b. quickening   2. a and b
   c. urinary frequency   3. a and c
   d. lightening   4. c and d
40. false labor contractions are most likely to:
   1. increase the period of labor
   2. be irregularly spaced and fail to cause dilatation of the cervix
   3. cause rupture of the placenta
   4. result in hemorrhage after delivery
41. Braxton-Hicks contractions are best described as:
   1. "false labor pains"
   2. the first fetal movements felt by the mother
   3. irregular uterine contractions which occur throughout pregnancy
   4. abnormally severe contractions of early labor
42. Morning sickness is more commonly experienced:
   1. during the second trimester of pregnancy
   2. during the first 3 months of pregnancy
   3. when the patient is hypertensive
   4. when salt is restricted from the diet

43. The pregnant woman is most likely to have frequency of urination:
    a. in the second trimester   1. all of these
    b. in the first trimester   2. all but a
    c. following lightening   3. a and d
    d. following quickening   4. b and c

44. The acute communicable disease that can cause severe deformities in the fetus if contracted early in pregnancy is:
    1. German measles
    2. scarlet fever
    3. gonorrhea
    4. tuberculosis

45. Placenta previa is a condition in which:
    1. the placenta adheres to the wall of the uterus
    2. the placenta lies low in the uterus and is against or completely covering the cervical opening
    3. the placenta separates from the uterine wall
    4. the placenta has two umbilical veins and only one umbilical artery

46. Excessive vomiting during pregnancy is known as:
    1. toxemia of pregnancy
    2. eclampsia
    3. morning sickness
    4. hyperemesis gravidarum

47. The toxic condition of pregnancy that is characterized by a rise in blood pressure, excessive edema, albuminuria, and, eventually, coma and convulsions is called:
    1. hyperemesis gravidarum
    2. eclampsia
    3. placenta previa
    4. abruptio placentae

48. Premature separation of the placenta from the uterine wall is called:
    1. an incomplete abortion
    2. a precipitate delivery
    3. abruptio placentae
    4. a stillbirth

49. An ectopic pregnancy is best defined as one which occurs:
    1. after the onset of menopause
    2. outside the uterus
    3. before the onset of menstruation
    4. in the fallopian tubes

50. The term "abortion" is best defined as:
    1. deliberate termination of pregnancy
    2. accidental removal of the products of conception from the uterus
    3. termination of pregnancy before the end of the third trimester
    4. expulsion of the products of conception before the fetus is viable

51. Rh factor incompatability:
    a. is found in 85% of white Americans   1. a and b
    b. may cause erythroblastosis in the fetus if the mother   2. c and d
       is Rh− and the fetus is Rh+   3. a and c
    c. may be treated with Rho-GAM if the Rh− woman   4. b and c
       is not sensitized to the Rh factor
    d. usually causes death of the unborn fetus

UNIT 2   LABOR AND DELIVERY

I. **Characteristics and Stages of Labor**
  A. Labor
   1. Combination of processes by which the fetus, the placenta, and the membranes are separated and expelled from the body of the pregnant woman after a period of approximately 280 days (40 weeks) gestation.
   2. The exact cause is not known; hormones thought to be a factor.
   3. A normal labor is one in which termination occurs naturally without complications or artificial aid.
   4. Premature labor or abortion—expulsion of the products of conception before the twentieth week of gestation; fetus is usually small and passes easily through the birth canal.
   5. Postmature labor—extension of pregnancy beyond the forty-second week of gestation. May yield a large fetus that causes difficulty during labor and delivery.
   6. Duration
     a. Varies, depending on
       1. Whether the labor is the first or subsequent one.
       2. Position of fetus in the uterus.
       3. Size of the fetus.
       4. Relative size of the maternal pelvis.
       5. Resistance of the soft tissues.
       6. Whether patient is tense or relaxed.
     b. Average is about 15 hours for first babies, and from 8 to 12 hours for succeeding ones.
     c. Labor extending beyond 24 hours is considered to be prolonged labor.
     d. Labor terminating within 3 hours after onset is termed "precipitate labor." (Not to be confused with precipitate delivery.)
   7. Stages
     a. First stage—stage of dilatation
       1. From the onset of labor until complete dilatation of the cervix occurs.
       2. Average length of time is from 8 to 12 hours.
     b. Second stage—expulsive stage
       1. From complete dilatation of the cervix until delivery of the baby.

   2. Lasts from a few minutes to an hour.
     c. Third stage—placental stage
       1. Placenta and membranes are separated and expelled from the body.
       2. Usually lasts only a few minutes and rarely more than an hour.
  B. Signs of approaching labor
   1. Lightening or dropping—descent of the presenting part into the pelvis.
     a. Usually takes place during last 2 weeks of pregnancy but may not occur until after the onset of labor.
     b. Allows the patient to breathe more easily and eat more without feeling full.
   2. Frequency of urination—due to pressure of the pregnant uterus on the urinary bladder.
   3. Loss of weight—due to changes in metabolism.
   4. False labor—also called Braxton-Hicks contractions; uterine movements that are not constant and do not cause dilatation of the cervix. Often mistaken for true labor.
   5. Show—vaginal discharge of blood-stained mucus. May occur several days prior to the onset of labor, but usually appears shortly after labor starts.
   6. Rupture of the membranes—may occur spontaneously and initiate labor, or artificially by the physician to stimulate regular contractions.
  C. Admission to hospital
   1. Physician has usually instructed the patient to come to the hospital as soon as labor is well established and contractions are regular.
   2. She probably has already had communication with him, and he may have made reservations for her.
   3. Husband may be sent to admission office to supply information needed there while patient is being prepared for delivery.
   4. Routine physical preparation (varies with individual institution)
     a. Nurse assists patient to disrobe and get into bed (bath is given if needed).
     b. Valuables are safeguarded.

c. Information is obtained as to:
   1. When contractions started.
   2. Their duration and frequency.
   3. Whether membranes are ruptured or intact.
   4. E.D.C. (expected date of confinement).
   5. Whether there have been previous labors.
d. Temperature, pulse, respiration, and blood pressure are taken.
e. Routine voided urine specimen is obtained if membranes are intact and there is not yet a bloody show.
f. Routine blood specimens for lab work may be drawn; tests may include CBC, VDRL, and blood type.
g. Fetal heart tones are checked for rate and rhythm. Normal range is 120–160 beats per minute.
   1. Manual fetoscope monitors FHT's intermittently.
   2. Monitors may be attached to the mother and fetus for continuous monitoring (Fig. 51).
h. Perineal area is shaved to insure cleanliness.
i. Cleansing enema is given only if ordered by the physician. Some reasons for *not* giving an enema are
   1. Vaginal bleeding other than show.
   2. Evidence of prolapsed cord.
   3. If patient is heavily sedated.
   4. Evidence of advanced labor. The patient may be allowed to go to the bathroom unless the physician or registered nurse feels it is contraindicated. After expulsion of the enema solution, the nurse should observe the contents and record in full.

j. Vitamin K preparation is seldom given since it is uncertain whether the fetus benefits from it in blood clotting.
k. It is usually considered unwise to use vaginal pads during labor, although underpads are used while patient is in bed.
l. Physician or nurse now may do a rectal or vaginal examination.
   1. Rectal — some institutions allow registered nurses to perform this examination if physician or intern is not readily available.
      a. Patient placed in lithotomy position and draped.
      b. Equipment needed — sterile glove and lubricating jelly.
      c. Sterile gauze square over vagina to protect from contamination.
   2. Vaginal — done by physician, intern, or registered nurse, according to hospital policy.
      a. Patient prepared as if for delivery.
      b. May be done in labor room or patient may be transferred to delivery room.
      c. Placed in lithotomy position and draped.
      d. Vaginal area, buttocks, and upper thighs are scrubbed with pHisoHex and sprayed with an antiseptic solution.
m. Results are recorded on the patient's chart.

5. Emotional support at time of admission
   a. Admission procedure may make a lasting impression on patient.
   b. This is a very special occasion in the life of the patient and her family.
   c. The nurse should receive the patient as she would a guest in her home.

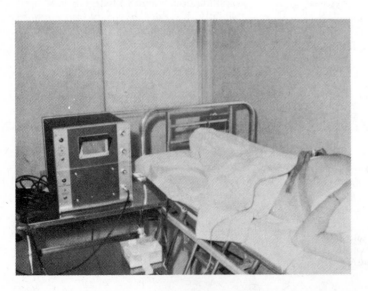

FIGURE 51. Monitoring the fetal heart. (From Bergin: *Nursing Clinics of North America,* 1:562, 1966.)

d. She should appear cheerful and enthusiastic.

e. If it is the patient's first admission to the hospital and time permits, familiarize her with her surroundings.

f. The nurse's attitude should relay confidence to her patient.

g. The patient should be addressed by her title and surname and every effort made to respect her individuality and privacy.

h. Simple explanations as to procedures to be done will eliminate fear of the unknown.

i. Never discuss the patient's condition within her hearing.

j. Every courtesy should be shown the patient's husband and family.

k. Proper nursing care will help to shorten the labor.

II. Nursing Care during Labor

A. First stage

1. Physical care—rest

a. A mild sedative may be given to allow for rest before hard labor begins.

b. Any position that insures comfort is permissible.

c. All measures should be taken to insure comfort and rest during this stage to conserve strength for labor.

d. Patient should be encouraged to rest between contractions.

e. Under no circumstances should she be permitted to "bear down" during the first stage.

f. Gown and linens are changed as often as necessary to keep the patient clean and dry.

2. Emotional support

a. The patient will look to the nurse for guidance and support.

b. She will gain much security by the knowledge that she will never be left alone.

c. Most institutions allow the husband to remain with his wife during this stage.

d. He may be allowed to help apply pressure to her lower back when the pain becomes more intense.

e. Progress reports to patient and family will relieve anxiety and help them feel a part of the situation.

3. Diet

a. Solid foods are withheld from the time true labor is established.

b. If a lengthy labor is expected, fluids by mouth are given in small quantities until hard labor commences.

c. I.V. fluids may be administered.

d. Thirst may be relieved by moistening tongue and lips at intervals with wet gauze.

4. Observations

a. The general appearance is noted to detect fatigue, restlessness, etc.

b. Movements of the fetus should be carefully noted.

c. A full bladder should be noticed and relieved.

d. Fetal heart tones should be checked every 30 mintues for rate and rhythm.

e. Contractions are checked at frequent intervals for frequency and duration. The consistency and size of the uterus should be carefully noted.

f. Vaginal discharges should be watched for amount and type, and it should be noted if amniotic fluid is escaping.

g. The patient's reaction to pain (facial expression, cries, signs of anxiety, etc.) should be noted as a guide to the type and amount of sedation to be given.

5. Positioning and activity

a. Activity increases the strength of contractions; in early labor the patient may be allowed to be ambulatory. Later, frequent changes of position in bed aid in the same fashion.

b. Controlled breathing exercises learned in classes for expectant parents promote relaxation and aid labor.

c. The bladder should not be allowed to become overdistended, as this retards labor and can cause incontinence or retention of urine following delivery. Catheterization is done only on the instructions of the physician.

d. No drug is given except on the written order of the attending physician.

B. Second stage

1. Signs indicating beginning of second stage

a. Change in patient's cry of pain.

b. Intensity; almost no relaxation between contractions.

c. Bulging of perineum.

d. Uncontrollable urge to bear down or to move her bowels.

e. Patient says she feels the baby coming.

2. Physical care

a. Transfer to delivery room.

b. Position on delivery table.

c. The perineal area, lower abdomen, and upper inner thighs are first scrubbed with soap and water, then sprayed with an antiseptic solution.

d. Sterile drapes are applied.

3. Emotional care

a. Remain with patient at all times.

b. Encourage her to bear down with her contractions.

c. Assure her that everything is going as it should.

4. Anesthesia

a. Local—injected into perineal area by

physician to reduce pain of episiotomy and its repair.

  b. Regional—mother remains awake for delivery.

    1. Saddle block—a low spinal which deadens area below umbilicus.

    2. Caudal—similar to saddle block but requires constant attention of anesthetist.

    3. Paracervical—local anesthetic injected near junction of vaginal and cervical walls. Interrupts impulses from uterus to spinal cord.

    4. Pudendal—local anesthetic for perineal tissues.

  c. General—administered by anesthetist; gas inhalation or intravenous injection. Causes state of unconsciousness.

  d. Natural—various methods used with the chief purpose being to make delivery a happy, natural experience. Local or regional anesthetics may be used in conjunction with principles of natural childbirth.

III. Delivery

  A. Process of normal delivery

    1. After sterile drapes are applied, the physician catheterizes the patient. (A distended bladder can obstruct the passage of the baby and cause trauma to the bladder.)

    2. Patient is encouraged to push with her contractions. If she is getting inhalation anesthesia, she may receive whiffs with each contraction.

    3. If needed, an episiotomy will be done just as the head begins to emerge through the vaginal outlet. This allows easier delivery of the head without tearing of the tissues of the perineum.

    4. As soon as the head is delivered, the physician suctions the baby's mouth and nose with a bulb syringe to remove mucus.

    5. The delivery is then completed after respiration is established. The baby is placed on the mother's abdomen and the cord clamped and cut. He is wrapped in a sterile cover and placed in an incubator.

  B. Third stage (expression of placenta)

    1. As the placenta shows signs of separating from the uterus, the physician gently expresses it and examines it carefully to make sure none has been retained in the uterus.

    2. The patient is given an injection of pituitary extract to insure a tightly contracted uterus. The nurse must watch the fundus closely for any change in size or consistency. If it should relax, gentle massage on the fundus will cause it to contract again.

    3. The physician then repairs the episiotomy; the nurse cleans the vulva and perineal area with an antiseptic solution; a sterile perineal pad is applied; and the patient is ready to be transferred to the recovery area.

  C. Immediate postpartum care

    1. Physical

      a. The fundus is checked frequently for size and consistency. It should remain tightly contracted and low in the pelvis.

      b. The lochia should be checked for amount and color. The appearance of the perineum should be noted; the physician may order an ice cap for the first 8–12 hours postpartum to prevent excessive swelling of the perineum.

      c. Since a full bladder can push the fundus up into the upper abdomen and cause hemorrhage, it should not be allowed to become overdistended.

      d. The patient should be allowed to rest; most hospitals restrict visitors in this area.

      e. Blood pressure, pulse, and respiration are checked frequently until well stabilized.

      f. She is allowed fluids, and may complain of hunger. In this case, a light diet is allowed.

    2. Emotional

      a. The patient is reassured as to her own and her baby's condition.

      b. She is allowed to see her baby when she recovers sufficiently from the anesthesia, and most hospitals allow the husband to visit at this time.

  D. Immediate care of the baby

    1. The infant is usually observed and evaluated for heart rate, respiratory rate, muscle tone, reflex irritability, and color at 1 and 5 minutes after delivery. A common tool for doing this is the Apgar scoring chart (Fig. 52).

    2. After being placed in the incubator immediately after delivery, the baby is properly identified. (Each institution has its own method.)

    3. Silver nitrate or penicillin drops are put into the baby's eyes.

    4. Most hospitals require footprints to be made for identification purposes, and if so, they are made at this time.

    5. The cord is checked to be sure it is clamped securely. It is usually thought unnecessary to apply a chemical to the stump or to cover it.

    6. The baby is then transferred to the nursery.

SIGN	0	1	2
I. Heart rate Strong and steady?	Not detectable	Slow (below 100)	Over 100
II. Respiratory effort Is the baby breathing frequently and regularly?	Absent	Slow, irregular	Good, crying
III. Muscle tone Is he kicking his feet and making fists?	Flaccid	Some flexion of extremities	Active motion
IV. Reflex irritability Does he cry lustily when a catheter is pushed up one nostril	No response	Grimace	Cry
or when he is prodded on the soles of his feet?	No response	Grimace	Cough or sneeze
V. Color Is he pink all over, or are his hands and feet bluish?	Blue, pale	Body pink, extremities blue	Completely pink

FIGURE 52.   Apgar Scoring Chart. (Bleier: *Maternity Nursing*. 3rd ed.)

IV. Complications of Labor and Delivery
A. Symptoms indicating fetal distress
1. A F.H.T. (fetal heart tone) count of less than 120 or more than 160 per minute.
2. The appearance of meconium in the vaginal discharge (except in breech presentation).
3. Hyperactivity of the fetus. This indicates the fetus is struggling for oxygen.

B. Symptoms indicating maternal danger
1. Vaginal bleeding in excess of a heavy show indicates a partially premature separation of the placenta or laceration of the cervix.
2. A rapid, irregular pulse and lowered blood pressure may be the first indication of hemorrhage as yet unseen.
3. Elevated blood pressure, headache, visual disturbances, extreme restlessness, and rapidly developing edema may be symptoms of toxemia.

4. A sudden cessation of contractions or a contraction that does not relax can result in conditions dangerous to mother and baby.
5. Hemorrhage immediately following delivery may be due to a relaxed uterus, and the nurse should be alert to this probability.

C. Operations in obstetrics
1. Forceps delivery—the use of forceps to aid in delivery of the head of the fetus. When used correctly by a skilled physician, it is entirely safe and can be life-saving for mother and baby.
2. Episiotomy—a surgical incision of the perineum to aid in delivery and prevent laceration.
3. Cesarean section—delivery of the fetus per abdominal and uterine walls. It is done when complications indicate a normal delivery is unsafe.

Questions

1. The first stage of labor includes the time from:
   1. the onset of labor until delivery of the infant
   2. the onset of labor until complete dilatation of the cervix
   3. delivery of the infant to delivery of the placenta
   4. the complete dilatation of the cervix until delivery of the infant

2. On admission to the obstetrical unit, the mother is interviewed for the following information:
   a. membranes intact or ruptured   1. all of these
   b. time contractions started   2. all but a
   c. frequency of contractions   3. all but b
   d. expected date of delivery   4. all but d

3. During the initial admission assessment of the mother, it would be best to:
   1. tell the father to go home as labor usually lasts a long time
   2. explain the admission procedure and reassure the father he will be allowed to see his wife as soon as it is completed
   3. send the father to the classes on care of the newborn
   4. ask him to wait in the waiting room

4. On admission to the obstetrical unit a vaginal examination is done. From this, the examiner is able to determine:
   a. fetal heart tones   1. all of these
   b. amount of cervical dilatation   2. all but d
   c. presenting part of the fetus   3. b and c
   d. time of impending delivery   4. c and d

5. On admission to the obstetrical unit, the mother is prepared by having the genital area shaved. The purpose of this procedure is to:
   1. provide a clean area for delivery
   2. allow for an easier delivery
   3. aid in dilatation of the cervix
   4. facilitate the application of perineal pads

6. Most obstetricians order an enema as soon as the patient is admitted. The reasons for this are to:
   a. empty the lower colon and rectum   1. a only
   b. insure a clean field for delivery   2. all but b
   c. stimulate contractions   3. c and d
   d. provide more space in the pelvis for easier   4. all of these
      delivery of the infant

7. Some valid reasons for not administering an enema to a patient would include:
   a. vaginal bleeding that is considered to be excessive   1. all of these
   b. advanced labor   2. all but d
   c. evidence of a prolapsed umbilical cord   3. b and c
   d. if the patient has had a bowel movement   4. c and d
      within the past 24 hours

8. The timing of contractions can best be accomplished by:
   1. placing the hand on the patient's abdomen
   2. noting the expression on the patient's face
   3. questioning the patient about the amount of pain she is having
   4. exposing the patient's abdomen and closely watching the rise and fall of the abdomen

9. In order to determine the frequency of uterine contractions most accurately, the nurse should:
   1. note the time interval between the onset of one contraction and the onset of the next for at least six consecutive contractions
   2. note the time elapsing between the end of one contraction and the onset of the next one
   3. note the time interval from the end of one contraction until the end of the next one
   4. count the number of contractions in a 10-minute interval

10. To determine the duration of the contractions, the nurse should:
    1. ask the patient to tell her how long each contraction lasts
    2. note the time interval from the onset of the contraction until relaxation of the uterus
    3. note the time interval between contractions
    4. record each contraction in a 10-minute period and divide the number of minutes by the number of contractions

11. The duration of labor depends on:
    a. the number of previous pregnancies and deliveries   1. all of these
    b. position of the fetus   2. a and d only
    c. size of the fetus in relation to the maternal pelvis   3. all but d
    d. the number of living children delivered by   4. b and c
       the mother

12. Overdistention of the urinary bladder should be avoided during labor primarily because it:
    1. may cause a sudden onset of eclampsia
    2. can retard labor
    3. may cause incontinence or retention following delivery
    4. may lead to a urinary infection

13. The fetoscope is a special instrument used to:
    1. listen to the fetal heart tones through the abdominal and uterine walls
    2. determine the length of the fetus
    3. measure the width of the maternal pelvis
    4. record the blood pressure of the mother at frequent intervals

14. The fetal and maternal monitor is used to record:
    a. fetal heart tones
    b. maternal blood pressure
    c. uterine contractions
    d. fetal position
    1. all of these
    2. all but d
    3. a and c
    4. a and d

15. Fetal distress during labor may be indicated by:
    a. a marked change in the rate of fetal heart tones
    b. irregularity of the fetal heart tones
    c. presence of meconium in the vaginal discharge in the absence of a breech presentation
    d. hyperactivity of the fetus
    1. all but c
    2. all of these
    3. b only
    4. d only

16. The normal rate of the fetal heart tones is:
    1. 90 to 200 per minute
    2. 120 to 200 per minute
    3. 120 to 160 per minute
    4. 60 to 90 per minute

17. Food and fluids are often withheld during active labor. Some factors influencing this include:
    a. peristalsis slows down during labor
    b. some medicines administered during labor cause nausea
    c. if vomiting occurs, there is danger of aspiration of food into lungs
    d. digestion slows down labor
    1. all of these
    2. all but b
    3. all but c
    4. all but d

18. Ambulation of the patient in labor is usually permitted:
    1. in early labor while membranes are intact
    2. in the presence of vaginal bleeding
    3. after sedation for discomfort
    4. between contractions

19. Some ways to add to the patient's comfort during the first stage of labor include:
    a. frequent changes of linens to insure a clean dry bed
    b. assisting her to change positions in bed
    c. allowing her to rest between contractions
    d. encouraging her to bear down with each contraction
    1. a and b
    2. c and d
    3. all of these
    4. all but d

20. In checking the perineum, the nurse notices a prolapsed cord. She should:
    a. observe the patient again in 15 minutes
    b. place in Trendelenburg or knee-chest position
    c. notify physician immediately
    d. monitor fetal heart rate frequently
    1. all of these
    2. all but a
    3. all but b
    4. all but d

21. Which of the following signs indicate the onset of the second stage of labor?
    a. an increase in the rate and intensity of contractions
    b. a bulging perineum
    c. an uncontrollable urge on the part of the patient to bear down
    d. a sudden cessation of contractions
    1. all of these
    2. a and b
    3. b and c
    4. all but d

22. During the second stage of labor the patient is encouraged to:
    1. pant rapidly between contractions
    2. bear down with each contraction and rest between contractions
    3. hold her thighs tightly together
    4. refrain from pushing with her contractions and relax as much as possible

23. In the majority of deliveries, when crowning occurs, the presenting part will be the:
     1. feet
     2. buttocks
     3. head
     4. shoulder

24. During delivery, when the umbilical cord emerges through the cervical opening before the presenting part emerges, there is danger of obstructing the flow of blood to the infant. This condition is called:
     1. a breech delivery
     2. a compound presentation
     3. an oblique presentation
     4. a prolapsed cord

25. The obstetrical operation that is done to enlarge the vaginal orifice is called:
     1. cesarean section
     2. episiotomy
     3. vaginal repair
     4. rupture of the membranes

26. Surgical enlargement of the vaginal orifice is performed:
     1. as the head begins to emerge through the vaginal outlet
     2. as the cervix begins to dilate
     3. after delivery of the head
     4. only as an emergency measure

27. The chief purpose of enlarging the vaginal orifice is to:
     1. prevent damage to the umbilical cord
     2. speed up the third stage of labor
     3. avoid the danger of infection
     4. prevent tearing of the tissues of the perineum

28. The birth of the newborn occurs in the:
     1. first stage
     2. second stage
     3. third stage
     4. fourth stage

29. The third stage of labor includes the time from:
     1. the onset of labor until delivery of the infant
     2. the onset of labor until complete dilatation of the cervix
     3. delivery of the infant to delivery of the placenta
     4. the complete dilatation of the cervix until delivery of the infant

30. After the placenta is expelled, the physician examines it thoroughly. The reason for doing this is to:
     1. determine if the entire placenta was delivered
     2. determine the presence of infection within the uterus
     3. obtain a sample for microscopic examination
     4. determine the presence of growths or tumors

31. A woman who has just delivered her first child is known as a:
     1. primipara
     2. primigravida
     3. multipara
     4. multigravida

32. Immediate postpartum care includes:
     a. frequent observation of the fundus for location, size, and consistency
     b. checking the mother's vital signs frequently
     c. constant massage of the uterus
     d. providing adequate rest for the mother

     1. all of these
     2. b only
     3. a only
     4. all but c

33. After delivery the uterus should be palpated for firmness. The fundus should be:
     1. soft and at the level of the umbilicus
     2. firm and two fingers below the umbilicus
     3. firm and at the level of the umbilicus
     4. firm and two fingers above the umbilicus

34. Lochia is the term used to describe:
    1. the fluid surrounding the fetus in utero
    2. the clear fluid secreted by the breasts during the first 24 hours after delivery
    3. the vaginal discharge following delivery
    4. the vaginal discharge secreted just before the second stage of labor
35. Immediately postpartum one would expect the lochia to be:
    1. bright red and in large amounts
    2. reddish-brown and profuse
    3. full of clots and particles of placental tissue
    4. yellowish-white and in large amounts
36. During this period the nurse must not allow the patient's bladder to become greatly distended. The main reason for this precaution is that:
    1. the bladder may have been weakened during labor and it may rupture
    2. the patient may void involuntarily and contaminate the birth canal
    3. a full bladder can push into the upper abdomen and lead to hemorrhage from the uterus
    4. an overdistended bladder may press against the suture line of the episiotomy and open the surgical wound
37. If the uterus is not felt at its proper location and is not of the proper consistency the nurse should suspect:
    1. that the bladder is overdistended
    2. that there is a second fetus or placenta within the uterus
    3. hemorrhage, even though there may be no external bleeding
    4. a collapse of the bladder
38. Hemorrhage following delivery is most often due to:
    a. abruptio placentae
    b. a relaxed uterus
    c. retention of a particle of the placenta or membranes
    d. spasms of the uterine muscles

    1. all but d
    2. all of these
    3. b and c
    4. d only

UNIT 3   THE PUERPERIUM

I. **Nursing during Puerperium**
  A. The puerperium or "lying in" is the period of 6 to 7 weeks following delivery during which the uterus returns to normal and lactation begins.
  B. Physiological changes
    1. Uterus
      a. Immediately following delivery, the uterus should be at, or below, the level of the umbilicus, well contracted, and in the midline.
      b. It decreases in size daily, until by the tenth day it can barely be felt behind the pubic bone.
      c. It returns to its normal prepregnant state (involution) in about 6 weeks.
    2. Lochia
      a. The discharge from the uterus immediately following delivery is bright red and called *lochia rubra*.
      b. Within a few days it is a reddish-brown color and is called *lochia serosa*.
      c. On about the tenth or twelfth day it becomes yellowish-white and is called *lochia alba*.
    3. Breasts
      a. First 2 or 3 days — secrete a thin, almost colorless liquid called *colostrum*.
      b. Lactation begins on the second to fourth day after delivery. Diet and emotional factors are believed to influence the quantity and composition of the milk.
    4. Return of menstruation
      a. Usually reestablished in non-nursing mothers in 6 to 8 weeks.
      b. Mothers who nurse their babies may not have a menstrual period for 4 to 6 months, or, in some, until they discontinue breast feeding. This, however, does not necessarily mean she does not ovulate; thus, she can become pregnant.
  C. Patient needs
    1. Physical
      a. Rest

        1. Very important immediately following delivery and can be insured by a clean dry bed, comfortable position, and quiet room.
        2. Daily rest periods should be encouraged.
        3. A good night's sleep is very important during this period to enable the mother to gain sufficient strength to care for her baby at home.
      b. Exercise
        1. Early ambulation is encouraged.
        2. The physician will instruct the patient about exercises to promote muscle tone of the abdomen.
      c. Cleanliness
        1. A daily bath is essential for comfort and to insure freedom from odors.
        2. After the patient is ambulatory, she may be permitted to shower.
        3. She may shampoo her hair at any time she feels it is needed.
        4. A tub bath is usually contraindicated for at least 2 weeks following delivery.
        5. She should be instructed in giving herself perineal care. An explanation as to why it is necessary to prevent infection will help to make her aware of its importance.
        6. Perineal pads should be changed as needed for comfort and cleanliness. She should be instructed to place and remove pads from front to back.
      d. Diet
        1. A well-balanced diet is essential to promote healing and insure good health.
        2. A nursing mother should have added amounts of milk (1½ quarts (1.4 liters) are recommended), lean meat, citrus fruits, green leafy vegetables, and liquids. Her physician may order vitamin supplements. She should avoid foods that produce gas.
      e. Breast care
        1. Breast feeding is encouraged, but

decision is to be made by the parents on advice of the physician. If asked for advice the nurse may stress the advantages of breast feeding.

2. Breasts are bathed first when the bath is given, with clean warm water and soap; wash one breast with gentle circular motion, starting with the nipple, and working outward. Dry with a clean towel and repeat the process for the second breast.

3. A good brassiere that gives adequate support will add to the patient's comfort and help prevent muscle stretching.

4. The physician will order an ointment to be applied to the nipples following breast feedings. This helps prevent soreness and cracking and promotes healing.

f. Elimination

1. Voiding may be difficult following delivery. The nurse must observe the patient closely to prevent an overdistended bladder which may cause uterine hemorrhage. Frequent voiding of small amounts may indicate inability to empty the bladder. Bathroom privileges may be allowed a few hours after delivery (with assistance).

2. A mild laxative or cleansing enema is usually ordered, if needed, to relieve constipation on the second or third day following delivery. Care should be taken to prevent injury to the perineum while inserting the colon tube. The patient should be instructed in perineal care following a bowel movement.

2. Emotional

a. Fatigue and discomfort following delivery may cause the new mother to be anxious about her own or her baby's well-being. The knowledge that she is in competent, skilled hands will bring some relief. Simple, matter-of-fact explanations to her questions will help, and the opportunity to handle and inspect the new baby will bring assurance of his healthy state.

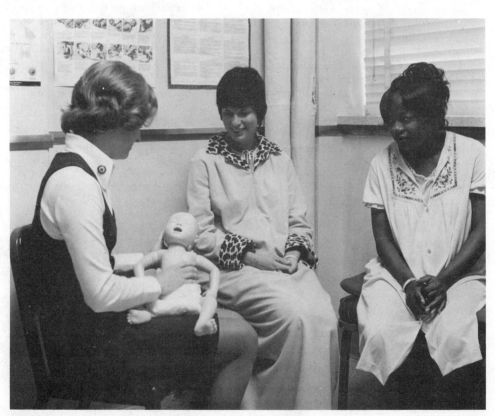

FIGURE 53.   The public health nurse, who may later visit the mother and infant at home, may also visit the new mother in the hospital to prepare her for taking care of herself and infant after going home. Note the cushions on the chairs for added comfort. (Courtesy of Carole Deegan, Director Patient Education Department, Medical Center of Central Georgia, Macon, Georgia. Photo by Terri Bryson, R.N.)

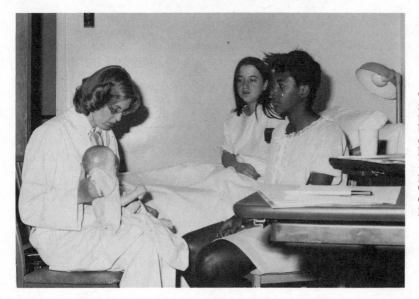

FIGURE 54. Providing an opportunity for new mothers to get together to discuss the normal characteristics of the newborn enables them to be aware of what to expect when they get home. (Courtesy Carole Deegan, Director Patient Education Department, Medical Center of Central Georgia, Macon, Georgia. Photo by Terri Bryson, R.N.)

Visits from her husband at this time also give comfort.

    b. Some patients experience a period of depression ("maternity blues") a few days following delivery. It is characterized by spells of crying for no apparent reason and usually distresses the patient very much. To let her cry it out, with the assurance that her feelings are more or less normal, is usually the wise course.

    c. Remember, the birth of each child is a very special event for the family and should be so considered by those in attendance.

II. Teaching the Patient (Fig. 53)

  A. Instructions concerning the mother

    1. Importance of rest, exercise, nutritive diet, and personal cleanliness.

    2. Necessity of adjustments when there is an older child in the home.

    3. Importance of reporting to her doctor any abnormal symptoms.

    4. Value of postpartum examination for her and her baby at 4 to 6 weeks after delivery.

    5. Reasons for refraining from marital relations and avoiding douches until after postpartum examination.

  B. Instructions concerning the baby

    1. How to handle the baby, and normal characteristics (Fig. 54).

    2. Bath demonstration (Fig. 55).

    3. How to prepare formula.

    4. How to hold the baby to feed him (Figs. 56 and 57).

    5. How and why to burp baby (Figs. 58 and 59).

FIGURE 55. The expression on the baby's face is engendered by the skill and confidence that the nurse exhibits in his care. (Davis, M. E., and Rubin, R.: *DeLee's Obstetrics for Nurses,* 17th ed., Philadelphia, W. B. Saunders Co., 1962.)

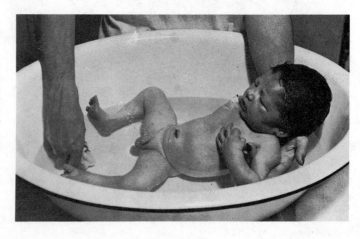

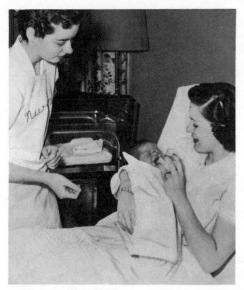

FIGURE 56.   Mother learns the art of feeding her baby. (Davis and Rubin: *DeLee's Obstetrics for Nurses.* 18th ed.)

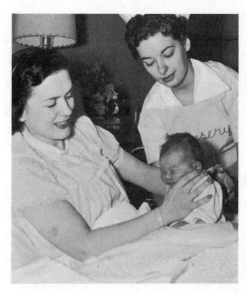

FIGURE 58.   The nurse helps with the "burping" technique. (Davis and Rubin: *DeLee's Obstetrics for Nurses.* 17th ed.)

6. Information concerning layette and how to dress for warm or cold weather.
7. Importance of playing with and cuddling him.
8. Instructions on care of navel cord and circumcision.
9. Importance of fresh air and sunshine.
10. Importance of early immunization.

III. **Discomforts and Complications of Puerperium**
  A. Afterpains
    1. Are usually more severe as baby nurses or following administration of *oxytocics* (drugs which stimulate uterine contractions).
    2. May require analgesic for relief.

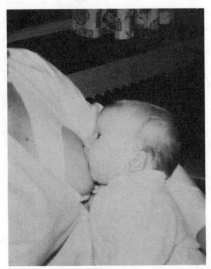

FIGURE 57.   Baby at breast. (Thompson: *Pediatrics for Practical Nurses.* 3rd ed.)

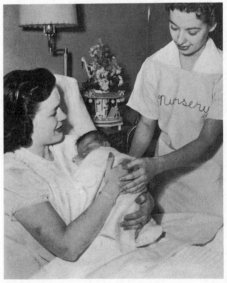

FIGURE 59.   Another method of holding and "bubbling" the baby. (Davis and Rubin: *DeLee's Obstetrics for Nurses.* 17th ed.)

B. Hemorrhoids
   1. Usually more severe following delivery.
   2. Sitz baths may help relieve pain, or the physician may order analgesic ointment, suppositories, or medicated packs.
C. Thrombophlebitis
   1. Usually occurs in veins of pelvis or legs.
   2. Bed rest with the limb immobilized and elevated, and heat applications are usually ordered. Patient may be required to wear elastic stockings on resuming activity.
D. Engorged breasts
   1. As lactation begins, the breast tissue becomes swollen and painful. This may occur even though the mother has had medication to suppress lactation. Breasts are not pumped, in this case.
   2. A breast binder or a brassiere that offers good support should be applied (Fig. 60).
   3. Nursing mothers usually gain relief as the baby nurses. Breasts are pumped immediately after nursing the baby, if ordered by the physician.
   4. Ice packs may be applied for relief of pain and to reduce swelling.
E. Puerperal infections
   1. Can be prevented by strict use of aseptic technique during labor and delivery.
   2. Never introduce any object into the birth canal of an obstetrical patient.
   3. Patients contracting an infection must be isolated, and nursing personnel cautioned of the danger of transmitting the disease to uninfected patients.
F. Hemorrhage
   1. May be caused by retained particle of placenta or flaccid uterus.
   2. May occur at any time, but frequently seen between sixth and tenth days following delivery.
   3. Physician must be notified and the source of bleeding determined.

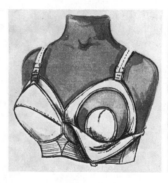
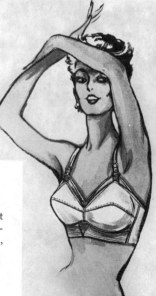

FIGURE 60.   Underlift nursing bra. Self-adjusting cups expand and contract without constriction. One motion unhooks top of cup for immediate access. Removable, moisture-proof protective shields. (Courtesy of Charma Bra Co., Inc., Clinical Research Division, New York.)

Questions

1. The puerperium is best defined as:
   1. the first 24 hours after delivery
   2. the first 24 hours before delivery
   3. the 6 to 7 weeks following delivery
   4. the first 5 days after delivery during which the mother is hospitalized

2. Which of the following changes take place during the puerperium?
    1. The uterus returns to its normal size and location, and lactation begins.
    2. The endometrium begins to undergo changes necessary for menstruation.
    3. Cervical dilatation takes place and the uterus begins to contract at regular intervals.
    4. The placenta begins to separate from the uterine wall and the cervix becomes completely dilated.
3. The term involution refers to:
    1. an increase in the size of the uterus to accommodate the growing fetus
    2. a sloughing off of the inner lining of the uterus
    3. the discharge of the ovum from the graafian follicle
    4. the return of the uterus to its normal prepregnant state
4. The purpose of applying dry heat to the perineum is to:
    a. promote healing
    b. relieve pain
    c. destroy bacteria
    d. decrease amount of lochia

    1. all of these
    2. a and b
    3. b and c
    4. c and d
5. Difficulty in voiding may occur due to swelling of the urinary meatus. Measures which would encourage the mother to void include:
    a. pouring warm water over the vulva
    b. catheterization as the only effective method
    c. running water in the sink
    d. instructing patient to void in warm sitz bath
    e. having no need for concern; she will void when necessary

    1. b only
    2. e only
    3. a, c, and d
    4. a and d
6. Lactation is the term used to describe:
    1. the first secretions of the breast following childbirth
    2. the secretion of milk by the breast
    3. a blood-tinged fluid sometimes secreted by the breasts of a primipara
    4. the manual expression of milk from the breast
7. The nursing mother should be taught the importance of cleanliness in the care of her breasts. To bathe the breast she should:
    a. use only sterile water and sterile cotton balls
    b. use warm water and soap, starting at the nipple and washing outward with a circular motion
    c. pat the breast dry
    d. sponge the breasts with alcohol or a mild boric acid solution

    1. a and d
    2. b and c
    3. a and b
    4. c and d
8. The nursing mother may not have a menstrual period for several months after delivery, or even until she discontinues breast feedings. She should be told that:
    1. ovulation is suppressed and pregnancy is impossible as long as breast feeding is continued
    2. breast feeding does not suppress ovulation and pregnancy is possible even though she continues breast feeding
    3. the uterus does not return to its normal size until after breast feeding is discontinued
    4. if the menstrual flow does not return in 2 months she should discontinue the breast feeding
9. The non-nursing mother will receive medication to suppress lactation. If she experiences some breast engorgement, the physician may order any of the following measures for her comfort:
    a. a mild sedative
    b. ice packs
    c. manual expression of milk
    d. a breast binder for support

    1. all of these
    2. all but a
    3. all but b
    4. all but c
10. The chief purpose of using a breast binder is to:
    1. immobilize the breasts downward against the chest wall
    2. increase the flow of milk
    3. reduce the size of the breasts
    4. support the breasts, holding them up and outward
11. Afterpains are caused by:
    1. trauma during labor and delivery
    2. contractions of the uterus as it attempts to regain its muscle tone
    3. constipation in the postpartum period
    4. a prolapsed uterus

12. Afterpains are more likely to be felt:
    a. when the baby nurses
    b. after a bowel movement
    c. by mothers who have had two or more deliveries
    d. following administration of oxytocic drugs such as ergotrate

    1. all of these
    2. d only
    3. all but a
    4. all but b

13. The patient should be taught to apply and remove perineal pads:
    1. from front to back
    2. from back to front
    3. with sterile forceps
    4. only after donning a pair of sterile gloves

14. When lochia has a foul smell, the nurse should:
    1. realize that this may be an indication of infection and report it immediately
    2. consider this to be normal during the first few days after delivery
    3. begin vaginal irrigations to reduce the odor and provide comfort for the patient
    4. discontinue the use of perineal pads for a few days

15. When administering an enema to a puerperal patient, it is most important for the nurse to:
    1. use a very small catheter
    2. administer no more than 100 ml. of solution
    3. be careful not to injure the perineum while inserting the tube
    4. insist that the patient administer it to herself, as she will need to know how before she goes home

16. The widely accepted practice that has greatly decreased the incidence of thrombophlebitis following childbirth is:
    1. early ambulation
    2. immobilization and elevation of the affected part
    3. the administration of antibiotics during the puerperium
    4. breast feeding of infants

17. The primary reason for cautioning mothers against taking douches or having marital relations until after the postpartum examination is:
    1. danger of rupturing the episiotomy wound
    2. reducing the danger of postpartum hemorrhage
    3. avoiding the possibility of introducing infection into the birth canal until healing is complete
    4. avoiding the danger of cystitis in the postpartum period

18. A woman pregnant for the second time, with one living child would be:
    1. Gravid II Para II
    2. Gravid II Para I
    3. Gravid I Para II
    4. Gravid I Para I

19. Identical twins:
    a. develop from a single fertilized ovum
    b. derive their food and oxygen from two separate placentas
    c. usually resemble each other very closely
    d. are always of the same sex

    1. all of these
    2. all but a
    3. all but b
    4. all but d

20. Fraternal twins are:
    1. developed from the same ovum
    2. a result of the fertilization of two separate ova
    3. always encased in the same amniotic sac
    4. nourished by the same placenta while in utero

21. A cesarean section may be done owing to:
    a. cephalopelvic disproportion
    b. placenta previa
    c. unsatisfactory progress in labor
    d. malpresentation

    1. all of these
    2. all but b
    3. all but c
    4. c only

22. Delivery, in the obstetrical sense, refers to:
    1. the actual birth of the infant
    2. the expulsion of the placenta
    3. the period from onset of labor until expulsion of the placenta
    4. removal of the infant and placenta by surgical means

UNIT 4   THE NEWBORN

I. **Nursing the Newborn Baby**
  A. The normal newborn baby
    1. Appearance
      a. Weight—7 to 7½ lbs. (3175 to 3402 grams).
      b. Length—20 to 21 inches (51 to 53 cm.).
      c. Color is dusky red with slightly blue-tinged extremities. As circulation improves the skin becomes slightly pink, and as the baby cries, vividly red.
      d. Head looks long and is large in comparison to rest of the body. The fontanels (soft spots) are open. The ears are creased or folded due to lack of hardened cartilage. The irides of Caucasian babies are usually blue with true color not determined until 3 to 6 months of age. Eyes do not track properly.
      e. The neck is small; thus the head seems to rest on the chest.
      f. The legs are pulled up onto the abdomen which protrudes somewhat.
      g. The hands are clenched into fists.
      h. Vernix caseosa may entirely cover body or be found only in body creases.
      i. Lanugo may be seen on back, shoulders, and forehead. Is especially evident in premature, but disappears in postnatal life.
      j. Sebaceous glands on face may be plugged with secretions and are called milia.
    2. Physiology
      a. Movements are disorganized but infant has good muscle tone.
      b. Is born with the sucking reflex, and is able to sneeze, cough, and cry.
      c. Is able to urinate and evacuate its bowels.
      d. The first bowel movements are dark green, thick, and sticky (meconium), but begin to change to yellow as he begins to take milk.
      e. In the first few days of life, he will lose about 10 per cent of his body weight, but will begin to regain it within a week.

      f. Respiration rate is between 40 and 60 per minute and irregular.
      g. Normal body temperature, taken rectally, is maintained near 99.6°F. (37.6°C). Because the temperature center is not fully developed, the environment must be regulated to help maintain body heat.
      h. The pulse rate ranges from 100 to 150 per minute and is irregular.
    3. Admittance to nursery
      a. A bland oil bath will remove the vernix caseosa very well, as will warm water and soap, if oil is contraindicated. At this time the baby's body is inspected thoroughly by the nurse.
      b. Temperature is taken rectally.
      c. He is weighed on admittance to the nursery and daily thereafter.
      d. Some institutions photograph and record footprints of newborn infants on admittance to the nursery for identification purposes.
      e. Length, and circumference of head and chest are measured.
      f. He is then dressed in diaper and shirt and placed in an incubator for a few hours or wrapped in a blanket and placed in his crib.
      g. For the first 24 hours he is watched closely for cyanosis. A sterile bulb syringe may be used to remove excess mucus from nose and throat.
    4. Physical needs
      a. Daily bath
        1. Serves to clean the skin and stimulate circulation.
        2. Procedure varies among institutions.
      b. Clothing
        1. Should be light and comfortable.
        2. Amount depends upon the temperature. Excessive clothing restricts the baby's movements and helps cause heat rash.
        3. Cotton clothes that launder well are preferable.

321

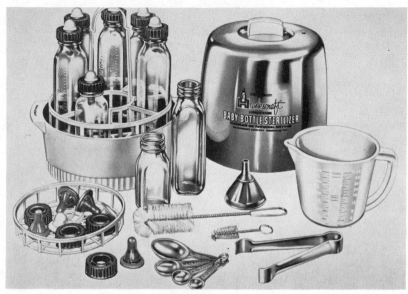

FIGURE 61.   Equipment for making formula in the home. (Courtesy Hankscraft Co., Reedsburg, Wis.)

c. Feeding
  1. Breast feeding
    a. Baby may be fed when he is hungry (demand feeding), or may be placed on a schedule of feeding every 3 or 4 hours.
    b. Instruct mother to begin nursing baby for 3 to 5 minutes at each breast, depending on the condition of the nipples and the desires of the baby. Nursing time may be increased to 20 minutes as the colostrum is replaced with "complete" milk.
    c. Warm water may be given between feedings.
    d. Mother should be instructed to "burp" her baby about halfway through the feeding, and again when he finishes.
    e. In some communities a group of mothers interested in promoting breast feeding have formed organizations to help the new mother. The La Leche League International is one such organization.
  2. Bottle feeding
    a. Physician chooses formula adequate for baby's needs.
    b. Holding him while feeding him gives a sense of security, and provides an opportunity for a pleasant contact between mother and baby.
    c. Strict sterilization methods are observed in preparing the formula

(Fig. 61). (Instructions for formula preparation methods are available to the mother from many sources. Some institutions provide instruction classes on the maternity unit.)
    d. Baby should be held upright for feeding and the bottle should be tilted so that the neck and the nipple are full to prevent air from being sucked into the stomach.
d. Sleep and exercise
  1. Normally, the newborn infant sleeps about 20 hours a day, waking only for feeding.
  2. He will gradually stay awake longer during the day but should sleep most of the night.
  3. Most babies seem to sleep on their abdomen, which is desirable since it allows for drainage if they regurgitate food or vomit.
  4. If possible, he should sleep in a room of his own but very near his parents.
  5. He provides some of his exercise by moving himself about, and more is provided in lifting and turning him.
5. Emotional needs
  a. The emotional needs of the newborn baby are met when his physical needs are met.
  b. He responds to the person caring for him, and feelings of security and well-being can be communicated to him in

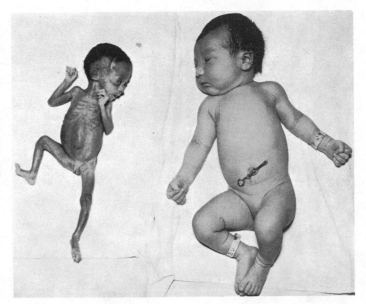

FIGURE 62. The premature baby, on the left, was 28 days old when this picture was taken. He lived and is normal. The baby on the right is a full-term newborn. (Davis and Rubin: *DeLee's Obstetrics for Nurses.* 17th ed.)

the manner of handling and holding him, and by the tone of voice.

c. Early in life he comes to feel his mother's presence and soon demands her attention.

6. Circumcision—surgical removal of foreskin of penis.

a. Is done with parents written consent. May be done in delivery room or the first or second day of life.

b. Petroleum jelly gauze may be applied until initial healing occurs.

II. The Premature Infant

A. Definition—weight is indicative of an infant's prematurity and physiological immaturity. A premature infant is now considered to be one who weighs 5 pounds, 8 ounces (2500 grams) or less at birth.

B. Characteristics of the premature infant (Fig. 62).

1. Poor control of body temperature, fatty tissue is very scant.

2. Difficulty with respiration.

3. Inability to handle infections of any kind.

4. Disturbances in nutrition, sucking reflex usually very weak or entirely absent.

5. Tendency to hemorrhage and develop anemia.

C. Initial care

1. Establish and maintain respiration. Placed in Isolette. Rockette and oxygen usually administered (Fig. 63). Oxygen

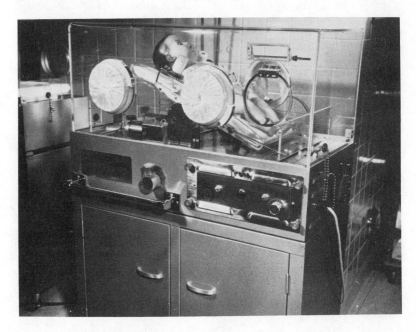

FIGURE 63. The Rockette, placed within the Isolette, is used for babies having respiratory and circulatory difficulties. (Bleier: *Maternity Nursing*, 3rd ed.)

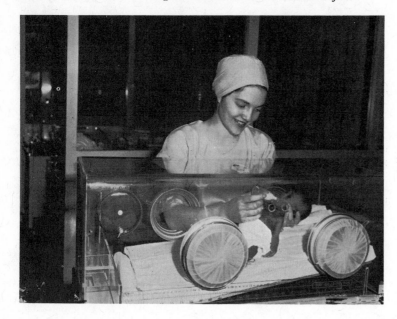

FIGURE 64. Premature baby is fed in the Isolette with special bottle. (Bleier: *Maternity Nursing*, 3rd ed.).

usually administered to increase the amount in tissues. Oxygen pressure (PO$_2$) of arterial blood is measured. When PO$_2$ is below 50 mm. Hg, cyanosis appears. When PO$_2$ is greater than 100 mm. Hg, retrolental fibroplasia, which results in blindness, occurs. Oxygen concentration within Isolette should be checked frequently by nurse with oxygen analyzer. Physician will order PO$_2$.

2. Maintain body temperature. Infant placed in Isolette and temperature kept between 80 and 90°F. (27 to 32°C).

3. Prevent exposure to infection by isolating premature infants, and handling them as little as possible. When necessary to handle the infant, gentleness is of primary importance.

4. Nutrition established at first by gavage if infant is unable to suck and swallow normally (Figs. 64 and 65). During feeding by bottle watch infant for vomiting, fatigue, or cyanosis.

D. Criteria for discharge
 1. Infant's condition: weight of 5½ pounds (2.5 kg.), freedom from infection.
 2. Plans for follow-up care.
 3. Ability of mother to care for infant, and home conditions to which infant will be exposed.

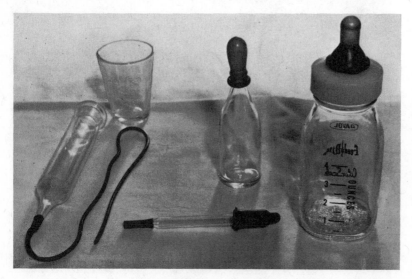

FIGURE 65. Equipment used for feeding the premature baby. Left to right: gavage equipment; medicine dropper feeder (note protective rubber tip on front); specially designed bottle with nipple (bottle holds 1½ ounces of formula); regular 4-ounce bottle with special nipple. (Bleier: *Maternity Nursing*, 3rd ed.)

III. **Signs and Symptoms of Illness in the Newborn Infant**
   A. Respiratory difficulty
      1. Characterized by
         a. Dyspnea (grunting respiration).
         b. Cyanosis.
         c. Retractions (pulling in of the chest wall on inspiration).
         d. Appearance of cyanosis when infant cries or nurses.
      2. May be due to
         a. Atelectasis (incomplete expansion of the lungs).
         b. Hyaline membrane disease.
         f. Brain injury.
         d. Congenital heart disease.
   B. Jaundice
      1. Physiological jaundice may be seen on the third or fourth day of life. Does not usually affect the baby's health.
      2. Erythroblastosis fetalis appears when there is an incompatibility between the red blood cells of the mother and those of her baby, the most frequent being incompatibility of the Rh factor. The characteristics of this disease are
         a. Early jaundice (within first 24 hours).
         b. Pallor.
         c. Edema.
         d. The treatment is phototherapy (Fig. 66) or exchange transfusion (Fig. 67).
         e. Prevention: Use of Rho-GAM injection within 72 hours of delivery if Rh-negative mother is not sensitized by the Rh factor.

IV. Trends in the care of infants at high risk (Fig. 68)
   A. Neonatology—the study and treatment of the sick newborn is developing as a specialized area.
   B. Services to provide early and maximum medical and nursing care for the infant at risk is being geographically regionalized.
   C. Special intensive care nurseries, including mobile intensive care units for the transfer of the distressed or sick newborn, are being made available to help each infant attain his best possible outcome.

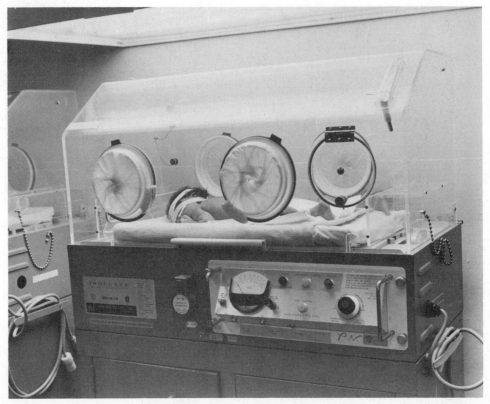

FIGURE 66.   The eyes of the newborn are covered during phototherapy treatment. (Courtesy of Carole Deegan, Director Patient Education Department, Medical Center of Central Georgia, Macon, Georgia. Photo by Terri Bryson, R.N.)

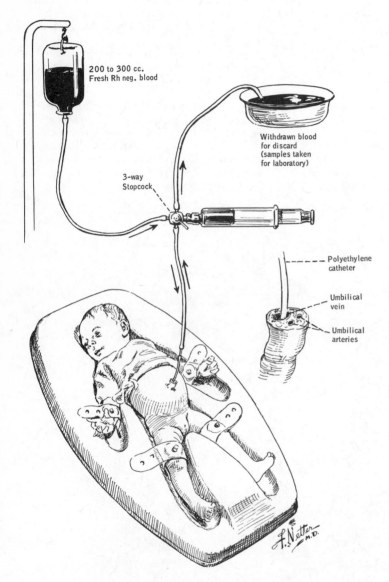

200 to 300 cc.
Fresh Rh neg. blood

Withdrawn blood
for discard
(samples taken
for laboratory)

3-way
Stopcock

Polyethylene
catheter

Umbilical
vein

Umbilical
arteries

FIGURE 67. Infant receiving exchange blood transfusion. (Bookmiller, M. M., Bowen, G. L., and Carpenter, D.: *A Textbook of Obstetrics and Obstetric Nursing*, 5th ed., Philadelphia, W. B. Saunders Co., 1967.)

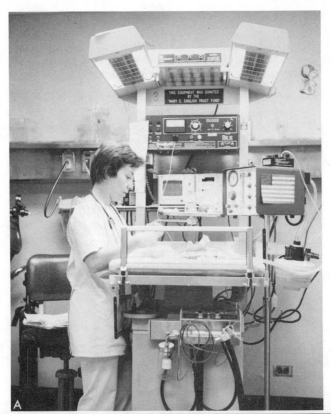

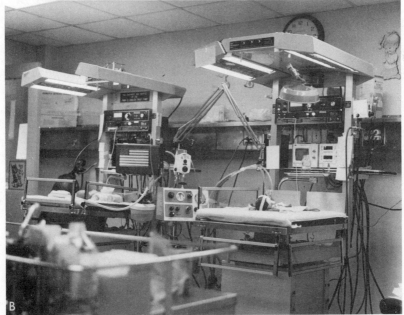

FIGURE 68. *A,* This infant in the Special Care Nursery receives continuous attention from his nurse, who specializes in neonatal nursing. *B,* Another view of the Special Care Nursery showing the extensive equipment available. (Courtesy of Carole Deegan, Director of Patient Education Department, Medical Center of Central Georgia, Macon, Georgia. Photo by Terri Bryson, R.N.)

Questions

1. The immediate care of the infant after delivery includes:
   a. suctioning of mucus from the nose and mouth
   b. establishing respiration and adequate ventilation of the lungs
   c. clamping and cutting the umbilical cord
   d. maintenance of body warmth

   1. all but b
   2. b and c
   3. c only
   4. all of these

2. All states in this country require the administration of 1 per cent silver nitrate or penicillin drops into the eyes of every newborn infant. The primary reason for this law is to:
   1. prevent syphilitic infection of the eyes
   2. prevent gonorrheal infection of the eyes
   3. avoid the development of retrolental fibroplasia
   4. avoid the development of congenital cataracts

3. Ophthalmia neonatorum is:
   1. a congenital heart defect
   2. gonorrheal infection of the conjunctiva
   3. formation of cataracts on the eyes of the newborn infant
   4. another name for congenital syphilis

4. Ophthalmia neonatorum is acquired by the infant:
   1. as a result of active syphilis in the mother
   2. through the placental barrier
   3. as a result of the administration of excessive amounts of anesthetic to the mother during labor
   4. during the birth process if the mother is infected with gonorrhea

5. Which of the following statements best describe the appearance of the newborn infant?
   a. the head is large in comparison to the body
   b. the neck is short and the abdomen protruding
   c. the fingers and toes are short and stubby
   d. the bones of the skull are joined together

   1. all of these
   2. a only
   3. b only
   4. all but d

6. The skin of the newborn is bright red because of the:
   1. irritation of the skin during delivery
   2. abundance of pigment that is characteristic of all newborn infants
   3. large number of RBC's present in his blood
   4. presence of anemia that is common to all newborns

7. The "soft spots" that can be felt in the newborn infant's skull are called the:
   1. suture lines
   2. fontanels
   3. parietal cavities
   4. occipital sutures

8. Plugged sebaceous glands on the nose and cheeks of the newborn are called:
   1. vernix caseosa
   2. milia
   3. lanugo
   4. mongolian spots

9. The thick, dark, green substance contained within the intestines of the fetus is called:
   1. Wharton's jelly
   2. amniotic fluid
   3. colostrum
   4. meconium

10. The movements of the newborn infant are jerky and poorly coordinated. This is primarily due to:
    1. hypersensitivity to cold
    2. immaturity of the nervous system
    3. poor muscle tone
    4. abnormal reflexes resulting from injury at birth

11. The physiological jaundice that is often seen on or about the third day of life is:
    1. indicative of an incompatibility of the maternal and infant blood
    2. due to improper care of the umbilical cord at birth
    3. the result of destruction of the excessive number of red blood cells present at birth
    4. a symptom of damage to the liver of the newborn infant
12. When the infant is admitted to the nursery, the cord stump is checked carefully for bleeding and then it is:
    1. covered with an abdominal binder
    2. left open to dry
    3. covered with Furacin dressings
    4. covered with wet sterile compresses
13. The respiratory rate of the normal newborn infant is:
    1. slow and regular while he is sleeping
    2. very hard to determine since the respirations are very shallow
    3. between 40 and 60 per minute and slightly irregular
    4. between 120 and 140 per minute
14. The pulse rate of the normal newborn is:
    1. 80 to 90   beats per minute
    2. 120 to 160 beats per minute
    3. 160 to 200 beats per minute
    4. 20 to 30   beats per minute
15. During his first few days of life, the newborn infant will normally lose:
    1. one half his birth weight
    2. about 25 per cent of his birth weight
    3. little or no body weight
    4. about 10 per cent of his birth weight
16. The newborn infant sleeps much of the time during the first few weeks of life. Normally he can be expected to:
    1. sleep continuously unless someone wakens him to feed him
    2. sleep all night if left undisturbed
    3. waken only when he needs to eat or announce some other discomfort
    4. sleep at very short intervals and stay awake at very short intervals
17. It is generally agreed that an infant should be fed:
    1. on a demand schedule when he becomes hungry
    2. every 4 hours even if he has to be forced to eat
    3. at least every 2 hours for the first 2 months of life
    4. at the convenience of the mother
18. The nurse should explain to the new mother who is bottle feeding her infant that she should hold him while he is taking the bottle. The reasons for this include:
    a. to keep him in an upright position and prevent air bubbles from forming in his stomach
    b. prevent aspiration in case he "spits up" some of his feeding
    c. allow for physical contact with his mother
    d. being sure of the exact amount taken at each feeding
    1. all of these
    2. all but b
    3. all but c
    4. all but d
19. Adequate sterilization of the formula is necessary to prevent gastrointestinal disturbances in the newborn infant. For the terminal method of sterilization, the mother should be taught to:
    1. wear rubber gloves and sterile gown while preparing the formula
    2. wash all the bottles in strong disinfectant before filling them with formula
    3. sterilize the formula after it has been poured into the bottles and the bottles are all sealed
    4. boil the formula in an open saucepan before each feeding
20. Usually a 24-hour formula is prepared once each day. Any formula left over at the the end of this time should be:
    1. mixed with a fresh supply and resterilized
    2. kept in the refrigerator until it can be used
    3. discarded because it may be detrimental to the infant
    4. slightly diluted and then resterilized

21. The mother who is breast-feeding her baby should be instructed in which of the following basics:
    a. cleanse nipples prior to each feeding
    b. limit nursing time to 2 to 3 minutes at each breast initially
    c. allow baby to nurse 15 to 20 minutes until he learns how to nurse
    d. assist baby to place nipple well into mouth

    1. all but a
    2. all but b
    3. all but c
    4. all but d

22. Some symptoms which would indicate distress in a newborn infant are:
    a. cyanosis
    b. grunting respirations
    c. jaundice within the first 24 hours after birth
    d. jaundice after the third day of life

    1. all of these
    2. all but d
    3. a and c
    4. b and d

23. A premature infant is best described as one who:
    1. has difficulty swallowing and sucking
    2. is born before completion of 9 months' gestation
    3. is physiologically immature
    4. weighs less than 5½ (2.5 kg.) pounds at birth

24. The premature infant has difficulty in maintaining normal body temperature. For this reason it is most important to:
    1. use only woolen clothing on the infant
    2. apply a hot water bottle to the infant's abdomen when his temperature falls below normal
    3. maintain a constant temperature between 80 to 90°F. (27 to 32°C.) within the Isolette
    4. set the thermostat within the nursery at 90°F (32°C.) and leave it there as long as the infant remains in the hospital

25. The premature infant is placed in an Isolette and administered oxygen primarily because:
    1. all premature infants have incomplete expansion of the lungs
    2. most premature infants have a respiratory disease at birth
    3. prematurity of an infant is characterized by difficulty with respiration
    4. most premature infants are born after excessive use of anesthesia during labor and are therefore heavily sedated

26. The arterial blood pressure (PO_2) of the newborn should not exceed:
    1. 20 mm. Hg
    2. 50 mm. Hg
    3. 70 mm. Hg
    4. 100 mm. Hg

27. Excessive arterial pressure (PO_2) in a premature infant has been found to be:
    1. a major factor in the development of anemia
    2. damaging to the lungs of the infant
    3. the cause of retrolental fibroplasia which produces blindness
    4. the cause of excessive destruction of red blood cells

28. The premature infant often must be fed by gavage during the first days of life because he:
    1. often has a very weak or absent sucking or swallowing reflex
    2. is unable to digest his food properly
    3. refuses to take a formula by mouth
    4. needs a larger amount of formula at each feeding than a normal infant

29. A very important aspect of nursing care in preventing infection and exhaustion in the premature infant is:
    1. feeding the infant on a demand schedule
    2. keeping the infant in an Isolette during the day
    3. handling the child as little as possible and with extreme gentleness
    4. eliminating routine bathing and checking the vital signs as required by a normal infant

30. A premature infant is discharged from the hospital when:
    a. his weight reaches 5½ pounds (2.5 kg.)
    b. he is able to take formula from a bottle
    c. his parents have been instructed in his care
    d. plans have been made for proper follow-up once he has been discharged

    1. b only
    2. a and b
    3. all but b
    4. all of these

In the following situations, all selections may answer the question or explain the condition, but only one is considered to be the *best* selection. Drawing on your knowledge of good health, nursing principles, courtesy, and tact, make the selection you feel best meets these standards.

Mrs. S. V., 24 years of age, is pregnant with her first child. On her first visit to her physician, she tells the nurse that she and her husband have moved here from another state and since she has no close relatives near to advise her, she looks to the nurse for help in planning for the coming child.

31. The nurse explains that a complete medical history is obtained from her to:
    1. fulfill the requirements of the state health department
    2. determine whether there are any conditions present that might present complications later to her or the baby
    3. add to statistics in research
    4. make sure she feels that the physician is interested in her as a person
32. While taking Mrs. S. V.'s medical history, she states her last menstrual period occurred November 16 to 20th. What is her expected delivery date?
    1. August 16
    2. August 23
    3. August 27
    4. September 16
33. Blood samples are taken for laboratory analysis. Mrs. S. V. wonders why. The nurse explains this is done:
    1. as a precaution in case a blood sample is needed at a time when it cannot be obtained
    2. only as a routine procedure
    3. to help determine her general state of health and to learn her blood type
    4. only in rare cases on special patients who may have a difficult labor and delivery
34. Mrs. S. V. is Rh negative. She asks if this means she will have a difficult pregnancy. What would the nurse's best reply be?
    1. You have an 85% chance of having no problems.
    2. No, but the baby will probably need an exchange transfusion soon after birth.
    3. We will be taking blood samples periodically to observe for any Rh factor problems that may arise.
    4. All pregnancies are difficult.
35. She asks how much weight she can expect to gain during her pregnancy. What would her physician tell her?
    1. A weight gain of 18 to 25 pounds (8.2 to 11.3 kg.) is expected, but more than this is excessive.
    2. It's best to remain on a strict diet to prevent any gain in weight
    3. The more you gain, the healthier your baby will be.
    4. As long as you have no swelling or high blood pressure you can gain as much as you like.
36. Mrs. S. V. is told there are certain symptoms that could be signs of danger, and must be reported to her physician. These are:
    a. any vaginal bleeding
    b. persistent vomiting or headaches
    c. marked swelling of her legs or feet
    d. leakage of water from the vagina
    1. a only
    2. d only
    3. all but b
    4. all of these
37. She asks the nurse if she should eat special kinds of food during her pregnancy. What would the nurse tell her?
    1. Eat whatever you want; it doesn't make any difference one way or the other.
    2. The smartest thing to do is eat as little as possible and not gain any weight.
    3. If you eat balanced meals, continue to do so, and drink at least a quart of milk a day.
    4. As long as you take vitamins you need not worry about your diet.
38. When told to return every 4 weeks, Mrs. S. V. asks why this is necessary as long as she feels well. What would she be told?
    1. It is psychologically good for the patient.
    2. By checking your blood pressure, weight, and urine often, most impending complications can be detected early; also, it offers you an opportunity to talk to your doctor about any question you may have.

       3. By checking patients often, the doctor can usually catch complications and correct them, thus eliminating unnecessary night calls.

       4. You probably need more attention than most of our patients.

39. Mrs. S. V. asks the nurse's opinion of whether she and her husband should attend the childbirth education classes. What would the best reply be?

       1. There's really no need since your doctor and I will tell you all you need to know.

       2. Do what you want, but the hospital policy will not allow your husband to be with you when you deliver anyway.

       3. They are helpful in preparing you and your husband for your pregnancy, delivery, and care of the baby.

       4. They're OK if you think you really want to know everything.

40. Conflicting emotions may face the pregnant woman. The nurse may be most supportive by:

    a. providing adequate explanations of procedures   1. all of these

    b. explain to Mrs. S. V. that she is not the   2. a and b
first woman to be pregnant nor the last   3. b and d

    c. answer Mrs. S. V.'s questions within the   4. a and c
limitations of her position

    d. asking her to direct all her questions to
her physician.

41. Several weeks later, Mrs. S. V. tells the nurse her clothes are tight and uncomfortable. She wonders if she should purchase maternity clothes. The nurse advises her:

       1. Yes, select clothes that are comfortable, attractive, and suited to the season. A good bra that offers support is a must. Low-heeled shoes will help prevent backache.

       2. It's a good idea to put off buying maternity clothes until you absolutely must. One gets so tired of wearing them as it is.

       3. You'll have to make that decision yourself, but since you'll only be wearing them for a short while, try to make do on as little as possible.

       4. Tight clothing helps you avoid gaining too much weight.

42. Mrs. S. V. calls one day and asks her physician if it is safe for her to water ski. What does he tell her?

       1. Yes, if you normally water ski a lot, it is all right to continue to do so.

       2. As long as you wear a life jacket there is no danger to you or the baby.

       3. That is hard to say. Some patients could water ski all day and not have any bad results from it, while others could even lose their babies because of it.

       4. No, that type of exercise is rather strenuous and an accident is likely.

43. Mrs. S. V. and her husband attend the expectant parents classes offered at the medical clinic and taught by her physician's nurse. While discussing amount and type of supplies for the baby, Mr. S. V. wonders if it is safe to use the diaper services that he has heard of. What would the nurse answer?

       1. Yes, they offer efficient, dependable, convenient service at reasonable cost. You can also feel sure the diapers have been thoroughly washed and sterilized.

       2. Yes, it is safe. Most parents are pleased with the service, but I personally feel that the mothers that use them are just too lazy to do their own work.

       3. I don't know a thing about them because I feel that care of babies' clothes is something that the mother should see to personally.

       4. If you have a washing machine it would be foolish to use a diaper service.

44. On one of her visits to the physician, Mrs. S. V. confesses that she is confused about the advisability of breast feeding. It seems friends have offered strong arguments for and against it. She asks the doctor for his opinion. What does he tell her?

       1. Actually, that is one subject I don't even discuss with the patient, since it really doesn't matter how the baby is fed, just so he gets enough of the right kinds of food.

       2. That is a decision you and your husband must make but we feel the baby gets a better start in life when breast fed. In addition to having a convenient, ready supply of milk available, it affords a feeling of closeness between mother and baby. However, when circumstances make nursing inconvenient or impossible, these needs can easily be met with the baby on bottle feedings.

3. I insist that all my patients breast feed their babies, and I doubt that you will find many physicians who will willingly accept the care of a young child that is not breast fed.
4. Breast fed babies are always stronger and healthier than those who are bottle fed.

45. During the seventh month of pregnancy, Mrs. S. V. complains of feeling fatigued in the afternoon. Also, her feet swell and this adds to the tired feeling, although the swelling is gone after a night's rest. On examination, her doctor finds no complications. What does he advise her?
1. I really don't think you need worry about this. It is just something that goes along with pregnancy, and will probably get worse before you reach term.
2. I can't find any reason for the symptoms you describe. However, to prevent needless worry for you and me, I think you should stay in bed from now until you deliver, except to go to the bathroom.
3. This is very serious and probably indicates a troublesome labor and delivery.
4. Everything is coming along normally, so I feel that what you need is to rest often during the day with your feet elevated, and avoid long periods of standing.

46. Mrs. S. V. is examined more often during her eighth month of pregnancy, and on one of these visits she asks her physician whether the baby would live, were she to deliver now. He tells her:
1. Don't you worry about that. If such a thing should happen, it would be out of your hands anyway.
2. Babies almost always die if born during the eighth month. For some reason they are able to live at 7 months, but not at 8.
3. Most babies are developed enough at 8 months to live and, with adequate care, do quite well.
4. If labor started now you probably would have a stillborn baby.

47. Mrs. S. V. mentions that she was given a baby shower and received 15 sleeper outfits size zero to 6 months. She asks, "How will I ever use them all?" What does the nurse suggest?
1. Exchange some for larger sizes or items you didn't receive but need.
2. It's not a good idea to exchange a gift someone has given you.
3. You'll have enough to change the sleeper with each feeding.
4. Someone must have had a sale on infant sleepers right before your shower.

48. She calls one day and tells her physician that she feels as if the weight of the baby has shifted and is resting low in her pelvis. She asks if this means she is in labor. What does he tell her?
1. I'm not sure, but I think you had better go on to the hospital now. This way you will feel safe and I won't be called unless it's necessary.
2. You have experienced what we call "lightening." The pregnant uterus, in preparing for labor, has settled low in the bony pelvis. This usually occurs about 2 weeks before labor starts, but should you experience any other symptoms, call me immediately.
3. No, you are not in labor. You will experience all sorts of uncomfortable and strange feelings from now until you deliver, so there's really no point in calling me again unless you are sure labor is well established.
4. It would be best if you stay off your feet until this condition subsides.

49. She asks how she is to know when to go to the hospital. What does he tell her?
1. Oh, that's one thing women know without being told. In fact, you will have to tell me when you are ready.
2. When your pains are occurring regularly every 15 minutes, or if the bag of waters breaks even in the absence of pains, then you must go to the hospital.
3. When you begin to feel you must bear down as if to move your bowels, you should go to the hospital.
4. As soon as you feel a contraction you should go to the hospital.

50. Five days before the estimated date of confinement, Mrs. S. V. enters the hospital. She is having contractions every 10 to 12 minutes. While being admitted, she tells the nurse she is having a vaginal discharge of blood-stained mucus. She asks if this is usual. What does the nurse tell her?
1. I will call your doctor because there is always a great danger of hemorrhage during labor, especially with the first baby.

    2. You may stop worrying about all that now; you are in good hands and we will take care of you.

    3. Yes, that is what we call the show. At the onset of labor, the mouth of the womb expels a mucus plug that has sealed it during pregnancy.

    4. I've never heard of such a thing but I'm sure you're all right.

51. Part of the admission procedure is a cleansing enema. Mrs. S. V. asks the nurse if this is necessary since she has had a bowel movement today. What does the nurse tell her?

    1. We always carry out the complete routine admission procedure regardless of whether it is necessary or not.

    2. Yes, the lower bowel needs to be completely empty during labor and delivery. A normal bowel movement does not adequately do this.

    3. I guess it will be all right to omit the enema this time. A normal bowel movement should have sufficiently emptied your colon.

    4. We will wait and ask the physician when he comes to examine you.

52. She tells the nurse she is very hungry and could eat a steak if her husband were allowed to bring it to her. What does the nurse tell her?

    1. I'm sorry, you can't have the steak now. You can have fluids, in small amounts, but your stomach must be empty of solids during the last stages of labor and delivery.

    2. Yes, tell him to bring it. You are going to need all the strength you can get before this is over.

    3. I can't stop you from eating whatever you want. Just don't hold us responsible if you aspirate some vomitus while under the anesthetic.

    4. If you are hungry we will order a regular diet from the hospital kitchen.

53. She asks the nurse how long it will be before the baby comes. What does the nurse tell her?

    1. There is no way of knowing; besides, you won't know a thing about it. Try to rest now.

    2. Really, Mrs. S. V., you would think you were just a child the way you ask questions. Can't you just trust us and relax?

    3. The length of labor varies with each patient, and it's hard to be accurate in predicting its length. Your doctor will be able to give a more satisfactory answer.

    4. That depends on how cooperative you are and the amount of drugs we have to give you.

54. While the nurse is checking the fetal heart tones, the patient asks if she could listen, too. What does the nurse answer?

    1. We feel that it's best that the patient not know anything about things such as that, since you don't know what it's all about and will only become frightened if anything goes wrong.

    2. You could, but if we're to stop and wait on you and explain everything you don't understand, we'll never have this baby.

    3. Yes, I'll place the instrument for you and you listen closely. You will hear a fairly rapid, regular beat. That's the baby's heart tones.

    4. It is against hospital policy to allow patients to use medical equipment.

55. As Mrs. S. V.'s labor progresses, she shows signs of discomfort but does not complain. Mr. S. V. remarks that he wishes he could do something to help. What does the nurse tell him?

    1. There's nothing anyone can do now but wait.

    2. You can help her by placing your hands on her lower back and gently pushing downward as the contraction gets harder, then relaxing the pressure as the contraction subsides.

    3. Except for being with her, there's really nothing you can do. It's better to remain as quiet as possible.

    4. Why don't you read aloud to her and distract her attention?

56. The patient asks the nurse if she shouldn't push with the pains so as to speed up labor. What does the nurse answer?

    1. No, at this stage you would only use up your strength by pushing. Try to relax and rest between contractions.

    2. Yes, the harder you push, the sooner the baby will come.

    3. It doesn't matter, you can if you want to.

    4. No, there is danger of rupturing the uterus or injuring your baby if you push now.

57. Mrs. S. V. becomes very hot and thirsty during this stage of labor. To relieve this discomfort it would be best for the nurse to:
    1. give her small sips of water and open the windows in the labor room
    2. apply an ice cap to the patient's forehead
    3. force fluids on the patient because these are symptoms of severe dehydration
    4. allow the patient to take small sips of water and bathe her face with a washcloth and cool water

58. As labor progresses Mrs. S. V. states that she has the feeling that her bowels are going to move. The nurse observes that the patient's perineum is bulging. She should know that:
    1. this indicates that the patient needs an enema
    2. the cervix has completely dilated and the patient will deliver soon
    3. the patient should be placed on a bedpan immediately
    4. a precipitate delivery is now inevitable since the infant is emerging through the birth canal

59. At this time the physician performs an amniotomy (rupture of the membranes). This procedure is done to:
    1. prevent tearing of the vaginal orifice
    2. prevent a postpartum infection
    3. slow down the process of labor
    4. hasten delivery

60. Mrs. S. V. is taken to the delivery room and an episiotomy performed. The chief purpose of this procedure is to:
    1. prevent tearing of the vaginal orifice
    2. decrease the size of the infant's head
    3. dilate the cervix
    4. rupture the amniotic sac

61. As soon as Mrs. S. V.'s baby boy is born his footprint is obtained and an identification bracelet is placed on his wrist. Identification of an infant is done:
    1. in the nursery after he is bathed and dressed
    2. after he is weighed
    3. as soon as he is admitted to the nursery
    4. in the delivery room before he is taken to the nursery

62. Mrs. S. V. is returned to her room and her husband allowed to visit her. They ask if they might see the baby. The nurse should:
    1. ask the nursery attendant to bring the baby to the mother's room for a short visit
    2. send the father to the nursery and have the mother wait to see her baby after she has had a good night's sleep
    3. express disapproval and take this opportunity to teach the parents the dangers of cross infection
    4. ask the father to bring the baby from the nursery to Mrs. S. V.'s room

63. As Mr. and Mrs. S. V. hold and inspect the baby for the first time, the nurse can reassure them that the following are normally seen in the newborn:
    a. sneezing   1. all of these
    b. jaundice present at birth   2. all but b
    c. milia   3. all but c
    d. hiccoughing   4. all but d

64. The next day Mr. S. V. visits his wife and tells the nurse that their baby had been placed in an incubator the day before, but is now in a crib like the other babies. He asks if this means that something was wrong at birth. The nurse should explain that:
    1. all babies are put in incubators and given oxygen for a while in case they have a respiratory infection
    2. a loss of blood when the cord is cut causes a deficiency of oxygen and some babies must be placed in an incubator
    3. the sudden change from the mother's body to the outside causes a drop in body temperature, and since the newborn infant's heat-regulating center is not yet fully developed, he is placed in an incubator until he is warm again
    4. many babies catch pneumonia when they are born, and the incubator is used to prevent chilling and the danger of such an occurrence

65. Mrs. S. V. has decided to nurse her baby, and when it is 24 hours old it is brought to breast. She is very willing to nurse her baby but has no idea how to go about it. The nurse advises her to:
    a. assume the position most comfortable for her
    b. always lie flat in bed to nurse the baby
    c. permit him to nurse only 3 to 5 minutes until her flow of milk has been established
    d. "burp" him as often as necessary
    e. always use a nipple shield

    1. a, c, and d
    2. c and e only
    3. a and b
    4. all but a

66. On the fourth day after her delivery the nurse finds Mrs. S. V. crying in her room. She says that nothing is wrong but she just can't stop crying. She tells the nurse she thinks she is losing her mind. What does the nurse answer to allay her fears best?
    1. I'm sure you are all right, but I'll call your physician and ask if he wants to call a psychiatrist to see you.
    2. There is always a possibility of psychosis after delivery. Have you had any episodes of depression like this before?
    3. You probably have the "maternity blues." Very often a mother feels depressed several days after her baby is born. You just cry it out and I'll be near and check on you if you need me.
    4. I really don't see that you have anything to cry about. You could have had a badly deformed baby and then I could understand this fit of depression.

67. As the nurse is preparing the baby for discharge on his fourth day of life, she makes the following observations. Which ones should she report immediately to the physician?
    a. enlarged breasts
    b. soft greenish-brown stool
    c. somewhat jaundiced skin
    d. lanugo on shoulders

    1. b and c
    2. c only
    3. all of these
    4. none of these

68. As Mrs. S. V. dresses the baby to go home, she notices a purulent discharge from the eyes. The nurse should:
    1. explain the discharge was probably due to Mrs. S. V. not washing her hands properly when feeding the baby, and instruct her in good handwashing
    2. explain the discharge is probably due to the silver nitrate that was instilled at birth, and that it will gradually disappear; instruct in proper cleaning of eyes
    3. notify the physician at once before discharged
    4. explain to Mrs. S. V. that she will have to leave the baby at the hospital until the condition is better

69. While preparing to go home, Mrs. S. V. asks the nurse if she could buy a tight girdle to wear to help flatten her abdominal muscles. What should the nurse answer?
    1. Yes, this is a must to help you regain muscle tone.
    2. The only way to flatten your abdomen is to lose a lot of weight.
    3. A girdle is all right, but you should take regular exercises to strengthen your abdominal muscles. Your physician will instruct you in these exercises.
    4. There isn't much that can be done to flatten the abdomen once it has been stretched during pregnancy.

Part XII
PEDIATRIC NURSING

I. **Normal Growth and Development**
  A. Each child grows and develops at his own rate. He should not be rushed into development beyond his own level.
  B. Growth is a continuous process, even though children do go through stages in which there are spurts of growth. The periods of rapid development are interspersed with "plateaus," during which periods there is little growth and development.
  C. Charts, graphs, and tables are useful only as guides. They do not mean that every child who is normal must conform exactly.
  D. Abnormal growth and development should be recognized early, and medical help and advice obtained.

II. **Periods of Growth and Development**
  A. Infancy—from birth to 1 year of age.
  B. Toddler—from 1 to 3 years of age.
  C. Preschool child—from 3 to 5 years of age.
  D. School child—from 5 to 12 years of age.
  E. Adolescence—from 12 to 20 years of age.

UNIT 1   THE INFANT AND THE TODDLER

I. **The Normal Infant**
  A. Basic needs
    1. Food; adequate nutrition.
    2. Warmth and comfort.
    3. Satisfaction of the sucking urge.
    4. Love and security.
  B. Demand feeding is not enough. Infant should have physical contact with the mother or nurse. At feeding time he should be cuddled and held. Bottle propping is dangerous and denies the infant needed contact with his mother or nurse.
  C. Warmth and comfort include being held and kept dry. Rhythmic rocking gives the infant a sense of security and love.
  D. Physical growth and development
    1. One month (Fig. 69)
      a. Infant sleeps 20 of 24 hours during first few months of life.
      b. Feeding includes breast milk or formula, with vitamins A, D, and C given as supplements.
      c. Gains about 6 ounces (170 gm.) per week for first 6 months.
      d. Gains about 1 inch (2.5 cm.) per month for first 6 months.
      e. Cries to announce needs.
      f. Allow to exercise arms and legs freely.
    2. Two months (Fig. 70)
      a. Posterior fontanel closes; infant has less difficulty focusing his eyes.
      b. First solid foods are usually given—fine cereals, strained fruits. Infant should be fed one food at a time to help him develop a taste for new foods.
      c. First DPT injection (immunization against diphtheria, whooping cough, tetanus). Oral poliomyelitis vaccine may also be given.
      d. Tears now formed.

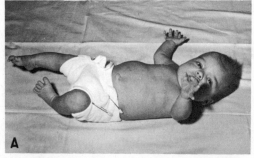
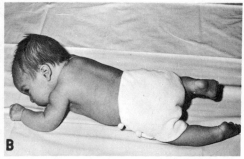
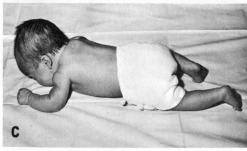

FIGURE 69. The 1-month-old infant. *A*, Random, generalized activity in response to stimulation. *B*, Makes crawling movements when prone on a flat surface. Pushes with toes. Holds hands in fists. *C*, Lifts head from the bed a short distance. Can turn head to the side when prone. (Marlow: *Textbook of Pediatric Nursing.* 4th ed.)

3. Three months (Fig. 71)
   a. Follows objects with his eyes.
   b. Cries less and takes short naps during the day.
   c. Strained meat added to diet.
   d. Coos and laughs aloud.
4. Four months (Fig. 72)
   a. Takes two to three naps daily; sleeps through night.
   b. Custard and simple puddings added to diet.
   c. Appearance of saliva.
   d. Second DPT immunization, second poliomyelitis vaccination.
5. Six months (Fig. 73)
   a. Birth weight should be doubled.

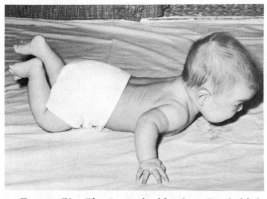

FIGURE 70. The 2-month-old infant. Can hold the head erect in midposition. Can lift the head and chest a short distance above the bed or table when lying on abdomen. (Marlow: *Textbook of Pediatric Nursing.* 4th ed.)

   b. May be weaned from breast or bottle to cup.
   c. Provide soft objects for chewing, such as teething ring.
   d. Diet includes yolk of egg; variety of fruits, meats, and vegetables.
   e. Lower incisor teeth begin to erupt.
   f. Grasps objects in hand and bangs them against floor.
   g. Gains about 4 oz. (113 Gm.) per week and ½ inch (1.3 cm.) per month during second 6 months.
   h. Third DPT immunization, third poliomyelitis vaccination.
6. Eight months (Fig. 74)
   a. Can be spoon-fed; can handle finger foods such as toast or crackers.
   b. Sleeps 11 to 13 hours each night.
   c. Says one or two words.
   d. Hitching (backward crawling) replaced with forward movement (crawling) by 10 months.
7. Twelve months (Fig. 75)
   a. Birth weight is tripled.
   b. Four upper incisors and two lower teeth have erupted.
   c. Drinks from a cup himself.
   d. Stands alone
   e. Has a vocabulary of about four words, including "ma-ma" and "da-da."
   f. Immunization against measles, rubella, and mumps. Tuberculin skin test also given.

II. **The Normal Toddler**
   A. General characteristics
      1. Has developed a mind and will of his own.

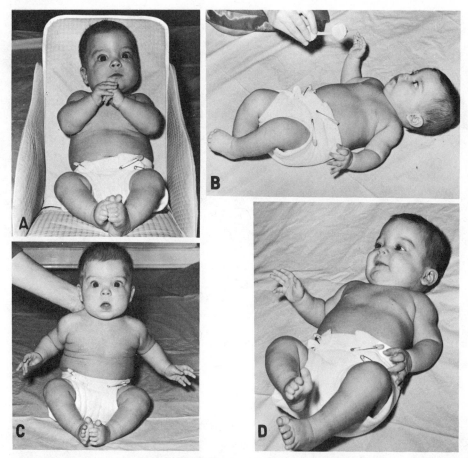

FIGURE 71.   The 3-month-old infant. *A*, Holds hands up in front and plays with fingers. *B*, Reaches for a shiny object, but misses it. *C*, Sits with support, back rounded, knees flexed. *D*, Smiles in response to mother's face and laughs aloud. (Marlow: *Textbook of Pediatric Nursing.* 4th ed.)

2. Likes to explore and is "into everything." Wants to feel, smell, and taste everything (Fig. 76).
3. Becomes negative and says "no" frequently; talks in short sentences by 2 years, vocabulary increases to about 900 words by the age of 3.
4. Anterior fontanel closes at about fifteenth month.
5. Acquires all 20 deciduous teeth by about 2½ years.
6. Progresses from playing by self to playing near children (parallel play) at 2 years, to playing with other children (cooperative play) at 3 years (Fig. 77).

B. Basic needs
   1. Love and security.
   2. Independence.
   3. Needs guidance in learning to talk, to walk, and to develop acceptable social habits.

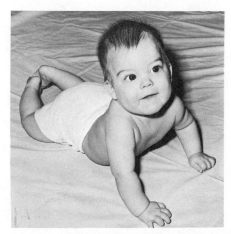

FIGURE 72.   The 4-month-old infant. Lifts head and shoulders at a 90-degree angle when on abdomen and looks around. Can hold head steady. Is increasingly aware of surroundings. Is socially inclined. (Marlow: *Textbook of Pediatric Nursing.* 4th ed.)

Text continued on page 343

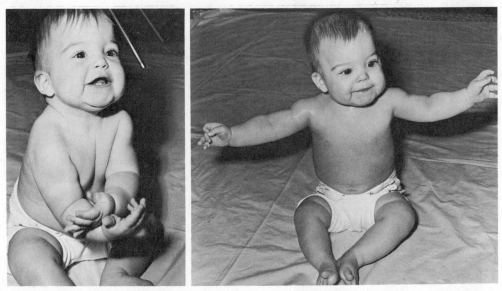

FIGURE 73.   The 6-month-old infant. *A*, Has two lower incisors. *B*, Sits momentarily without support. Holds arms out for balance. (Marlow: *Textbook of Pediatric Nursing.* 4th ed.)

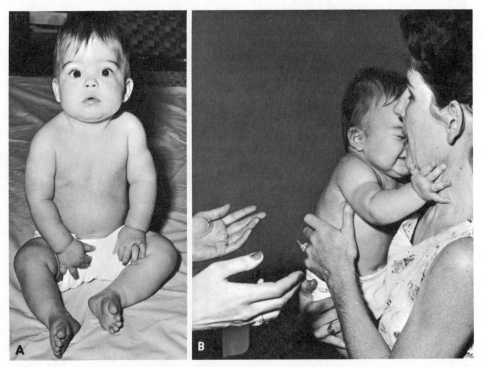

FIGURE 74.   The 8-month-old infant. *A*, Sits alone steadily. Has increased interest in activity in environment. *B*, "Eight months' anxiety." Greets strangers by turning away and crying. (Marlow: *Textbook of Pediatric Nursing.* 4th ed.)

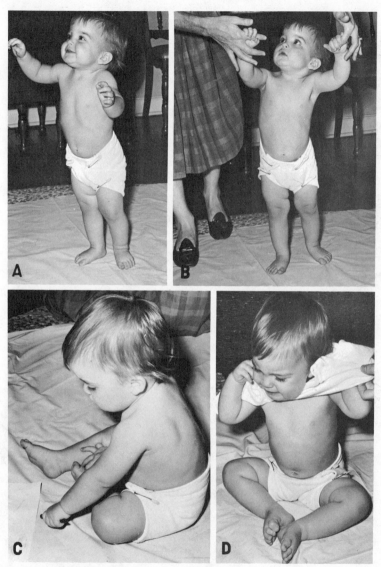

FIGURE 75.   The 12-month-old infant. *A*, Stands alone for a moment or possibly longer. *B*, Walks with help. *C*, Holds a crayon adaptively to make a stroke and can mark on a piece of paper. *D*, Cooperates in dressing. Puts arm through sleeve. (Marlow: *Textbook of Pediatric Nursing.* 4th ed.)

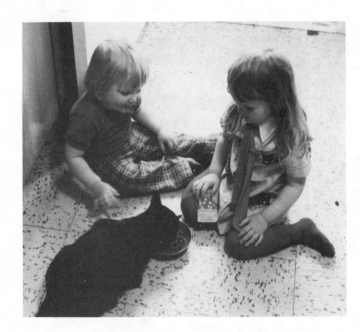

FIGURE 76.   Toddlers are curious about pets and love to watch them eat—and possibly share in their food. (Photo by Reginald Muhl.)

FIGURE 77.   "Reading" story books is a favorite pastime for toddlers. (Photo by Reginald Muhl.)

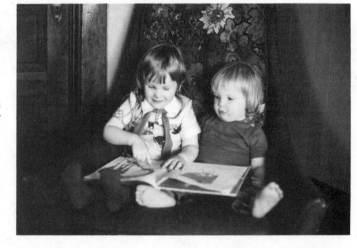

4. Self-concept developing.
C. Immunization—DPT and poliomyelitis booster at 18 months of age.
D. Toilet training may be attempted at the end of the first year but it should not be rushed.
 1. Bowel control is usually accomplished by 18 months of age.
 2. Bladder control is more difficult and should be established by 2 years. Bed-wetting (enuresis) may continue into the third year.
 3. During illness the child may regress to infantile behavior. Scolding or showing strong disapproval may be harmful and child should be treated with patience and understanding.
E. Safety measures
 1. Toys painted with lead paint are dangerous because the toddler tends to put everything into his mouth and he may swallow some of the paint.
 2. Precautions with poisons; accident prevention (Figs. 78 and 79).

III. Congenital Disorders
A. Congenital heart disease
 1. A defect in the structure of the heart or major blood vessels leading to and from the heart. Results from improper development during fetal life. Believed to be associated with infections in the mother during pregnancy.
 2. Major types (Fig. 80).
 3. Symptoms (Fig. 81).
 4. Treatment—surgical correction whenever possible.
B. Cleft lip
 1. Incomplete closure of the upper lip.
 2. Symptoms are obvious at birth.
 3. Treatment—surgical repair, usually within the first few months of life.
  a. Feeding before surgery may require the use of a special nipple or syringe.
  b. Nursing care following surgery
   1. Infant is restrained to prevent injury to the suture line (Fig. 82).
   2. Infant is positioned on his back or side, never on his abdomen until operative site is completely healed.
C. Cleft palate
 1. Incomplete closure of the roof of the mouth. May involve the soft palate or the hard palate and nose. Sometimes accompanied by cleft lip.
 2. Treatment is surgical repair, usually postponed until at least 10 months of age.

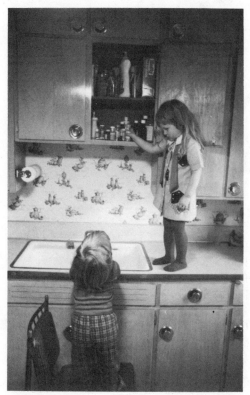

FIGURE 78.   Climbing to high places may result in falls and also in getting into things which can be harmful. (Photo by Reginald Muhl.)

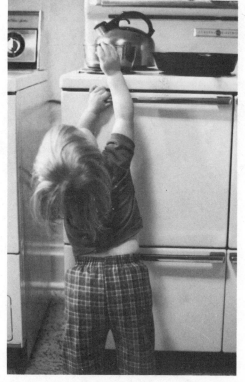

FIGURE 79.   A toddler may try to see what's cooking on the stove and possibly burn himself. Always turn handles toward back of stove. (Photo by Reginald Muhl.)

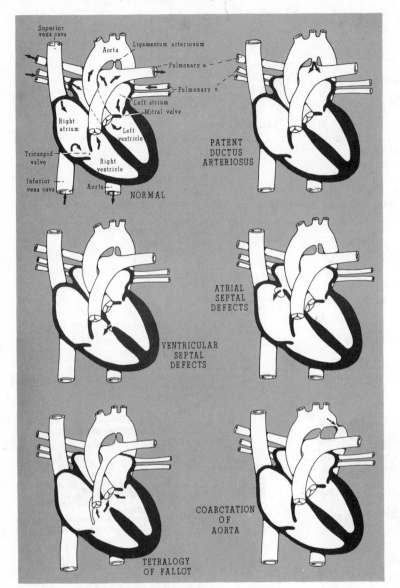

FIGURE 80.   Normal heart and common congenital defects. (Jacob and Francone: *Structure and Function in Man.* 3rd ed.)

Infants	Children
1. Dyspnea	1. Dyspnea
2. Difficulty with feeding	2. Poor physical development
3. Stridor or choking spells	3. Decreased exercise tolerance
4. Pulse rate over 200	4. Recurrent respiratory infections
5. Recurrent respiratory infections	5. Heart murmur and thrill
6. Failure to gain weight	6. Cyanosis
7. Heart murmurs	7. Squatting
8. Cyanosis	8. Clubbing of fingers and toes
9. Cerebrovascular accidents	9. Elevated blood pressure
10. Anoxic attacks	

FIGURE 81.   General signs and symptoms of congenital heart abnormalities. (NSF Education Service, Ross Laboratories.)

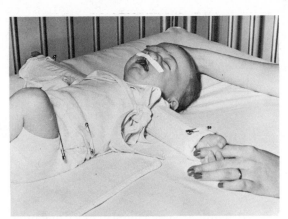

FIGURE 82. Appearance of a 2-month-old infant after repair of a cleft lip. A Band-Aid is used to hold the suture line together. Elbow restraints prevent the infant from rubbing his face. The mother remained with this child throughout his hospitalization. (Marlow: *Textbook of Pediatric Nursing.* 4th ed.)

    a. Before surgery the infant has difficulty feeding because he cannot suck. Special feeder is often used.
    b. Speech defects may result if speech therapy is not instituted.
    c. Postoperative care
       1. Arm restraints are necessary.
       2. Activities are restricted to quiet play; crying is to be avoided.
       3. Mouth must be kept clean and free from irritation.
       4. Diet restricted to fluids until sutures are removed. Do not give child straws or small objects he may put into his mouth.

D. Hydrocephalus
    1. Characterized by an increased accumulation of cerebrospinal fluid within the ventricles of the brain, resulting in an increase in the size of the head.
    2. Nursing care of the child with hydrocephalus requires frequent changing of position of the head as well as the body. Pressure sores on the head are a constant threat.
    3. Malnutrition common in these infants. During feeding the infant should be held in the arms and the head should be well supported.
    4. Surgical correction with shunt operation may be done. Prognosis has improved with newer drugs and surgical techniques.

E. Spina bifida
    1. A congenital defect of the spine in which portions of the bony spine may be completely or partially lacking.
      a. Meningocele—protrusion of the meninges through the spinal defect.

      b. Meningomyelocele—protrusion of the meninges and spinal cord through the spinal defect.
    2. Treatment of meningocele consists of surgical removal of the sac and closure of the tissues. Meningomyelocele is extremely difficult to treat because of the involvement of the spinal cord.
    3. Nursing care is aimed at preventing infection or injury to the sac. Infant requires same tender loving care, adequate nutrition, and skin care as a normal infant.
    4. Hydrocephalus often accompanies spina bifida.

F. Down's syndrome (mongolism)
    1. A congenital defect of the embryo, caused by chromosomal abnormalities, most often occurring in infants born of mothers over the age of 35.
    2. Characteristics of the mongoloid (Fig. 83).

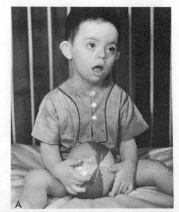

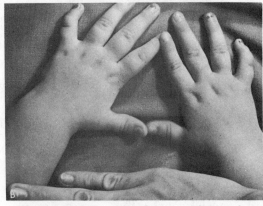

FIGURE 83. Down's syndrome. *A,* The muscles are underdeveloped, the joints are loose, and the child can assume unusual positions comfortably for prolonged periods. *B,* The hands are short and thick, and the little finger is curved. (Courtesy of Dr. Ralph V. Platou and the American Academy of Pediatrics. From Marlow: *Textbook of Pediatric Nursing.* 4th ed.)

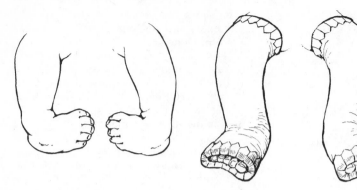

FIGURE 84. Bilateral talipes equinovarus before and after application of the plaster casts. Adhesive petals have been placed around the ends of the casts. (Marlow: *Textbook of Pediatric Nursing.* 4th ed.)

a. Characteristic appearance includes round face, low-set ears, upward slanting eyes, flat nose, protruding tongue, short fingers.

b. Mongoloids develop slowly and seldom reach a mental age above 7 years.

c. Resistance to infection is poor; congenital umbilical hernia and heart defects are common.

G. Club foot

1. Characterized by one or both feet turned outward or inward (Fig. 84).

2. Treatment should start early with the use of casts and splints to hold feet in correct position. Surgery is indicated if conservative treatment is ineffective or treatment is delayed until after 2 years of age.

3. Nursing care focuses on physical care of children in casts and emotional support to a child undergoing a long period of frequent hospitalizations.

H. Cystic fibrosis

1. Congenital disease inherited as recessive trait from both parents.

2. Characterized by changes in exocrine glands, with the sweat glands producing large amounts of salty sweat and the mucous glands secreting thick mucus. Affects all parts of body, but especially lungs and pancreas.

3. Treatment

a. Respiratory relief aimed at preventing infections and thinning thick secretions.

b. Dietary management aimed at providing high-calorie diet with supplementary vitamins and pancreatic enzymes.

4. Nursing care individualized according to severity of condition.

I. Phenylketonuria (PKU)

1. Inherited as a recessive trait from both parents.

2. Characterized by faulty metabolism of phenylalanine, an amino acid. A high concentration in the blood results in severe, irreversible retardation.

3. Early detection through blood and urine tests on the newborn are required in many states.

4. Treatment consists of close dietary management and use of Lofenalac diet, a synthetic food which provides protein for growth and repair.

5. Prognosis good if detected early and proper dietary management followed.

J. Sickle cell disease

1. An inherited defect in hemoglobin formation causing red blood cells to become fragile and sickle-shaped.

2. Symptoms caused by lumping together of malformed cells, causing obstruction of vessels, destruction of RBC's, and infarcts in various areas of body due to disrupted blood supply. Organs most often affected include spleen, heart, kidneys, lungs, GI tract, joints, and brain.

a. Severe pain in affected part.

b. Fever.

c. Vomiting.

d. Convulsions, coma.

e. Jaundice apparent two to three days past crisis.

3. Treatment consists of supportive measures such as protection from infection and blood transfusions. During a crisis, treatment is aimed at relief of pain, control of fever, and adequate fluids.

IV. **Upper Respiratory Infections in the Infant and Toddler**

A. One of the most common disorders in children. More serious because of the small size of the air passages, which easily become obstructed with mucus.

B. Symptoms are more severe than in older children and adults; temperature may be very high and lead to febrile convulsions; gastrointestinal disturbances such as vomiting and diarrhea frequently accompany respiratory infections in infants and toddlers.

C. Nursing care

1. Provide rest by keeping infant in a quiet environment.

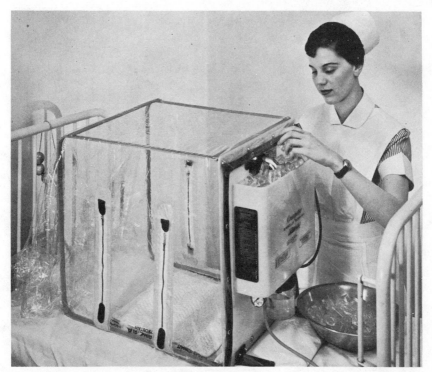

FIGURE 85. Croupette. The trough at the back of the Croupette is filled with ice and tap water to the level indicated. (Air-Shields, Inc., Hatboro, Pa.)

2. Fluid intake is increased but infant will have difficulty sucking and swallowing when nasal passages are obstructed. Should be fed very slowly and allowed periods of rest while taking fluids from the bottle.
3. Humidity. Extra moisture may be provided by croup tent or Croupette (Figs. 85 and 86).
   a. If croup tent is used, care must be taken to protect infant from burns by steam or the nozzle of vaporizer. Croup tent provides warm, moist air.
   b. Croupette provides cool, moist air, and is especially helpful if the infant has an elevated temperature. Oxygen may be administered in the Croupette; otherwise the dia-pump must be attached to provide fresh air within the tent.
   c. Mattress is protected with rubber sheet and the linens and clothes of the infant are changed as needed to keep him dry and avoid chilling.
4. Nose drops are frequently used to clear nasal passages. During this procedure the infant may be restrained with mummy restraint. (Fig. 87).
   a. Infant is held so that the head is lower than the shoulders during the administration of the drops. This

position is maintained for one or two minutes after drops are instilled.
   b. Upper lip should be protected from excoriation by the irritating nasal discharge. Cold cream or petrolatum may be used.
5. Medication by mouth should be given from a spoon or medicine dropper. Pills and tablets are crushed and mixed with water or syrup. Never force medication (especially oily ones) into the mouth of a child.
D. Complications of respiratory infection
1. Otitis media—one of the most common complications of an upper respiratory infection because of the location and position of the eustachian tube in infants and small children (Fig. 88).
   a. Definition—an inflammation of the middle ear.
   b. Symptoms include elevated temperature and earache. Small infants may pull at the ear to indicate that it is painful.
   c. Treatment and nursing care include use of antibiotics to control infections and measures to reduce pain.
   d. Older children should be taught to blow the nose with the mouth open. Closing one nostril while blowing the nose is dangerous because it spreads

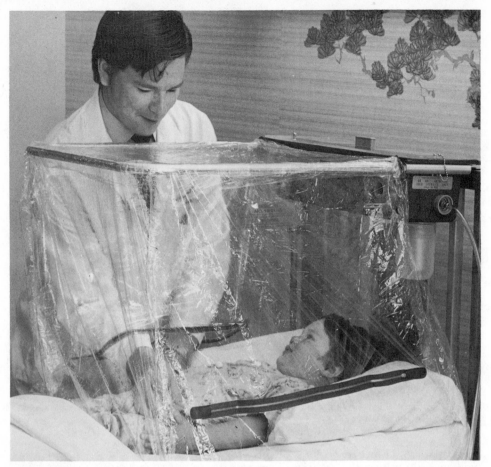

FIGURE 86.

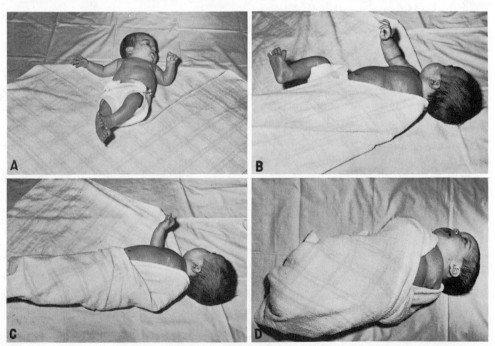

FIGURE 87.   Mummy restraint. *A,* One corner of a small blanket is folded over. The infant is placed on the blanket with his neck at the edge of the fold. *B,* One side of the blanket is pulled *firmly* over one shoulder. *C,* The remainder of that side of the blanket is tucked under the opposite side of the infant's body. *D,* The procedure is repeated with the other side of the blanket. The blanket should be pinned in place. (Note: When applying a mummy restraint, be certain that the extremities are not forced into an uncomfortable position.) (Marlow: *Textbook of Pediatric Nursing.* 4th ed.)

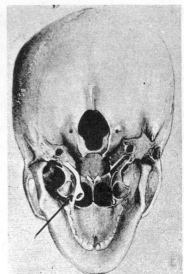

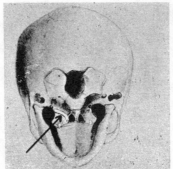

FIGURE 88. Diagram showing the position and direction of the eustachian tube in the infant and adult. The infant's eustachian tube is shorter, wider, and straighter. (Jeans, Wright, F. H., and Blake, F. G.: *Essentials of Pediatrics.* 6th ed., Philadelphia, J. B. Lippincott Co., 19 .)

infection from the nasopharynx to the middle ear.

2. Interstitial pneumonitis
   a. Involvement of the lung tissues.
   b. Symptoms include severe dyspnea, cyanosis, cough, and fever.
   c. Treatment is symptomatic
      1. Increased humidity to thin bronchial secretions.
      2. Administration of oxygen to relieve cyanosis.
      3. Antibiotics to control infection and sedatives to encourage rest.
      4. Patient is very seriously ill. Encourage fluids; monitor vital signs closely. Antipyretic drugs to reduce fever may be ordered.
3. Febrile convulsions
   a. Frequently accompany the elevated temperature produced by upper respiratory infections. Occur in infants and small children because of immaturity of the nervous system at this age.
   b. Measures to reduce body temperature include use of antipyretic drugs, alcohol sponges, and cool tap water enemas.
      1. Do not use more than 300 cc. of solution unless otherwise ordered by the physician.
      2. Rectal tube is inserted only 2 to 4 inches (5 to 10 cm.).
      3. Position of the infant or toddler (Fig. 89).

V. Croup (Acute Spasmodic Laryngitis)
A. Spasms of the muscles of the larynx produce partial respiratory obstruction.

B. Attacks occur at night and are frightening to the child and his parents; however, uncomplicated croup rarely, if ever, is fatal. Hyperactive, nervous children are affected more often than quiet ones.
C. Symptoms include a typical "barking" cough and dyspnea. A high-pitched, rasping noise is heard with each inspiration of

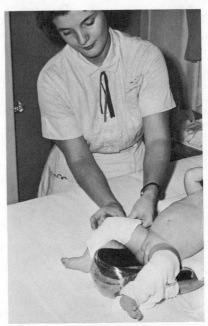

FIGURE 89. Positioning the infant for an enema. A pillow is placed under the infant's head and back. The buttocks are placed upon the bedpan, which has been covered with a folded diaper to protect the infant's back. The legs are restrained in position with a diaper brought under the bedpan and pinned over the legs. (Marlow: *Textbook of Pediatric Nursing.* 4th ed.)

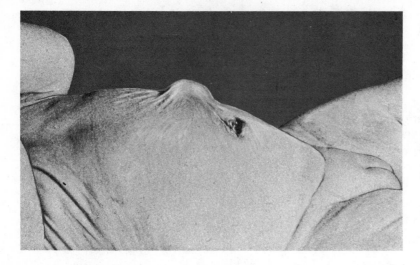

FIGURE 90. Poor skin turgor. The skin has lost its elasticity, owing to severe dehydration. (Courtesy of Dr. Ralph V. Platou and the American Academy of Pediatrics. From Marlow: *Textbook of Pediatric Nursing.* 4th ed.)

air. Child appears to be struggling for breath.

D. Treatment is mostly symptomatic and aimed at reducing laryngeal spasms.
   1. High humidity with warm moist air is important (see page 347).
   2. Emetics are given to induce vomiting, as this is effective in reducing the laryngeal spasms.
   3. Sedatives, such as phenobarbital, are given to relax the child and produce sleep.
   4. The secretions from the nose and throat of a child with croup are *not* highly contagious as in other respiratory diseases.

VI. **Vomiting and Diarrhea**
   A. Vomiting—result of sudden contractions of muscles of stomach and diaphragm. Diarrhea—passing of frequent unformed stool.
   B. These conditions produce a severe disturbance in the electolyte balance and the infant is dehydrated very quickly (Fig. 90).
   C. Treatment is aimed at replacing fluids and minerals lost through vomiting and diarrhea.
      1. Intravenous therapy—usually in scalp vein (Fig. 91).
      2. Hypodermoclysis also used to administer fluids (Fig. 92).
   D. Nursing care
      1. Infant is restrained as necessary during fluid therapy to prevent dislodgment of the needle. Position should be changed often and the limbs exercised passively whenever possible. Restrained parts are checked often for circulatory obstruction.
      2. Special mouth care is important because of dehydration and restriction of fluids by mouth as long as vomiting is present. Cold cream applied to the lips will help

prevent drying and cracking.
   3. Infant should be given a pacifier to satisfy the sucking urge while fluids and foods are being withheld.
   4. An elevated temperature frequently accompanies this condition; special measures may be needed to control febrile convulsions.
   5. Urinary output should be recorded as to frequency and apparent concentration of the urine since the output cannot be measured in most cases.
   6. Collection of urine specimens for laboratory analysis requires special container (Fig. 93).

VII. **Infantile Eczema**
   A. Definition—an inflammation of the skin. The exact cause is not known but it seems to have a familial tendency. Infant is oversensitive to certain substances in his diet or environment.
   B. Symptoms—vesicles that weep and form a dry crust; severe itching produces irritability and loss of sleep.
   C. Treatment and nursing care
      1. Mostly symptomatic to relieve discomfort. If allergen is known it is removed from the diet or environment.
      2. Ointments may be applied to relieve itching and irritation of the skin.
      3. Elbow cuff restraints are used to reduce scratching of the lesions. These restraints simply prevent the child from bending his elbow; they should not restrict exercise and physical activities (Fig. 94).
      4. Fingernails are kept short; cotton socks may be placed over the hands and feet to reduce scratching.
      5. Soothing emollient baths are given to reduce itching and control irritation of the skin.

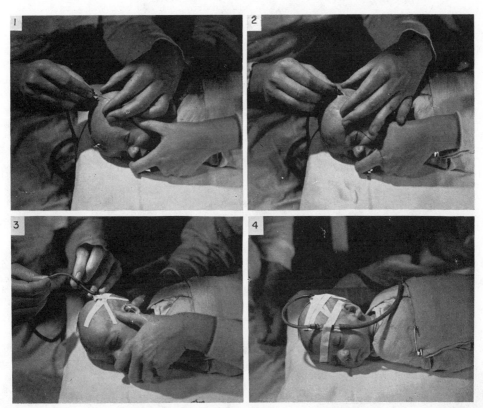

FIGURE 91. Arrangement for long-continued drip of intravenous fluids to a baby. *1*, The child is mummied. Small needle, carrying a soft rubber connector, being inserted into vein. *2*, Needle in vein. *3*, Needle strapped into place with adhesive tape. *4*, The rubber connector attached to the infusion apparatus. With an arrangement of this sort, infusion can be continued for many hours. When the child is put back in his crib, sandbags can be placed in front of the forehead and behind the occiput to limit movements of the head. With this sort of continuous infusion in the scalp the baby should not be fed by mouth. There is too much danger of vomiting and aspiration, since the child cannot move his head adequately to clear the throat. (Gross, R. E.: *The Surgery of Infancy and Childhood.*)

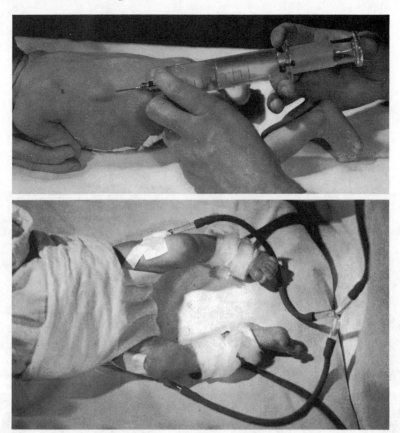

FIGURE 92.   Hypodermoclysis into *(A)* tissues of back of a small baby, given with a needle and syringe. *B,* Common method of giving hypodermoclysis in thighs of babies. The ankles are restrained. Needles are inserted and strapped to each thigh. (Gross: *The Surgery of Infancy and Childhood.*)

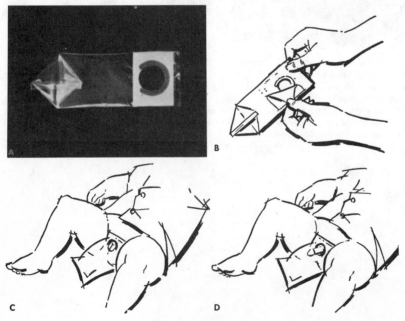

FIGURE 93.   Sterilon's pediatric urine collector for use with both sexes. *A,* Urine collector bag. *B,* Removing paper backing exposing adhesive surface. *C,* On the female, the round opening in the bag is placed so as to cover the upper half of the external genitalia. *D,* On the male, the penis is projected through the round opening in the bag. (Thompson: *Pediatrics for Practical Nurses.* 3rd ed.)

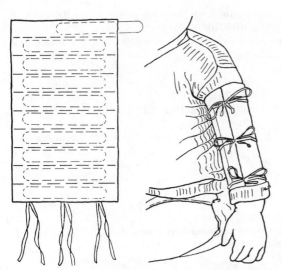

FIGURE 94. *Left*, Elbow cuff restraint. Elbow cuff for use in treatment of eczema. *Right*, Elbow cuff applied. (Blake, F. G., and Wright, F. H.: *Essentials of Pediatric Nursing.* 7th ed., Philadelphia, J. B. Lippincott Co., 1963.)

VIII. Leukemia

A. More than half the cases of childhood leukemia occur in children under the age of 5.

B. Acute leukemia is more common in children than adults.

C. Nursing care is similar to that for adults with leukemia (see Part VII, Unit 8).

1. Emotional support for the parents is extremely important, as there is no cure for leukemia.

2. Extreme care must be taken to avoid injury to the mucous membranes of the mouth or rectum because of a tendency to hemorrhage. Rectal temperatures, if taken, must be done with gentleness.

3. Observation and recording of bleeding from the body orifices.

4. Child will be extremely irritable and uncomfortable most of the time. His mother or father should be allowed to stay with him whenever possible to comfort him and prevent loneliness and grief in the child.

Questions

Mrs. Wise is a young neighbor of yours who has recently given birth to a girl, Jane. This is her first child and, being an only child herself, she has had very little experience with infants and small children. Mrs. Wise is very apprehensive about caring for her infant and looks to you, a practical nurse, for advice and assistance.

1. Mrs. Wise is concerned because Jane, at 1 month, sleeps so much of the day. You should tell her that infants:
   1. sleep all day and stay awake most of the night until they get on a regular schedule
   2. should have only a brief nap during the day, even if you have to force them to stay awake
   3. need at least 12 hours of sleep out of every 24
   4. usually sleep about 20 hours out of every 24 during the first month of life

2. Mrs. Wise received as a gift a bottle prop and she wants to use it during the day to prop the baby's bottle while she is too busy to stop and feed her. Bottle propping is:
   1. considered dangerous because the infant may aspirate some of the formula while sucking or he may get air in his stomach
   2. a safe and time-saving practice for busy mothers
   3. all right if the mother is sure the infant has a good cough reflex
   4. better than holding the infant while he takes his formula because he can take the formula more slowly when the bottle is propped

3. Mrs. Wise wants to cuddle and rock Jane but she is afraid she will become spoiled if she does this. Mrs. Wise should be told that:
   1. all babies like to be held and it is best not to start cuddling and rocking them unless you intend to continue catering to their every wish
   2. physical contact with the mother is a basic need of the infant; if rocking and cuddling are not carried to extreme they are not harmful and are actually necessary to a child's sense of security
   3. infants do not need physical contact with another human because they are not aware of their environment at this age

    4. if she had other children she would know that a young mother has enough to do without stopping to pay attention to an infant

4. When Mrs. Wise took Jane to the pediatrician for her first visit, the infant was given an injection. Mrs. Wise asks you what a "DPT shot" is. The best answer to this question would be:
   1. immunization against all childhood diseases
   2. the first poliomyelitis shot
   3. the letters DPT stand for diphtheria, tetanus, and pertussis; a DPT shot immunizes Jane against these three diseases
   4. this injection is given to determine Jane's susceptibility to pertussis and tuberculosis

5. Pertussis is the medical name for:
   1. lockjaw
   2. tuberculosis
   3. infantile paralysis
   4. whooping cough

6. The first dose of oral poliomyelitis vaccine may be given:
   1. only after the infant is 6 months old
   2. at 2 months of age
   3. as soon as the infant is weaned
   4. only when the infant is 1 year old

7. Jane was placed on baby cereals and strained fruits. These foods are usually started:
   1. when the infant begins teething
   2. at 2 months to 3 months of age
   3. at 6 months of age
   4. after the infant is weaned

8. When new foods are started, it is best to:
   1. give only the new food and formula for the first few feedings after it is started
   2. mix the new food with one the child has already developed a liking for
   3. feed the infant one type of food at a time so he can develop a taste for each food
   4. mix each new food with the formula so the taste of the food will be disguised

9. Strained meat is usually added to the diet at:
   1. 6 weeks
   2. 3 months
   3. 6 months
   4. 1 year

10. Most infants, when placed on their abdomen, are able to lift the head and chest at a 90-degree angle by the age of:
    1. 2 months
    2. 4 months
    3. 2 weeks
    4. 6 months

11. By the time Jane is 3 months old she should be able to:
    1. see objects only as shapes and shadows
    2. focus her eyes on objects and enjoy watching mobile toys placed over her crib
    3. distinguish between light and dark only
    4. focus her eyes only momentarily

12. When Jane visited the pediatrician at 5 months, Mrs. Wise was expecting her to receive a smallpox vaccination. When she did not, Mrs. Wise inquired. What would the best answer be?
    1. We now wait until the age of 1 year to give it.
    2. Smallpox immunization is no longer routinely given to children in the United States.
    3. The world is free of smallpox so there is no need to immunize against it.
    4. Since Jane has an upper respiratory infection, we will wait until she is over that before immunizing her for smallpox.

13. Jane weighed 6 pounds (2.7 kg.) at birth. By the time she is 6 months old she should weigh about:

      1. 21 pounds (9.5 kg.)
      2. 8 pounds (3.6 kg.)
      3. 12 pounds (5.5 kg.)
      4. 26 pounds (11.8 kg.)

14. When Jane was almost 5 months old she began to drool excessively. At this time it would be best to:
      1. give her something soft to chew on because she is probably teething
      2. take her to the pediatrician because this indicates difficulty in swallowing
      3. place her on a limited number of fluids per day until the drooling subsides
      4. take her off baby foods and allow her to eat from the table

15. Mrs. Wise asks you when it would be safe to let Jane drink from a cup. Most infants may be weaned from bottle or breast to a cup at:
      1. 6 weeks
      2. 6 months
      3. 18 months
      4. 2 years

16. Motor development in an infant progresses from the head downward. A normal child can usually grasp objects, hold them in his hands, and play with them at:
      1. 6 weeks
      2. 2 months
      3. 6 months
      4. 1 year

17. Sitting alone momentarily is usually accomplished by the age of:
      1. 2 months
      2. 6 months
      3. 1 year
      4. 18 months

18. Jane will enjoy feeding herself finger foods by the time she is 8 months old. Mrs. Wise should be advised to allow Jane to feed herself:
      1. toast or crackers
      2. raw vegetables
      3. bananas
      4. corn on the cob

19. Most infants are able to crawl by the time they are:
      1. 2 months old
      2. 6 months old
      3. 10 months old
      4. 18 months old

20. Mrs. Wise has a friend who told her that her baby was able to walk alone at 10 months. Jane is able to take only a few steps with help at this age and Mrs. Wise is afraid that something is wrong. What could you tell Mrs. Wise to reassure her best?
      1. Your friend is exaggerating. No baby is able to walk alone at 10 months.
      2. Jane is probably slightly retarded, but she will no doubt outgrow this in time.
      3. Every child develops at his own rate. Most children don't begin walking alone until they are 12 months or older.
      4. Perhaps Jane has a mild case of cerebral palsy. If she doesn't walk soon you should tell your pediatrician.

21. The infant can verbalize about four words, including "ma-ma" and "da-da," at about:
      1. 6 months
      2. 8 months
      3. 10 months
      4. 12 months

22. At the age of 14 months Jane has learned to use the toilet for bowel movements, but she still has difficulty controlling her bladder. Mrs. Wise is very anxious to train Jane and she wonders if she should not spank Jane every time she wets her pants. As a practical nurse you should know that:
      1. Jane probably has a urinary disorder that is causing difficulty in toilet training
      2. firm discipline is all that is needed because Jane could use the toilet if she really wanted to

3. any child who has good bowel control should also have good bladder control
4. toilet training should not be rushed; at 14 months of age Jane should not be expected to have perfect bladder control

23. In establishing toilet training, it is best if the mother or nurse will:
    1. praise the child when he has success rather than punish him when he has an "accident"
    2. remind the child about every hour during the day that he will have an accident if he doesn't try to use the toilet
    3. leave the child in diapers until he is completely in control of his bowels and bladder
    4. withhold some favorite food at meals or deny the child a favorite toy until he cooperates and stops wetting his pants

24. The age of "exploring" and showing a desire to find out about the world around him usually begins when a child:
    1. begins walking
    2. is able to speak in sentences
    3. is old enough to enter school
    4. is able to focus his eyes properly

25. At this age of exploring it is most important for the mother to be aware of:
    1. safety hazards such as poisons, medicines, steaming percolators, etc., which may be within reach of the child
    2. the need for teaching the child good table manners
    3. the danger of spoiling the child with too much love and affection
    4. extreme jealousy toward other children in the family or neighborhood

26. In selecting a toy for an 18-month-old, which of the following would be most appropriate for the age?
    a. tricycle   1. a and c
    b. pull toy that makes noise   2. b and c
    c. bright colored mobile   3. a and d
    d. wooden pegs and hammer   4. b and d

27. The child has a complete set of deciduous teeth at the age of:
    1. 1½ years
    2. 2 years
    3. 2½ years
    4. 3 years

The following questions refer to congenital disorders.

28. Congenital defects in the structure of the heart are believed to be:
    1. caused by poor prenatal care during pregnancy
    2. due to an inherited deficiency in the fetus
    3. associated with infections, such as measles, in the mother during the first trimester of pregnancy
    4. caused by improper care during the first few weeks of the infant's life

29. Not all congenital heart defects are obvious at birth. Symptoms of such a defect in older children include:
    a. dyspnea on the slightest exertion   1. all of these
    b. an abnormally slow pulse rate   2. b only
    c. poor physical development   3. a and d
    d. fatigue out of proportion to the amount 4. all but b
       of exercise taken

30. In recent years the correction of many congenital heart defects has been made possible through:
    1. the discovery of drugs which prevent the occurrence of these defects
    2. the development of surgical techniques for open heart surgery
    3. improvements in the nutrition of newborn infants
    4. prevention of conception in women who are likely to transmit the disease through defective genes

31. Incomplete closure of the upper lip is referred to as:
    1. cleft lip
    2. hydrocephalus
    3. cleft palate
    4. spina bifida

32. Surgical closure of the upper lip is usually done:
    1. at the age of 5 years
    2. after the child becomes aware of his deformity
    3. immediately after birth, before discharge from the hospital
    4. within the first few months of life
33. Immediately after surgical repair of the cleft lip it is most important to prevent injury to the operative area. This is best accomplished by:
    1. keeping the patient heavily sedated
    2. keeping the infant lying on his abdomen with his head turned to the side
    3. restraining the infant's arms and refraining from placing him on his abdomen
    4. giving the child a pacifier so he will not put his fingers or thumb into his mouth
34. Cleft palate involves the roof of the mouth. In addition to feeding problems, this condition also causes:
    1. deafness
    2. speech defects which require speech therapy
    3. mental retardation
    4. paralysis of the throat
35. Feeding problems in these infants are usually overcome by:
    1. administering fluids by vein until surgery can be performed
    2. using a specially designed nipple or syringe
    3. giving feedings through a Levin tube
    4. feeding the child through a gastrostomy tube
36. The term used to describe an increased accumulation of cerebrospinal fluid within the ventricles of the brain is:
    1. anencephalus
    2. microcephalus
    3. hydrocephalus
    4. hypercephalus
37. After the insertion of a shunt to drain the accumulating cerebrospinal fluid within the brain, the nurse must observe the infant for signs of occlusion of the shunt and thus increasing intracranial pressure. Which of the following symptoms indicate increasing intracranial pressure?
    a. increasing irritability
    b. decreasing pulse
    c. increasing blood pressure
    d. increasing appetite
    e. decreasing blood pressure

    1. all of these
    2. a, c, and d
    3. b, d, and e
    4. a, b, and c
38. A congenital defect of the spin through which the meninges protrude and are encased in a soft sac is called:
    1. occult spina bifida
    2. meningocele
    3. meningomyelocele
    4. hydrocephalus
39. Surgical correction of a meningomyelocele is extremely difficult, primarily because:
    1. the spinal cord is involved
    2. this condition occurs only in premature infants
    3. the brain tissues are severely damaged
    4. affected children have no resistance to infection
40. The characteristics of a child with Down's syndrome include:
    a. slanted, Oriental eyes
    b. protruding tongue
    c. very short legs and arms
    d. usually born of a mother over the age of 35

    1. all of these
    2. a only
    3. all but c
    4. d only
41. In selecting a toy for a child with Down's syndrome it is best to:
    1. consider ages of other children in the family
    2. consider mental age rather than chronological age
    3. consider chronological age rather than mental age
    4. avoid giving toys to the retarded, as they are unable to play with them properly

42. Johnny, age 3 months, has bilateral club feet, which are being treated with Denis Browne braces. He is extremely fussy due to an upper respiratory infection, and his mother asks if she might remove the brace until Johnny feels better. What would your best reply be?
    1. Of course, a week or two won't make any difference to Johnny's feet.
    2. Absolutely not or he'll have to have surgery to correct his foot problem.
    3. Even though Johnny doesn't feel well, it would be best to continue the use of the brace on his feet.
    4. If you let Johnny get by without his braces now, he'll fuss every time you try to put them on.
43. Cystic fibrosis is characterized by:
    a. changes in endocrine glands
    b. changes in exocrine glands
    c. respiratory involvement
    d. unusually salty sweat
    1. all of these
    2. all but a
    3. all but b
    4. all but c
44. The organ of the digestive system most often involved in cystic fibrosis is:
    1. pancreas
    2. stomach
    3. gallbladder
    4. liver
45. Untreated PKU is characterized by:
    1. large amounts of sugar in the blood and urine
    2. severe irreversible mental retardation
    3. large accumulations of fluid in brain
    4. sac protruding from spinal cord
46. The infant with PKU is unable to properly metabolize phenylalanine, which is a(n):
    a. amino acid
    b. sugar
    c. fat
    d. protein
    1. a only
    2. b only
    3. a and c
    4. a and d

Ricky, age 18 months, is admitted to the hospital with a severe upper respiratory infection. He is dyspneic, slightly cyanotic, and has a temperature of 102.8° F. (39.3° C.). The physician has ordered a Croupette with oxygen.

47. The Croupette is:
    1. a plastic tent designed so that the air within the tent is kept warm and moist
    2. prepared by placing a blanket or sheet over the sides of the crib and placing a steam kettle nearby
    3. a plastic tent designed to provide cool moist air for the patient to breathe
    4. a very small oxygen tent designed for administration of oxygen to infants
48. If oxygen had not been ordered with the Croupette, it would be necessary for the nurse to:
    1. attach a dia-pump to the Croupette when setting it up
    2. fold the lower end of the tent up over the top to provide fresh air for the infant
    3. keep the chamber at the back of the Croupette empty
    4. remind the physician that oxygen must always be used with a Croupette
49. While Ricky is in the Croupette the nurse must be sure to:
    1. keep the oxygen flow at no more than 4 liters per minute
    2. change the bed linens and Ricky's gown as often as necessary to keep him dry and comfortable
    3. establish a continuous drainage from the ice chamber as the ice melts
    4. restrain him so he cannot change position in bed or sit up
50. Upper respiratory infections are more serious in infants than in adults chiefly because:
    1. infants have no ability to build up an immunity to diseases
    2. most infants cannot be given antibiotics
    3. the air passages of an infant are very small and are easily obstructed with mucus
    4. infants cannot be given a well-balanced diet and therefore have very poor resistance to infections
51. When nose drops are administered to an infant the nurse should:

    1.   hold the infant so that his head is lower than the rest of the body, and maintain that position for several minutes after the drops are given
    2.   hold the infant in a sitting position during the procedure and for several minutes thereafter
    3.   place the infant on his abdomen immediately after the drops are given so as to establish drainage
    4.   keep the infant on his side during and after the administration of the drops

52.   If an infant has difficulty breathing through his nose while taking liquids from a bottle, it is most important for the nurse to:
    1.   withhold the feedings until his nasal passages are completely clear
    2.   feed the infant by gavage
    3.   give the formula to the infant while he is lying on his abdomen
    4.   feed the infant very slowly and allow him periods of rest during the feeding

53.   Cold cream or petrolatum should be applied to the upper lip of an infant when:
    1.   he has fever blisters
    2.   there is bleeding from the gums
    3.   there is a nasal discharge which is irritating to the upper lip and nasal openings
    4.   nose drops are not allowed by the physician

54.   Mummy restraints for infants and small children may be used whenever it is necessary to perform certain procedures or treatments. In this type of restraint:
    1.   the infant's arms are wrapped in gauze and tied to the side of the crib
    2.   the infant is wrapped in a folded sheet or blanket and his arms are held immobilized against his body
    3.   tongue blades are taped to his arms to prevent bending at the elbows
    4.   the infant's arms are taped to his body

55.   Whenever a medication in the form of a pill or tablet is ordered for an infant or small child, the nurse should:
    1.   dissolve the medication in milk or formula
    2.   crush the pill or tablet and mix it with water or syrup
    3.   instruct the patient to chew the pill or tablet
    4.   instruct the patient to hold the pill or tablet in his mouth until it is dissolved

56.   When giving oral medications to Ricky it would be best for the nurse to use a:
    1.   paper cup
    2.   small baby bottle
    3.   glass that can be sterilized after use
    4.   spoon or medicine dropper

57.   Ricky is to receive Tempra syrup 60 mg. for temperature over 101° F. (38.3° C.). The label on the Tempra bottle reads "2 gr. per 5 cc." How much Tempra do you give?
    1.   2.5 cc.
    2.   5 cc.
    3.   10 cc.
    4.   60 cc.

58.   Sometimes Ricky cried and refused to take his oral medication. When this occurs it would be best if the nurse:
    1.   forced the medication between his lips because he must have the medication on time
    2.   asked his mother to give it when she comes to visit each night
    3.   held Ricky's nose until he opened his mouth to breathe or cry and then put the medication in his mouth
    4.   calmed Ricky by holding him and talking to him until he stopped crying and then gave him the medication

59.   Otitis media is a common complication of upper respiratory infections in children of Ricky's age. The term otitis media refers to:
    1.   an inflammation of the middle ear
    2.   juvenile pneumonia
    3.   an inflammation of the nasal sinuses
    4.   vomiting and diarrhea in infants

60.   Otitis media occurs frequently in infants primarily because:
    1.   infants are unable to cough up the mucus collecting in the bronchi
    2.   the sinuses of an infant are not fully developed

3. the infant's eustachian tube is shorter, wider, and straighter than that of an adult
4. the digestive system of an infant is not fully developed and is easily irritated

61. Interstitial pneumonitis refers to:
1. inflammatory involvement of the lung tissues
2. permanent dilatation of the alveoli of the lung
3. a congenital defect in the lungs
4. improper expansion of the lungs in a newborn infant

62. The most common symptoms of interstitial pneumonitis are:
1. vomiting and diarrhea
2. severe dyspnea and cyanosis
3. production of profuse sputum and persistent cough
4. severe headache and stiff neck

63. The morning after his admission to the hospital Ricky's temperature was 104.2° F. (40.1° C.). A temperature this high frequently produces febrile convulsions in infants primarily because:
1. the nervous system of an infant is not fully developed
2. it is extremely difficult to lower the body temperature of an infant
3. many infants have a predisposition to epilepsy
4. the meninges and tissues of the brain are easily infected in infants

64. Ricky started on ampicillin 250 mg. The label on the bottle reads "125 mg. per 5 cc." How much do you give him?
1. 2.5 cc.
2. 5 cc.
3. 10 cc.
4. 25 cc.

65. Ricky's physician ordered a cool tap-water enema to lower his temperature. When giving an enema to Ricky the nurse should use:
1. at least 1 quart (1 liter) of tap water
2. no more than 300 cc. of tap water
3. about 750 cc. of tap water
4. no more than 3 ounces (85 Gm.) of tap water

66. When administering an enema to an infant or small child, the rectal tube is inserted:
1. 2 to 4 inches (5 to 10 cm.)
2. at least 8 inches (20 cm.)
3. about ¾ of an inch (2 cm.)
4. not more than 1 inch (2.5 cm.)

67. The best position for an infant receiving an enema is:
1. on his abdomen with a quilted pad under his hips
2. lying on his back with his buttocks on a small bedpan and pillow under his head and back
3. lying on his left side with the knees drawn up and a diaper folded between his legs
4. on his left side with a pillow under his head and shoulders

68. Ricky improved with treatment and was discharged from the hospital. His mother was told to keep him quiet at home during his convalescence. An important factor in providing rest for Ricky would be:
1. giving him a mild sedative every 4 hours
2. providing a quiet environment and keeping noise and confusion in the home at a minimum
3. placing him in a darkened room and entering only when it is time to feed him
4. allowing him to stay with his mother as she performs her household chores so that he won't feel alone and become frightened

The following questions refer to various disorders of the infant and toddler.

69. Croup is characterized by:
1. an infection of the pharynx
2. spasms of the larynx with partial obstruction of the respiratory tract
3. contractions of the trachea which can be fatal if a tracheotomy is not performed immediately
4. an inflammation of the lung tissues and severe cyanosis

70. The cough of a child with croup is best described as:
    1. deep and moist
    2. nasal in quality and productive of rusty sputum
    3. extremely painful and nonproductive
    4. "barking," with a high-pitched, rasping noise each time a breath is taken
71. Attacks of croup occur most often:
    1. at night, and in children who are hyperactive and nervous
    2. after meals, and in mentally disturbed children
    3. during the day, when the child is active and excited
    4. at night, and in children who are quiet and well adjusted
72. If a croup tent is devised by placing a blanket or sheet over a crib, the covering should be arranged so that the crib is:
    1. covered on all sides, with the top open
    2. covered on the top only, with the sides left open
    3. completely covered on top and sides
    4. covered on top and sides about halfway, with the rest of the crib left open
73. The croup tent provides:
    1. oxygen to relieve dyspnea
    2. warm moist air
    3. cool moist air
    4. cool dry air to dry up nasal secretions
74. Emetics are sometimes used to reduce laryngeal spasms in croup. These drugs are given primarily to:
    1. dry up bronchial secretions
    2. produce sleep
    3. induce vomiting
    4. thin the bronchial secretions and dilate the bronchi
75. A sedative that is frequently given to produce sleep and relaxation in a child with croup is:
    1. aspirin
    2. morphine sulfate
    3. scopolamine
    4. phenobarbital
76. Even though croup does involve the respiratory system, the nurse should know that:
    1. the child with croup always has complications involving the nervous system
    2. the nasal and bronchial secretions from a child with croup are not highly contagious
    3. a common complication of croup is congestive heart failure
    4. the disease is usually transmitted through contaminated food or water
77. Vomiting and diarrhea are very serious in an infant primarily because:
    1. the infant loses vital electrolytes and becomes severely dehydrated very quickly
    2. they tend to become chronic and lead to ulcerative colitis in later life
    3. there is no satisfactory treatment for this condition in children
    4. complications caused by vomiting and diarrhea may produce severe damage to the heart
78. Intravenous therapy in an infant is usually administered through:
    1. the femoral vein
    2. a large vein in the arm
    3. a scalp vein
    4. an abdominal vein
79. Hypodermoclysis refers to:
    1. removal of fluid from the spine
    2. administration of fluids into the subcutaneous tissues
    3. administration of fluids via a Levin tube
    4. removal of fluids from the tissues
80. When an infant is not allowed fluids by mouth for a period of time, it is most important for the nurse to:
    1. give special mouth care and apply cold cream or petrolatum to the lips to prevent cracking
    2. carefully measure the infant's urinary output and record in cubic centimeters

3. collect a daily urine specimen and send it to the laboratory

4. restrain the infant's arms so he will not suck his thumb while he is hungry

81. When an infant is restrained for administration of fluid therapy, the nurse must be sure to:

    1. immobilize the infant in one position until the fluids are discontinued
    2. change the infant's position often and passively exercise the limbs of the infant
    3. remind the infant's mother that she must not allow the infant to change positions because the needle may become dislodged
    4. avoid changing the infant's gown or bed linen until the fluids are discontinued

82. When caring for an infant who is severely dehydrated, the nurse should realize that:

    1. she cannot record the exact amount of urine voided, but she should record the number of times the infant voids
    2. it is impossible to keep a record of urinary output for an infant
    3. an indwelling catheter is always inserted so that an accurate account can be made of the urinary output
    4. physicians are concerned only with fluid intake and are not interested in the infant's urinary output

83. Collection of a urine specimen from an infant or small child is best accomplished by:

    1. using a small emesis basin to collect the urine
    2. strapping the infant to a bedpan until he voids
    3. sitting the infant on a small chamber pot until he voids
    4. applying a specially designed collection device to the infant and removing it immediately after he voids

84. Infantile eczema is:

    1. caused by *Staphylococcus aureus*
    2. a parasitic skin disease
    3. a result of sensitivity to a certain substance
    4. caused by unsanitary conditions in the infant's home

85. Elbow cuff restraints are designed so that:

    1. tongue blades can be inserted into pockets sewn in the restraints
    2. the entire upper body and arms are immobilized
    3. an infant cannot move his arms away from his body
    4. the lower extremities of the infant are held immobile

86. Elbow cuff restraints are used in many skin diseases primarily because they:

    1. keep the child quiet
    2. prevent walking and crawling, which predispose the lesions to infection
    3. do not have to be removed periodically to permit exercising the limb and checking for circulatory obstruction
    4. prevent the child from bending his elbows and scratching the skin lesions

87. Leukemia in children is:

    1. usually of the chronic type
    2. rarely fatal, and progresses very slowly
    3. most often acute, and progresses rapidly
    4. curable, whereas it is incurable in adults

88. Extreme care should be taken in handling the child with leukemia, primarily because:

    1. he is subject to convulsions in the early stages of the disease
    2. bleeding from the body orifices and under the skin is quite common
    3. any activity is liable to elevate the body temperature drastically
    4. paralysis may result if the child is not handled properly

89. When caring for a child with leukemia the nurse must realize that:

    1. the parents of the child will require comfort and moral support throughout the child's illness
    2. most children with leukemia prefer to be left alone
    3. there is no pain or discomfort associated with leukemia
    4. children with leukemia are very quiet and easy to care for

UNIT 2   THE PRESCHOOL CHILD

I. Normal Growth and Development
A. Basic needs
1. Identification with parent of the same sex.
2. Socialization with others his age (Fig. 95).
3. At this age child should be taught safety measures and ways to avoid accidents, which are the major cause of death between the ages of 1 year and 19 years of age.
B. Dental care is important at this age. The deciduous (baby) teeth pave the way for the permanent teeth. If neglected, the deciduous teeth may cause crowding and displacement of the permanent teeth.
C. Further immunization against childhood diseases such as diphtheria, whooping cough, tetanus, poliomyelitis, and smallpox.
D. Adequate nutrition at this age may present problems because the child is more interested in other things in his environment.
1. Simple foods are preferred.
2. Too much stress should not be placed on table manners at this age.
3. Children tend to imitate the eating habits of older brothers and sisters and parents.

II. Disorders of the Preschool Child
A. Cerebral palsy
1. Definition—cerebral palsy refers to a group of disorders that affect the motor control centers of the brain.
2. Can be caused by many factors, including injury at birth, anoxia, subdural hemorrhage, or infection of the brain or meninges.
3. Symptoms may range from mild difficulty in control of the muscles to a severe handicap. Defects in speech, sight, and hearing may complicate the condition. Mental retardation may or may not accompany cerebral palsy.
4. Treatment and nursing care
   a. There is no cure for this disorder.
   b. The objective of treatment is to help the child utilize his remaining functions and adjust to his handicap.
   c. Physical therapy is employed and

measures must be taken to prevent deformities, such as contractures and muscular atrophy.
B. Tonsillitis and adenoiditis
1. Definition—an inflammation of the tonsils and adenoids. These are located in the pharynx and are composed of lymphoid tissue.
2. Symptoms—severe sore throat and elevated temperature. In chronic cases the tonsils and adenoids are greatly enlarged.
3. Treatment
   a. Usually conservative at first. Antibiotics are used to control infection; general hygienic measures to improve the child's general health.
   b. Surgery is indicated if the tissues cause obstruction to swallowing or breathing, or if there are recurrent episodes of sore throat and respiratory infection.
   c. Preoperative nursing care
      1. Blood tests and urinalysis are done. Bleeding time and clotting time are checked.

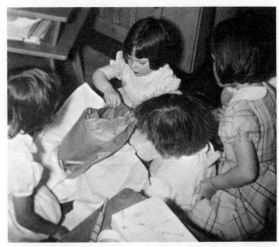

FIGURE 95. Socialization is an important phase for the preschool period. Children begin to understand the meaning of friendship. (Thompson: *Pediatrics for Practical Nurses*, 3rd ed.).

2. Child should be told in advance that he is to be hospitalized. If possible, his mother should allow him to participate in preparation for his stay in the hospital; for example, she may let him help pack his suitcase. If he wishes to bring a favorite toy or book to the hospital this wish should be granted because it will help him adjust to separation from his home and family.
3. Foods and fluids are withheld before surgery.
4. Any elevated temperature or other signs of an infection should be reported promptly, as this may prohibit surgery.

d. Postoperative care
1. Child is placed on his abdomen or partly on abdomen and partly on side with knee of upper leg flexed to facilitate drainage and prevent aspiration of mucus or blood into the lungs.
2. Hemorrhage is a constant danger and the child is watched closely for signs of bleeding from the mouth. Frequent swallowing and restlessness may also indicate bleeding from the operative site. The vital signs are checked regularly.
3. An ice collar will reduce swelling and discomfort and help prevent hemorrhage.
4. Small amounts of liquids are given by mouth after the child has re-acted, if there is no vomiting. Milk and synthetic fruit juices are least irritating.
5. During the convalescent stage the child should have adequate rest and some restriction of activities. Soft bland foods are given until healing is complete.

C. Communicable diseases
1. Immunizations have helped reduce the incidence of these diseases, but they are still a major cause of illness in children.
2. The mother should be told that an immunization record should be kept on each child as soon as immunizations are begun (Table 17).
3. Symptoms and incubation periods for common communicable diseases (Table 18).
4. Tests for susceptibility to a particular disease include the Schick test for diphtheria, the Dick test for scarlet fever, and the tuberculin test for tuberculosis.
5. Nursing care of the child with a communicable disease requires isolation until he is no longer considered to be a source of infection (see Part IX).
   a. Diversional activities for the child should be interspersed with periods of rest.
   b. Toys, books, etc. brought into the isolation unit must be decontaminated or burned to prevent the spread of disease to others.

Table 17. Immunization Record: Recommended Schedule for Active Immunization of Normal Infants and Children*

2 months	DTP[1]	TOPV[2]
4 months	DTP	TOPV
6 months	DTP	TOPV
1 year	Measles[3]	Tuberculin test[4]
	Rubella[3]	Mumps[3]
1½ years	DTP	TOPV
4–6 years	DTP	TOPV
14–16 years	Td[5] and thereafter every 10 years	

*Recommended by the American Academy of Pediatrics in *Report of the Committee on Infectious Diseases*, 1975, p. 3 (red book).

[1]DTP – diphtheria and tetanus toxoids combined with pertussis vaccine.

[2]TOPV – trivalent oral poliovirus vaccine. This recommendation is suitable for breast-fed as well as bottle-fed infants.

[3]May be given at 1 year as measles-rubella or measles-mumps-rubella combined vaccines.

[4]Frequency of repeated tuberculin tests depends on risk of exposure of the child and on the prevalence of tuberculosis in the population group. The initial test should be at the time of, or preceding, the measles immunization.

[5]Td – combined tetanus and diphtheria toxoids (adult type) for those more than 6 years of age in contrast to diphtheria and tetanus (DT), which contains a larger amount of diphtheria antigen. Tetanus toxoid at time of injury. For clean, minor wounds, no booster dose is needed by a fully immunized child unless more than 10 years have elapsed since the last dose. For contaminated wounds, a booster dose should be given if more than 5 years have elapsed since the last dose.

Table 18.   Common Communicable Diseases

DISEASE	FIRST SIGNS	INCUBATION PERIOD	PREVENTION	LENGTH OF CONTAGIOUS PERIOD	MANAGEMENT
Chickenpox	Mild fever followed in 36 hours by small raised pimples which become filled with clear fluid. Scabs form later. Successive crops of pox appear.	2–3 weeks. Usually 14–16 days.	None. Immune after one attack.	6 days after appearance of rash.	Usually not serious. Trim fingernails to prevent scratching. Diluted alcohol or a solution of baking soda and water may ease itching.
German measles (3-day measles)	Mild fever, sore throat, or cold symptoms may precede fine rose-colored rash. Enlarged glands at back of neck and behind ears.	2–3½ weeks. Usually 18 days.	Vaccine can be given to provide immunity.	Until rash fades. About 5 days.	Not a serious disease, complications rare; give general good care and keep baby quiet. Avoid exposing any woman who is, or might be, in the early months of pregnancy unless she is sure she has had the disease.
Measles	Mounting fever; dry cough; running nose and red eyes for 3 or 4 days before rash, which starts at hairline and spreads down in blotches. Small red spots with white centers in mouth (Koplik's spots) may occasionally be seen before rash.	1–2 weeks. Usually 10 or 11 days.	Vaccine can be given to provide immunity. A baby not vaccinated if exposed can be given gamma globulin to lighten or prevent measles.	Until 5 days after the rash has appeared.	May be mild or severe with complications of a serious nature; follow doctor's advice in caring for a child with measles, as it is a most treacherous disease. If other children who have not had the disease are exposed, ask the doctor about protective inoculations for them.
Mumps	Fever; headache; vomiting; glands near ear and at jawline ache, and these develop painful swelling. Other parts of body may be affected also.	14–28 days. Usually around 18 days.	Vaccine can be given to provide immunity.	Until all swelling disappears.	Keep child in bed until fever subsides; indoors unless weather is warm.

DISEASE	FIRST SIGNS	INCUBATION PERIOD	PREVENTION	LENGTH OF CONTAGIOUS PERIOD	MANAGEMENT
Roseola	High fever for 2 or 3 days which then falls to normal before appearance of a fine rash or large pink blotches on back and stomach or sometimes the whole body. Child may not seem very ill despite high fever (103–105°F.), but he may convulse.	Not fully known.	None. Usually affects children from 6 months to 3 years of age.	Until the child seems well.	No special measures except rest and quiet. Force fluids during fever.
Strep throat (septic sore throat) and scarlet fever (scarlatina)	Sometimes vomiting and fever before sudden and severe sore throat. If followed by fine rash on body and limbs, it is called scarlet fever.	1–7 days. Usually 2–5 days	Antibiotics may prevent or lighten an attack if doctor feels it wise.	7–10 days. When all abnormal discharge from nose, eyes, throat has ceased.	Frequently less severe than formerly; responds to antibiotics, which should be continued for full course to prevent serious complications.
Whooping cough	At first seems like a cold with low fever and cough which changes at end of second week to spells of coughing accompanied by a noisy gasp for air which creates the "whoop."	5–21 days. Usually around 10	Give injections of vaccine to all children in infancy; if an unvaccinated child has been exposed, the doctor may want to give a protective serum promptly.	At least 4 weeks.	Child needs careful supervision of doctor throughout this taxing illness.

(Adapted from United States Department of Health, Education, and Welfare: *Infant Care*, 1963, pp. 80–82, and *Your Child from One to Six*, 1962, pp. 82–83.)

Questions

1. At the preschool age children should begin to:
    1. withdraw from others and show a desire to be left alone
    2. enjoy the socialization of others their own age
    3. revert to infantile behavior until they have adjusted to school
    4. require extensive physical care such as bathing and clothing because they cannot do these things for themselves
2. Mothers should be told that preschool children:
    1. are not old enough to learn safety rules, and require constant supervision
    2. are not prone to accidental injury or death
    3. rarely experience accidental injury
    4. are capable of understanding simple rules which will prevent many accidents
3. Most of the children of preschool age:
    1. eat well and present no nutritional problems
    2. have excellent table manners
    3. present some eating problems, chiefly because they are more interested in other things
    4. refuse to eat whenever they want attention from their parents
4. The eating habits of a preschool child are usually:
    1. copied from other members of the family
    2. not important, because nutrition at this age does not affect the child's health
    3. well established before he is 2 years old and cannot be changed
    4. learned from his friends
5. Children of preschool age:
    1. do not require dental care for their deciduous teeth because they will soon lose them
    2. should receive regular dental care because the permanent teeth can be affected by decay in the deciduous teeth
    3. should be examined by a dentist at least once before their permanent teeth begin to erupt
    4. cannot be expected to brush their teeth; therefore, dental care should be postponed until school age
6. Some basic principles of discipline for the preschool child include:
    a. being consistent in disciplining
    b. one parent should be primarily responsible for the discipline
    c. spankings are the only form of discipline a preschooler understands
    d. rewarding of good deeds is effective
    e. discipline should be given at the time of the incident

    1. a, b, and c
    2. b, c, and d
    3. a, d, and e
    4. all but b

Marion Taylor, age 5, has had repeated episodes of sore throat and tonsillitis. She has begun to lose weight and is less fully developed than other children of her age. She breathes through her mouth and snores in her sleep. Her pediatrician has referred her to a surgeon for evaluation and possible surgery for removal of the tonsils and adenoids.

7. The tonsils and adenoids are important in localizing infections primarily because they are:
    1. located below the trachea
    2. composed of lymphoid tissue
    3. a part of the digestive system
    4. not easily infected
8. Surgical removal of the tonsils and adenoids is indicated when:
    a. an inflammation of these organs first develops
    b. a child has a tendency to develop streptococcal infections of the throat

    1. b only
    2. all but c
    3. b and c
    4. c and d

      c. these organs enlarge and cause an ob-
          struction to swallowing or breathing
      d. there are persistent and recurring
          episodes of inflammation in these organs

9. Marion's mother was told by the surgeon that the child would be scheduled for surgical removal of her tonsils and adenoids the following week. Mrs. Taylor should:
    1. avoid talking about the surgery in Marion's presence because she will be frightened and uncooperative if she knows what is going to take place
    2. tell Marion that she is going on a "trip" to the hospital and it will be a very pleasant experience for her
    3. prepare Marion for the ordeal by telling her that it will be very painful and unpleasant but there is nothing else to do but get it over with
    4. tell Marion about the proposed surgery the day before admission and emphasize the good points, such as that she will feel much better and not have a sore throat often when her tonsils are removed

10. Marion will probably accept her hospitalization better if she is:
    1. told that she will be given medicine to make her sleep so she won't know what is going on while she is there
    2. allowed to help pack her own suitcase and choose the toys or books she wishes to take along
    3. not told about the hospital visit until just before time to leave home
    4. warned that she must cooperate with the doctors and nurses or they will have to give her "shots" to help her get well

11. Upon her admission to the hospital Marion was visited by the laboratory technician who needed to obtain a sample of blood. Marion asked the nurse if the technician was going to hurt her. What would the best answer to the child's question be?
    1. Of course not. You won't feel a thing.
    2. I don't know. But even if she does you must not complain.
    3. It will probably hurt a little bit, but we are doing this because we want to take very good care of you while you are staying with us.
    4. Yes, it will hurt, but we have to know your blood type because you may get very sick and need a blood transfusion after your tonsils are taken out.

12. If Marion asks what they are going to do with her blood sample after it is taken, what would it be best to tell her?
    1. The technician is going to take it to the laboratory and examine it carefully so we will know exactly what we need to do to help you get well.
    2. I can't explain that to you because you are too little to understand.
    3. They are going to take it to the laboratory and do experiments on it.
    4. They will keep it in case something goes wrong while you are having your tonsils removed.

13. Before Marion goes to surgery it is very important that the nurse keep an accurate record of the child's temperature and vital signs, primarily because:
    1. any change in the vital signs would indicate the need for immediate surgery
    2. an elevated temperature or change in vital signs may indicate an infection which would prohibit surgery until the infection subsided
    3. hemorrhage before surgery is quite common in cases of chronic tonsillitis
    4. the child may need intravenous fluids or a blood transfusion before surgery if the vital signs are not within normal range

14. Immediately after surgery it would be best to place Marion:
    1. in Fowler's position
    2. on her back
    3. on her abdomen
    4. in lithotomy position

15. The most common complication in the postoperative period is:
    1. loss of speech
    2. hemorrhage
    3. abdominal distention
    4. loss of hearing

16. Which of the following may indicate bleeding from the operative site after Marion's surgery?
    1. elevated temperature
    2. flushed face and loss of consciousness
    3. tarry stools
    4. frequent swallowing and restlessness
17. Which of the following would be most beneficial in reducing swelling and discomfort in the operative site?
    1. frequent suctioning to remove blood and mucus
    2. an ice collar
    3. a hot water bottle to the neck
    4. frequent throat irrigation
18. When liquids by mouth are allowed it would be best to give Marion:
    1. lemonade
    2. fresh orange juice
    3. milk or synthetic fruit juices
    4. hot tea or coffee
19. The evening of her operative day Marion became restless and wanted to get out of bed. It would be best for the nurse to:
    1. allow Marion's mother to hold the child in her lap and rock her for a while
    2. tell Marion to quit acting like a baby, and that a big girl 5 years old should be ashamed to sit in her mother's lap
    3. permit Marion to run about the halls so she will sleep better at night
    4. restrain Marion to keep her from sitting up or getting out of bed
20. When Marion was discharged from the hospital her mother was told to keep her on a bland diet. Mrs. Taylor asks you what a "bland diet" is. What would your best answer be?
    1. Nothing but liquids such as fresh fruit juices are allowed.
    2. A diet that is soft and easy to swallow and does not contain any spices or strong seasonings.
    3. One that contains absolutely no salt or pepper.
    4. It is very complicated and difficult to follow. If you have time it would be best to try to find a dietitian who can explain it to you.

The following questions refer to communicable diseases in children.

21. Which of the following statements best describes the incidence of communicable diseases in children?
    1. Immunizations against communicable diseases have resulted in the elimination of these diseases in the lives of children.
    2. Communicable diseases are a necessary part of every child's life and the sooner they catch them the better off they will be.
    3. Communicable diseases are never serious and only those that cause serious illness require immunization.
    4. Immunizations have reduced the incidence of communicable diseases but they are still a major cause of illness in children.
22. Before a child starts to school he should receive:
    1. immunization against cholera
    2. DPT injections, even though he may have had them when he was an infant
    3. his fourth smallpox vaccination
    4. DPT injections only if he did not receive them in his infancy
23. Complications of chickenpox include:
    1. central nervous system involvement
    2. hearing loss and deafness
    3. loss of eyesight acuity
    4. no serious complications known
24. The itching accompanying chickenpox can best be relieved by:
    1. bathing the lesions in a solution of baking soda and water
    2. applying 95 per cent alcohol to the sores
    3. bathing the lesions in a solution of vinegar and water
    4. removing the scabs by vigorously scrubbing the lesions with soap and water

25. German measles is also referred to as:
    1. scarlet fever
    2. 3-day measles
    3. red measles
    4. roseola
26. German measles are especially serious if contracted:
    1. by a pregnant woman
    2. before the age of 1
    3. by a preadolescent
    4. not a serious problem at any time
27. Vaccine may now be given to provide artificial immunity against:
    a. German measles   1. all of these
    b. chickenpox   2. all but a
    c. measles   3. all but b
    d. mumps   4. all but d
28. The incubation period for mumps is:
    1. 2 to 4 weeks
    2. 1 to 5 days
    3. 2 to 4 months
    4. 1 week
29. A "strep" throat that is accompanied by a fine rash on the body and limbs is called:
    1. measles
    2. scarlet fever
    3. roseola
    4. glandular fever
30. The communicable disease that affects the parotid glands near the ear and jaw is called:
    1. mumps
    2. measles
    3. glandular fever
    4. infectious mononucleosis
31. The child with whooping cough:
    1. is not severely ill
    2. does not require medical treatment
    3. may become physically exhausted, and needs careful medical supervision
    4. usually requires hospitalization and intensive nursing care
32. The child with mumps must be considered to be a source of contagion until:
    1. his temperature returns to normal
    2. at least 1 month has elapsed since the onset of symptoms
    3. all swelling disappears
    4. the rash has completely disappeared
33. The Shick test is done to determine an individual's susceptibility to:
    1. scarlet fever
    2. tuberculosis
    3. tetanus
    4. diphtheria
34. When providing diversional activities for a child in isolation, it must be remembered that:
    1. these children are always on absolute bed rest
    2. any articles brought into the unit must be washable or capable of being sterilized or they will have to be destroyed when the child is no longer a source of contagion
    3. the room must always be darkened and the child's eyes must be protected whenever he has any communicable disease
    4. most children enjoy reading for hours on end

UNIT 3   THE SCHOOL AGE CHILD

I. Normal Growth and Development

A. Child is ready to face reality and wishes to engage in tasks in the real world around him.

B. School is an important part of the child's life.

C. At age 6, the temporary teeth loosen and the incisors are replaced by permanent teeth.

D. Each night 10 to 12 hours of sleep are needed. Sleep and rest are necessary to normal growth and development.

E. Table manners improve as the child grows older.

F. This is a relatively healthy period of life.

II. Disorders of the School Age Child

A. Rheumatic fever—highest incidence in children between 5 and 15 years of age.

   1. Definition—a systemic disease which is characterized by destruction of connective tissue. It is especially damaging to the heart. Rheumatic fever is associated with infections caused by *hemolytic streptococci*.

   2. Symptoms include joint pain, chorea (a nervous disorder), and inflammation of the membranes, valves, or muscle of the heart.

     a. The joint pains of rheumatic fever are not to be mistaken for what is loosely called "growing pains." The shoulders, knees, and ankles are usually involved and arthritis subsides in one joint, only to appear in another. There may be swelling of the joint and discoloration.

     b. Chorea is also called St. Vitus' dance. It is characterized by involuntary motion of the muscles. Stress or emotional excitement may aggravate the condition.

     c. Involvement of the heart is serious and produces symptoms of dyspnea, chest pain, low-grade fever, increased pulse and respiratory rate, and heart murmur.

     d. Skin eruptions—small red raised circles appearing as wavy red lines on trunk and abdomen.

     e. Cutaneous nodules at the back of head, along spine may appear for weeks or months.

   3. Treatment and nursing care are aimed at relieving symptoms and providing complete physical and mental rest to avoid complications.

     a. Medications include aspirin for control of joint pain, steroids as anti-inflammatory agents, and antibiotics to prevent further bacterial infection.

     b. Heart medications such as digitalis or one of its derivatives are given to slow and strengthen the heartbeat.

     c. Absolute bed rest is necessary as long as the symptoms persist and the sedimentation rate is above normal.

      1. While on bed rest, the child must be properly positioned to prevent orthopedic deformities and postural defects.

      2. Special attention is given to the skin to prevent breakdown.

      3. Small frequent feedings are necessary to avoid overburdening the heart and circulatory system and to provide adequate nutrition.

      4. School work is continued when the physician permits. A visiting teacher assists the child and teaches him on a regular daily basis until he is able to return to school.

      5. Hobbies or other activities to interest the child while he is on bed rest must be geared to the child's interests and talents.

     d. During the convalescent stage the child's progress is followed very closely by the physician. Emphasis is placed on what the child *can* do rather than what he cannot do or is not allowed to do.

B. Diabetes mellitus

   1. Characterized by a deficiency of insulin which is necessary to metabolize carbohydrates.

   2. Juvenile diabetes (appearance of symptoms in childhood) occurs in about 5% of cases and is more serious and difficult to treat than if symptoms occur later.

   3. Onset of symptoms is rapid.

     a. Easily fatigued.

     b. Polydipsia (excessive thirst)

     c. Polyuria (increased urine output)

     d. Hyperorexia (increased appetite)

     e. Glycosuria (sugar in urine)

4. Diabetes in children is controlled with insulin and diet and regulation of exercise.
5. The child over 7 years of age can usually be taught to administer his own insulin.
6. Exercise lowers the blood sugar and decreases the need for insulin. This may present difficulties if the exercises are not planned according to mealtime and the type of insulin taken. Generally, it is considered best to recommend mild exercise before meals and more strenuous sports after meals.
7. Education of the child and his parents in regard to diet, administration of insulin, and prevention of complications is the same as for older diabetics.
C. Appendicitis
  1. Characterized by an inflammation of the lining of the appendix due to an obstruction of the opening into the cecum.
  2. Symptoms include abdominal tenderness, low-grade fever, vomiting, and elevated white blood count.
  3. Treatment
    a. Surgical removal—appendectomy.
    b. Preoperative nursing care
      1. Blood tests and urinalysis done to observe WBC.
      2. Close observation of vital signs.
      3. Bed rest—ice bag may be ordered to involved area to reduce pain and decrease peristalsis.
      4. Food and fluids withheld.
      5. Avoid giving laxatives or enemas.
    c. Postoperative care
      1. In uncomplicated cases, care is basic with recovery rapid.
      2. If appendix has ruptured, generalized peritonitis may make child very ill. Antibiotics, parenteral fluids, gastric suction, and abdominal drains may be necessary.

Questions

Ann is a 6-year-old patient who has been admitted to the hospital for diagnostic tests. She has lost weight recently, has been running a low-grade fever, and complains of having pains in her arms and legs. Her admission diagnosis was possible rheumatic fever.

1. When Ann was being admitted to the hospital, she told the nurse that her front "baby" tooth was loose and seemed about to fall out. The practical nurse should know that:
    1. the loss of several teeth often accompanies high fevers
    2. teeth often become loose when a child has rheumatic fever
    3. most children begin to lose their temporary teeth at about 6 years of age
    4. Ann probably is suffering from some type of nutritional deficiency
2. The type of pain most often associated with rheumatic fever:
    1. involves the muscles, and results from involuntary muscle spasms
    2. is usually located in the joints, and tends to migrate from one joint to another
    3. is never associated with swelling or any other indication that the disease is present
    4. usually produces total paralysis in the lower limbs
3. Rheumatic fever is associated with:
    1. infections caused by the hemolytic streptococcus
    2. violent injury to one of the limbs
    3. viral infections of the respiratory tract
    4. bacterial infections of the bones
4. Ann's condition was diagnosed as rheumatic fever and she was placed on absolute bed rest. What would be the best way to explain this to Ann?
    1. You must stay in bed or you will damage your heart and that can kill you.
    2. Your doctor has told us to keep you in bed and we will do it even if we have to tie you down.
    3. We want you to stay in bed and rest all the time. We will do everything for you, even give you a bath in bed and bring your meals to you so you can get well soon.
    4. You must be very quiet in your room. The doctor wants you to rest whenever you get tried so you won't have any complications.

5. Sometimes rheumatic fever is characterized by a nervous disorder in which there is involuntary motion of the muscles. This condition is referred to as:
   1. cerebral palsy
   2. chorea
   3. neuralgia
   4. arthritis

6. Ann's physician ordered aspirin to be given her every 4 hours. Salicylates such as aspirin are given in the treatment of rheumatic fever primarily because these drugs:
   1. destroy the bacteria causing the disease
   2. keep the body temperature below normal
   3. prevent involvement of the heart
   4. relieve joint pain

7. The most serious complication of rheumatic fever is:
   1. involvement of the heart
   2. permanent paralysis
   3. disintegration of the joints
   4. mental deterioration

8. While Ann is in the acute stage of her illness she should be given:
   1. liquids only
   2. only two meals a day
   3. double servings on her tray
   4. small, frequent feedings

9. As Ann's condition improved she was allowed more physical activity. When explaining the change in her routine it would be best to:
   1. emphasize the things she is permitted to do rather than the things she cannot do
   2. warn Ann that too much activity may cause complications which would make her seriously ill
   3. stress the importance of rest, because she will need to avoid strenuous exercise for the rest of her life
   4. tell Ann that she must realize that even though she can get out of bed for a while each day she will never be able to play like other children

10. Barbara is a 13-year-old patient admitted to the hospital for a diagnostic work-up for possible diabetes mellitus. Symptoms of diabetes mellitus include:
    a. urinary retention
    b. polydipsia
    c. increase in appetite
    d. easily fatigued
    1. all of these
    2. all but a
    3. all but b
    4. all but d

11. Diabetes mellitus is:
    1. much milder in children than in adults
    2. more severe in children, and has a more rapid onset
    3. very common in children, but they usually outgrow it
    4. an acute disease that usually is fatal when it occurs in children

12. In diabetes mellitus, carbohydrates are inefficiently metabolized due to a deficiency of:
    1. sugar
    2. thyroxin
    3. insulin
    4. amino acids

13. The parents of diabetic children should know that:
    1. children under the age of 14 cannot be allowed to give their own insulin
    2. exercise lowers the blood sugar and decreases the need for insulin
    3. children are best treated with oral substitutes for insulin
    4. a diabetic child cannot participate in any type of sport or active play

14. Diabetes mellitus can be controlled with a proper combination of:
    a. diet
    b. insulin
    c. exercise
    d. education
    1. all of these
    2. all but a
    3. all but c
    4. all but d

15. The early adolescent experiences stress and some emotional difficulty in social adjustment primarily because:
    1. he is usually unprepared for coping with social experiences
    2. his physical growth is much more rapid than his emotional and social development

3. he has reached the peak of physical growth but is not yet ready for adult responsibilities
4. he is more concerned with himself than with others in his age group

16. One of the most outstanding features of early adolescence is:
    1. development of secondary sex characteristics
    2. ability to cope with social situations involving members of the opposite sex
    3. lack of emotional instability or social conflict
    4. mental development reaches a plateau

17. The prime of physical growth and development is usually reached between the ages of:
    1. 12–14 years
    2. 14–16 years
    3. 16–18 years
    4. 18–20 years

18. The major cause of death during the adolescent years is:
    1. rheumatic heart disease
    2. malignancy, particularly the lymphomas
    3. accidents
    4. venereal disease

19. Carole, age 14, is admitted to the hospital with the following symptoms: severe abdominal pain, vomiting, and a fever of 101° F. (38.3° C). She is diagnosed as being in sickle cell crisis. Sickle cell crisis is the result of:
    1. malformed cells clumping together, causing capillary obstructions
    2. an infection in the blood
    3. failure of the person to follow his diet
    4. white blood cells attacking red cells

20. The treatment of sickle cell crisis is:
    1. surgical removal of the sickle-shaped cells
    2. surgical removal of the defective bone marrow which is producing the cells
    3. supportive therapy of the presenting symptoms
    4. large doses of chemotherapy

21. Carole is in severe pain. She has Demerol 60 mg. ordered. Using the ampoule "Demerol 100 mg. per 2 cc," how much Demerol will she receive?
    1. 0.6 cc.
    2. 1.0 cc.
    3. 1.2 cc.
    4. 1.5 cc.

22. Terry, age 15, is admitted with possible appendicitis. Which of the following are "typical" symptoms of appendicitis?
    a. low-grade fever
    b. abdominal pain over umbilicus, moving to right side
    c. nausea and vomiting
    d. abnormal-looking red blood cells

    1. all but a
    2. all but c
    3. all but d
    4. all of these

23. The physician ordered ice packs to the abdominal area. The reason for this is to:
    a. prevent spread of infection
    b. reduce fever
    c. decrease comfort
    d. slow down peristalsis

    1. a and c
    2. b and d
    3. a and d
    4. c and d

24. It is most important for the nurse to keep close observation of a patient suspected of having an acute appendicitis. Which of the following should be reported immediately?
    a. a loose stool
    b. requests for fluids to drink
    c. complaints of increasing abdominal pain
    d. temperature of 104.2° F. (40.1° C.)

    1. a and c
    2. b and d
    3. b and c
    4. c and d

25. The symptoms of appendicitis are similar to other conditions. Therefore the physician must take a careful history and physical examination to make an accurate diagnosis, but delay of surgical intervention of a "hot" appendix could result in rupture of the appendix with the complication of:
    1. pericarditis
    2. hepatitis
    3. pancreatitis
    4. peritonitis

UNIT 4   THE ADOLESCENT

I. **Adolescence**—the developmental stage between 12 and 20 years. Physical development is much more accelerated than emotional and social development.
   A. Early adolescence
      1. Physical development—girls grow more rapidly between the ages of 11 and 13; boys grow more rapidly from 13 to 15.
         a. Reproductive organs become functional—puberty.
            1. Males—production of spermatozoa and testosterone by testes.
            2. Females—maturation of ova in ovary with onset of menstruation. First menstrual period called menarche.
         b. Secondary sex characteristics develop.
            1. Male—voice changes; growth of hair on face, chest, in pubic area, and axillae; skin changes; increase in height and weight, with broadening of chest.
            2. Female—enlargement of breasts, thighs, and hips; voice changes, growth of pubic and axillae hair, skin changes.
            3. Glands—oil and perspiration become more active with increasing hormonal activity, often resulting in appearance of acne.
      2. Emotional-social development.
         a. Emotional problems may arise as a result of the stress of adjusting to sexual maturation, achievement of the male or female role, and the search for values, ideals, and identity.
         b. Physical activity and mobility give opportunity to work out aggressive feelings, gain control over feelings of helplessness, and relieve tension.
         c. More comfortable with members of own sex while engaging in activities with both sexes.
         d. Females may be more mature than males in early adolescence.
   B. Middle adolescence
      1. Physical maturity reached at about 16 or 17 years of age.
      2. Emotional-social development.
         a. Increasingly independent of any one person; has friends with both sexes.
         b. Anxious for approval from peers or "gang." Feels a need to be accepted by others in age group but is resentful of prying adults.
         c. Begins dating; may "go steady."
         d. Wishes to be treated as an adult. Is making transition from child to adult, but may find responsibilities and expectations of adulthood somewhat frightening.
   C. Late adolescence—ages 18 to 20
      1. Considered the prime of physical health.
      2. Emotional-social development.
         a. Developing capacity to care and share with one individual—intimacy.
         b. Time for decision-making that will affect the future.

II. **Health Concerns of the Adolescent**
   A. Major cause of death is accidents, which are also responsible for many serious injuries.
   B. Venereal disease is becoming epidemic, posing a serious threat to the health and welfare of this age group.
   C. Unwanted pregnancies underscore the need for sex education for the adolescent.
   D. Smoking, alcohol, and drugs pose serious temptations for use, especially with pressure from peer groups to conform.
   E. Health difficulties associated with maturation.
      1. Acne vulgaris
      2. Menstrual irregularities
      3. Nutritional concerns

III. **Nursing the Adolescent**
   A. The older adolescent wants to be consulted and included in plans for his care and treatment. He resents being "treated like a child" but may regress to more childlike behavior during an illness.
   B. Need for socialization and contact with his peer group are very important.
   C. Limitation of movement causes frustration, poor self-image, loss of self-esteem, and feelings of extreme anxiety and anger.
   D. During convalescence there may be playful violation of rules. Teasing and mock sexual overtones can be expected. The nurse should accept the show of affection as a sign of gratitude and remain polite and understanding.

Questions

1. Ralph Thomas is a 16-year-old who has been admitted to the hospital with a diagnosis of bilateral pneumonia. He is very ill and has been placed on bed rest and is receiving oxygen. Ralph's parents are divorced and his mother is an alcoholic. When planning nursing care for Ralph, it would be best to:
    1. assume that his parents will not be cooperative or interested in what is being done for Ralph
    2. accept the fact that Ralph will not be able to participate in or understand any plans made for his care
    3. encourage Ralph to express his wishes and opinions in regard to plans made for his care
    4. concentrate on gaining the interest and cooperation of his mother who must learn to accept some responsibility for his care

2. As Ralph's condition improved he was allowed visitors. One evening as you attempted to enter Ralph's room to give a medication, you find that the door is closed and a chair propped against it so that you cannot open it. There are several teenagers visiting with Ralph. Which of the following statements best explains the reason for the "locked" door?
    1. Adolescents are by nature rebellious and Ralph and his friends are protesting hospital rules and regulations.
    2. It is very likely that Ralph and his friends are engaging in some harmful or immoral activity in their room and do not want to be seen.
    3. Ralph probably has a grudge against you and other members of the nursing staff and wants to do something to show his hostility toward you.
    4. Adolescents tend to be more comfortable in their own peer group and resent adults who appear to be prying into their personal affairs.

3. After you have persuaded one of Ralph's friends to let you into the room, it would be most appropriate for you to:
    1. ask his friends to leave and tell them they cannot come back to visit Ralph
    2. reprimand Ralph for his childish behavior and tell him that you are going to report his actions to the supervisor
    3. administer the medication without comment and, as you leave, close the door, assuring Ralph that he need not "lock" the door and you will always knock before entering his room
    4. ask Ralph why the door was closed and tell him that it is against hospital rules for the door to a patient's room to be locked

4. During his confinement to bed Ralph often had fits of temper and used abusive language when speaking to the nurses. Which of the following statements best explains Ralph's behavior?
    1. He probably has had very little discipline at home and is behaving as he usually does when he is well.
    2. Limitation of movement has produced in Ralph extreme frustration and feelings of anxiety and anger that he must express in some way.
    3. Most adolescents cannot cope with situations in which they become dependent on others for their personal care.
    4. Ralph has developed an intense dislike and lack of respect for females because of the way his mother has treated him during his childhood.

5. In spite of Ralph's demands that he be treated as an adult, there are times when he acts very childish and apparently enjoys being "babied." Which of the following best explains Ralph's behavior?
    1. Ralph is probably a very immature 16-year-old who does not have the emotional and social development expected of one his age.
    2. Ralph is enjoying being babied because he has never received enough attention from his mother.
    3. It is not unusual for an adolescent who is ill to regress to more childish behavior at times.
    4. Ralph is acting this way to get more attention and he must not be encouraged to continue behaving in this way.

6. As Ralph's illness improved he became easier to talk with and he seemed to enjoy your company. One day he makes a very suggestive remark and playfully pats you on the thigh. You should respond to this by:
    1. explaining to Ralph that this type of behavior will not be tolerated and he must never say or do anything like this again
    2. ignoring his words and actions, considering them typical of boys of his age
    3. being more careful of your behavior and trying to avoid being with Ralph any more than is absolutely necessary
    4. recognizing his behavior as a sign of affection and gratitude for the care you have given him

BIBLIOGRAPHY

American Academy of Pediatrics: *Report of the Committee on Infectious Diseases.* Evanston, Illinois, American Academy of Pediatrics, 1975.

American National Red Cross: *First Aid Textbook.* New York, Doubleday, 1957.

Asperheim, M.K.: *Pharmacology for Practical Nurses,* 4th edition. Philadelphia, W.B. Saunders, 1975.

Beland, I.L., and Passos, J.Y.: *Clinical Nursing,* 3rd edition. New York, Macmillan, 1975.

Bethea, D.C.: *Introductory Maternity Nursing,* 2nd edition. Philadelphia, J.B. Lippincott, 1973.

Bleier, I.J.: *Maternity Nursing: A Textbook for Practical Nurses,* 3rd edition. Philadelphia, W.B. Saunders, 1971.

Brooks, S.M.: *Integrated Basic Science,* 2nd edition. St. Louis, C.V. Mosby, 1966.

Brunner, L.S., and Suddarth, D.S.: *Textbook of Medical-Surgical Nursing,* 3rd edition. Philadelphia, J.B. Lippincott, 1975.

Buch, C.H.: *Personal and Vocational Relationships for Practical Nurses,* 2nd edition. Philadelphia, W.B. Saunders, 1966.

Committee on Trauma, American Academy of Orthopedic Surgeons; *Emergency Care and Transportation of the Sick and Injured.* Menasha, Wisconsin, George Banta, 1971.

Crawford, A.L., and Buchanan, B.P.: *Psychiatric Nursing,* 3rd edition. Philadelphia, F.A. Davis, 1970.

Culver, V.M.: *Modern Bedside Nursing,* 8th edition. Philadelphia, W.B. Saunders, 1974.

Dienhart, C.M.: *Basic Human Anatomy and Physiology,* 2nd edition. Philadelphia, W.B. Saunders, 1973.

Domonkos, A.: *Andrew's Diseases of the Skin,* 6th edition. Philadelphia, W.B. Saunders, 1971.

Du Gas, B.W.: *Kozier–Du Gas' Introduction to Patient Care,* 2nd edition. Philadelphia, W.B. Saunders, 1972.

Duncan, G.G.: *A Modern Pilgrim's Progress with Further Revelations for Diabetics,* 2nd edition. Philadelphia, W.B. Saunders, 1967.

Falconer, M.W., Ezell, A.S., Patterson, H.R., and Gustafson, E.A.: *The Drug, The Nurse, The Patient,* 5th edition. Philadelphia, W.B. Saunders, 1974.

French, R.M.: *The Nurse's Guide to Diagnostic Procedures,* 4th edition. New York, McGraw-Hill, 1975.

Frobisher, M., and Fuerst, R.: *Microbiology in Health and Disease,* 13th edition. Philadelphia, W.B. Saunders, 1973.

Fuerst, E.V., Wolf, L., and Weitzel, M.H.: *Fundamentals of Nursing,* 5th edition. Philadelphia, J.B. Lippincott, 1974.

Guyton, A.C.: *Basic Human Physiology: Normal Function and Mechanisms of Disease.* Philadelphia, W.B. Saunders, 1971.

Hamilton, M.P.: *Basic Maternity Nursing,* 3rd edition. St. Louis, C.V. Mosby, 1975.

Hamilton, M.P.: *Basic Pediatric Nursing,* 2nd edition. St. Louis, C.V. Mosby, 1974.

Harmer, B.: *Textbook of the Principles and Practices of Nursing,* 5th edition. New York, Macmillan, 1955.

Hymovich, D.P.: *Nursing of Children: A Family-Centered Guide for Study,* 2nd edition. Philadelphia, W.B. Saunders, 1974.

Ingalls, A.J., and Salerno, M.C.: *Maternal and Child Health Nursing,* 3rd edition. St. Louis, C.V. Mosby, 1975.

Irving, S.: *Basic Psychiatric Nursing,* Philadelphia, W.B. Saunders, 1973.

Jacob, S.W., and Francone, C.A.: *Structure and Function in Man,* 3rd edition. Philadelphia, W.B. Saunders, 1974.

Johnston, D.F., and Hood, G.: *Total Patient Care,* 4th edition. St. Louis, C.V. Mosby, 1976.

Keane, C.B.: *Essentials of Nursing: A Medical-Surgical Text for Practical Nurses,* 3rd edition. Philadelphia, W.B. Saunders, 1974.

Kerr, A.: *Orthopedic Nursing Procedures,* 2nd edition. New York, Springer, 1969.

Luckmann, J., and Sorensen, K.C.: *Medical-Surgical Nursing: A Psychophysiologic Approach.* Philadelphia, W.B. Saunders, 1974.

Marlow, D.R.: *Textbook of Pediatric Nursing,* 4th edition. Philadelphia, W.B. Saunders, 1973.

Mason, M.A.: *Basic Medical Surgical Nursing,* 3rd edition. New York, Macmillan, 1974.

Memmler, R.L.: *The Human Body in Health and Dis-*

ease, 3rd edition. Philadelphia, J.B. Lippincott, 1970.

Miller, B.F., and Keane, C.B.: *Encyclopedia and Dictionary of Medicine and Nursing.* Philadelphia, W.B. Saunders, 1972.

Nave, C.R., and Nave, B.C.: *Physics for the Health Sciences.* Philadelphia, W.B. Saunders, 1975.

Newton, K., and Anderson, H.: *Geriatric Nursing,* 5th edition. St. Louis, C.V. Mosby, 1971.

Rapier, D.K., Koch, M.J., et al.: *Practical Nursing,* 4th edition. St. Louis, C.V. Mosby, 1970.

Robinson, A.M.: *Working with the Mentally Ill,* 4th edition. St. Louis, C.V. Mosby, 1971.

Shackelton, A.D.: *Practical Nurse Nutrition Education,* 3rd edition. Philadelphia, W.B. Saunders, 1972.

Shafer, K.N., et al.: *Medical-Surgical Nursing,* 6th edition. St. Louis, C.V. Mosby, 1975.

Smith, D., and Germain, C.P.: *Care of the Adult Patient,* 4th edition. Philadelphia, J.B. Lippincott, 1975.

Stevens, M.K.: *Geriatric Nursing for Practical Nurses,* 2nd edition. Philadelphia, W.B. Saunders, 1975.

Sutton, A.L.: *Bedside Nursing Techniques in Medicine and Surgery,* 2nd edition. Philadelphia, W.B. Saunders, 1969.

Thompson, E.D.: *Pediatrics for Practical Nurses,* 3rd edition. Philadelphia, W.B. Saunders, 1976.

U.S. Department of Health, Education, and Welfare: *Isolation Technique for Use in the Hospital.* Washington, D.C., U.S. Government Printing Office, 1970.

Wood, L.A.: *Nursing Skills for Allied Health Services.* Philadelphia, W.B. Saunders, 1972 (Vols. I and II) and 1975 (Vol. III).

INDEX

ANSWER SECTION
FOR
SAUNDERS REVIEW
FOR
PRACTICAL NURSES

The blank answer sheets on the following pages are perforated so that after a test has been completed it can be removed and handed in to the instructor if that is desired.

The pages showing the correct answers, which follow the blank answer sheets, are also perforated so they can be removed if the instructor wishes.

In any event, the student should carefully and thoughtfully answer the questions in a test before checking the correct answers. When a student has made a mistake, the place in the text where the correct answer is explained can be found by consulting the index.

DIRECTIONS: Read each question and its numbered answers. When you have decided which answer is correct, blacken the corresponding space on this sheet with the special pencil. Make your mark as long as the pair of lines, and move the pencil point up and down firmly to make a heavy black line. If you change your mind, erase your first mark completely. Make no stray marks; they may count against you.

SAMPLE:

1. Chicago is

1—1 a country
1—2 a mountain
1—3 an island
1—4 a city
1—5 a state

STUDENT NAME

DATE

START HERE AND WORK ACROSS →

1 2 3 4
5 6 7 8
9 10 11 12
13 14 15 16
17 18 19 20
21 22 23 24
25 26 27 28
29 30 31 32
33 34 35 36
37 38 39 40
41 42

STUDENT NAME

DATE

START HERE AND WORK ACROSS →

STUDENT NAME_____

DATE_____

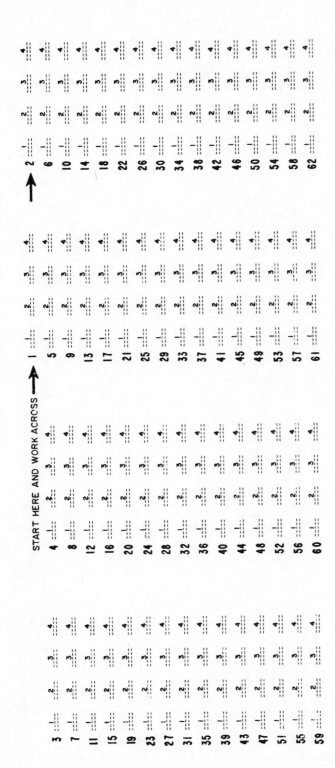

START HERE AND WORK ACROSS →

STUDENT NAME_____

DATE_____

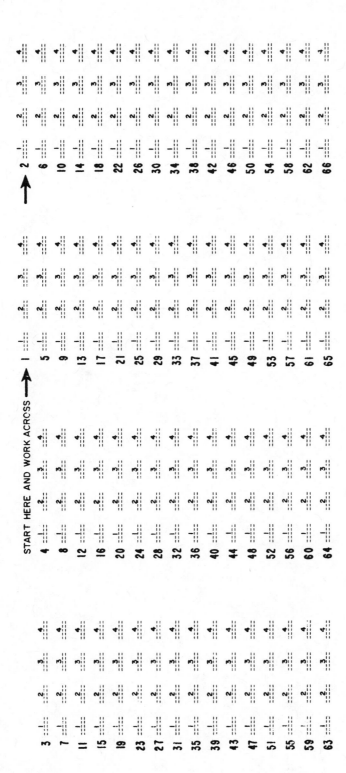

START HERE AND WORK ACROSS

STUDENT NAME

DATE

START HERE AND WORK ACROSS →

413

102 106 110 114 118 122 126

101 105 109 113 117 121 125

100 104 108 112 116 120 124

99 103 107 111 115 119 123

STUDENT NAME

DATE

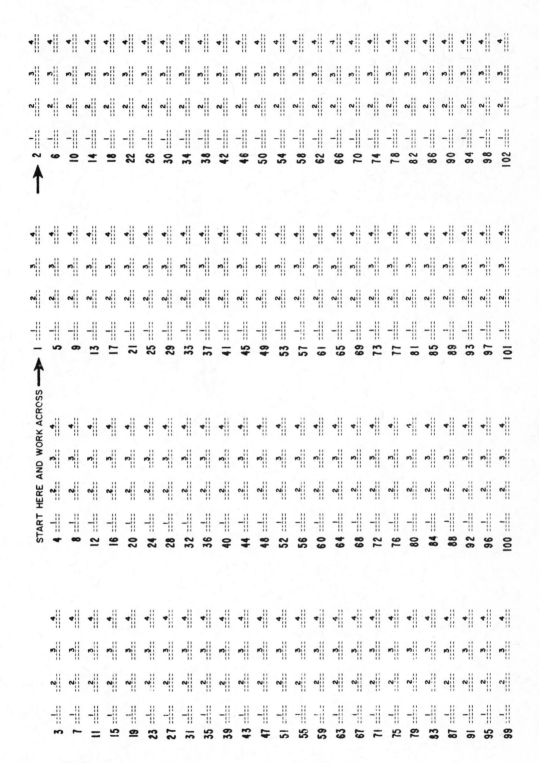

START HERE AND WORK ACROSS →

STUDENT NAME

DATE

START HERE AND WORK ACROSS

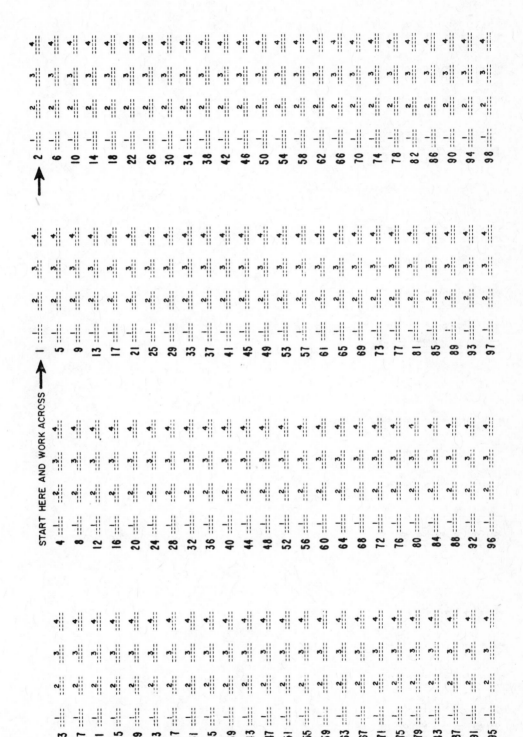

102 106 110 114 118 122 126

101 105 109 113 117 121 125

100 104 108 112 116 120 124

99 103 107 111 115 119 123

STUDENT NAME_____

DATE_____

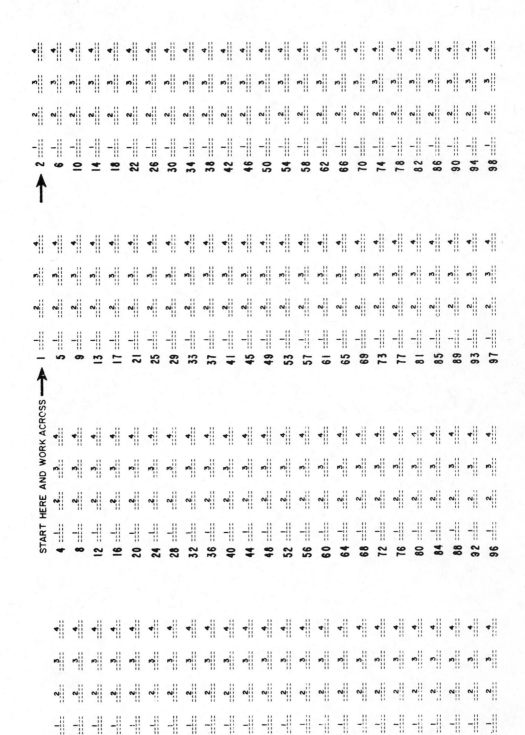

START HERE AND WORK ACROSS →

102 106 110 114 118 122 126 130

101 105 109 113 117 121 125 129

100 104 108 112 116 120 124 128

99 103 107 111 115 119 123 127

STUDENT NAME

DATE

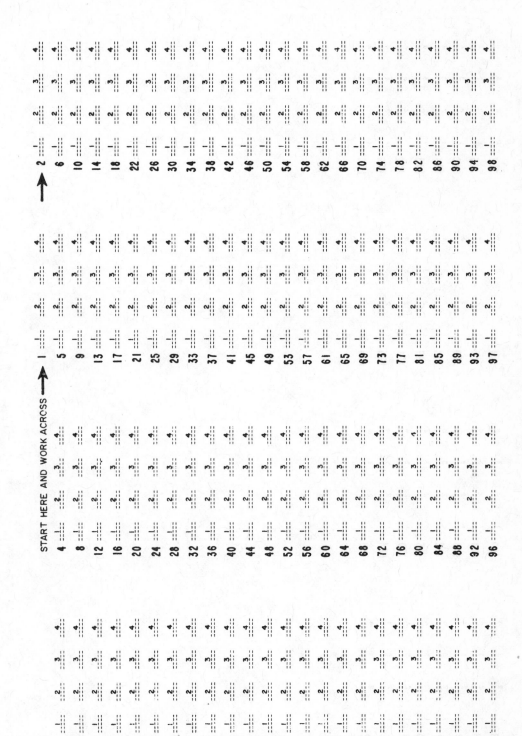

START HERE AND WORK ACROSS →

102 106 110 114 118 122 126 130

101 105 109 113 117 121 125 129

100 104 108 112 116 120 124 128

99 103 107 111 115 119 123 127

STUDENT NAME

DATE

START HERE AND WORK ACROSS →

1 2 3 4 5 6 7 8 9 10 11 12 13 14 15 16 17 18

STUDENT NAME

DATE

START HERE AND WORK ACROSS

1 2 3 4
5 6 7 8
9 10 11 12
13 14 15 16
17 18

STUDENT NAME______________________________

DATE______________________________

START HERE AND WORK ACROSS →

3	1	2	3	4	4	1	2	3	4	→ 1	1	2	3	4	→ 2	1	2	3	4
7	1	2	3	4	8	1	2	3	4	5	1	2	3	4	6	1	2	3	4
11	1	2	3	4	12	1	2	3	4	9	1	2	3	4	10	1	2	3	4
15	1	2	3	4	16	1	2	3	4	13	1	2	3	4	14	1	2	3	4
19	1	2	3	4	20	1	2	3	4	17	1	2	3	4	18	1	2	3	4
23	1	2	3	4	24	1	2	3	4	21	1	2	3	4	22	1	2	3	4
27	1	2	3	4	28	1	2	3	4	25	1	2	3	4	26	1	2	3	4
31	1	2	3	4	32	1	2	3	4	29	1	2	3	4	30	1	2	3	4
35	1	2	3	4	36	1	2	3	4	33	1	2	3	4	34	1	2	3	4
										37	1	2	3	4	38	1	2	3	4

STUDENT NAME________________

DATE________________

START HERE AND WORK ACROSS →

		1 ::1:: ::2:: ::3:: ::4::	→ 2 ::1:: ::2:: ::3:: ::4::
3 ::1:: ::2:: ::3:: ::4::	4 ::1:: ::2:: ::3:: ::4::	5 ::1:: ::2:: ::3:: ::4::	6 ::1:: ::2:: ::3:: ::4::
7 ::1:: ::2:: ::3:: ::4::	8 ::1:: ::2:: ::3:: ::4::	9 ::1:: ::2:: ::3:: ::4::	10 ::1:: ::2:: ::3:: ::4::
11 ::1:: ::2:: ::3:: ::4::	12 ::1:: ::2:: ::3:: ::4::	13 ::1:: ::2:: ::3:: ::4::	14 ::1:: ::2:: ::3:: ::4::
15 ::1:: ::2:: ::3:: ::4::	16 ::1:: ::2:: ::3:: ::4::	17 ::1:: ::2:: ::3:: ::4::	18 ::1:: ::2:: ::3:: ::4::
19 ::1:: ::2:: ::3:: ::4::	20 ::1:: ::2:: ::3:: ::4::	21 ::1:: ::2:: ::3:: ::4::	22 ::1:: ::2:: ::3:: ::4::
23 ::1:: ::2:: ::3:: ::4::	24 ::1:: ::2:: ::3:: ::4::	25 ::1:: ::2:: ::3:: ::4::	26 ::1:: ::2:: ::3:: ::4::

STUDENT NAME

DATE

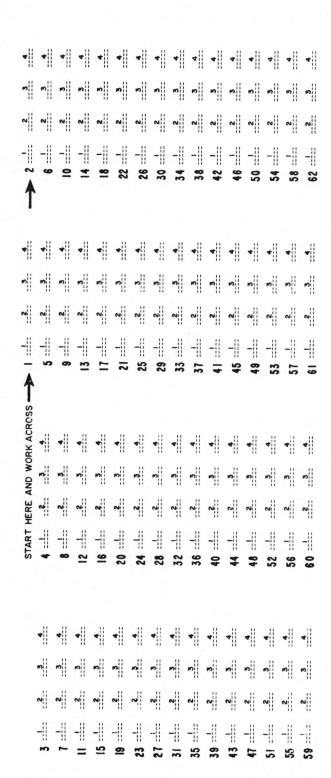

START HERE AND WORK ACROSS →

STUDENT NAME

DATE

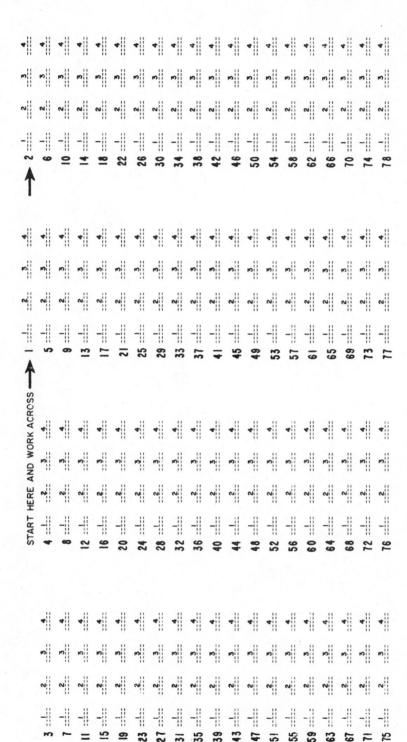

START HERE AND WORK ACROSS →

STUDENT NAME

DATE

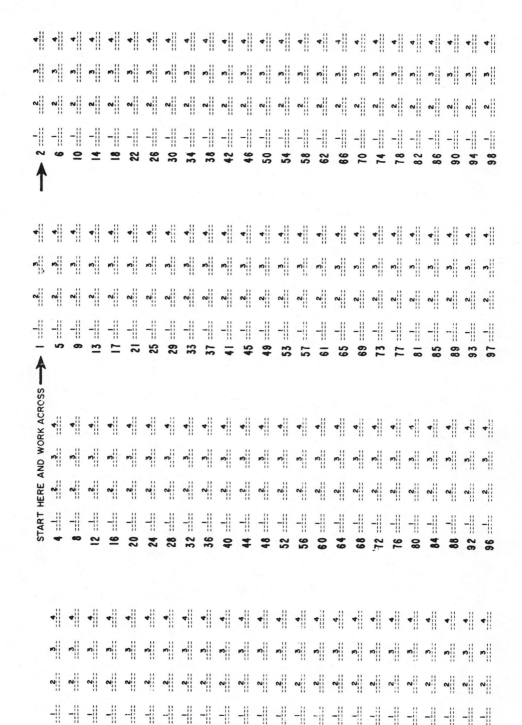

START HERE AND WORK ACROSS

102 106 110 114 118

101 105 109 113 117

100 104 108 112 116

99 103 107 111 115

STUDENT NAME

DATE

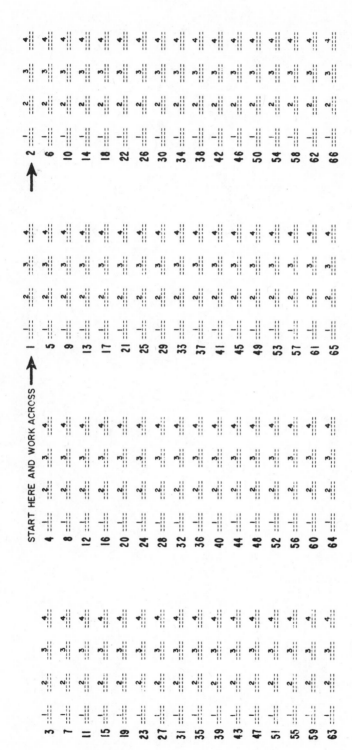

START HERE AND WORK ACROSS →

STUDENT NAME

DATE

START HERE AND WORK ACROSS →

↑

1   2   3   4
5   6   7   8
9   10 11 12
13 14 15 16
17 18 19 20
21 22 23 24
25 26 27 28
29 30

STUDENT NAME

DATE

START HERE AND WORK ACROSS →

STUDENT NAME

DATE

START HERE AND WORK ACROSS →

STUDENT NAME

DATE

START HERE AND WORK ACROSS

1 2 3 4
5 6 7 8
9 10 11 12
13 14 15 16
17 18 19 20
21 22

STUDENT NAME____________________

DATE____________________

START HERE AND WORK ACROSS →

1 1 2 3 4	2 1 2 3 4	3 1 2 3 4	4 1 2 3 4
5 1 2 3 4	6 1 2 3 4	7 1 2 3 4	8 1 2 3 4
9 1 2 3 4	10 1 2 3 4	11 1 2 3 4	12 1 2 3 4
13 1 2 3 4	14 1 2 3 4	15 1 2 3 4	16 1 2 3 4
17 1 2 3 4	18 1 2 3 4	19 1 2 3 4	20 1 2 3 4
21 1 2 3 4	22 1 2 3 4	23 1 2 3 4	24 1 2 3 4
25 1 2 3 4	26 1 2 3 4	27 1 2 3 4	28 1 2 3 4
29 1 2 3 4	30 1 2 3 4		

STUDENT NAME

DATE

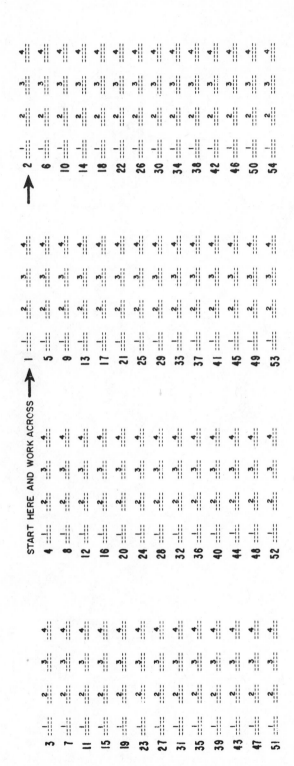

START HERE AND WORK ACROSS →

STUDENT NAME

DATE

START HERE AND WORK ACROSS

1 2 3 4 5 6 7 8 9 10 11 12 13 14 15 16 17 18 19 20 21 22 23 24 25 26 27 28 29 30

STUDENT NAME

DATE

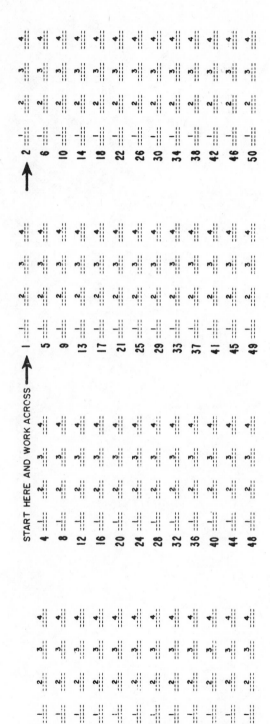

START HERE AND WORK ACROSS →

STUDENT NAME_____

DATE_____

START HERE AND WORK ACROSS →

STUDENT NAME

DATE

START HERE AND WORK ACROSS

STUDENT NAME

DATE

START HERE AND WORK ACROSS →

STUDENT NAME

DATE

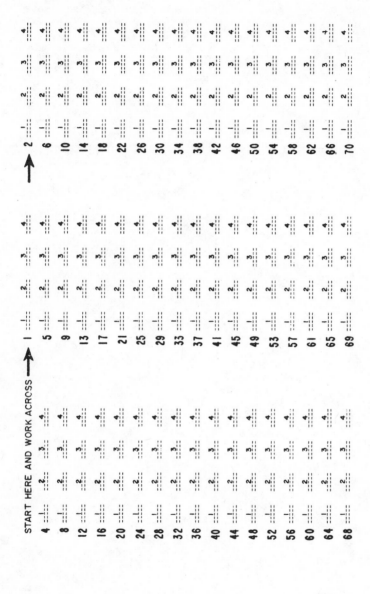

START HERE AND WORK ACROSS

STUDENT NAME

DATE

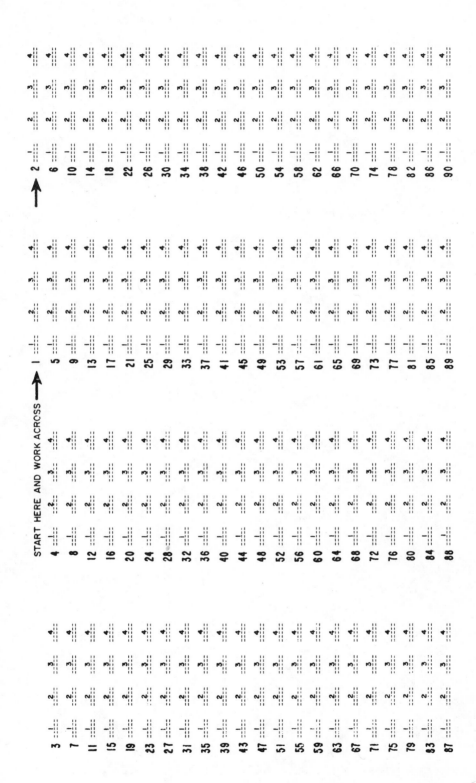

START HERE AND WORK ACROSS →

STUDENT NAME

DATE

START HERE AND WORK ACROSS →

STUDENT NAME

DATE

START HERE AND WORK ACROSS →

STUDENT NAME

DATE

START HERE AND WORK ACROSS →

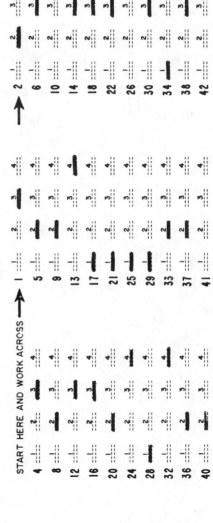

PART I   Personal Hygiene and Community Health   (pp. 1 to 6)

START HERE AND WORK ACROSS

PART II   Personal and Vocational Relationships   (pp. 7 to 14)

START HERE AND WORK ACROSS

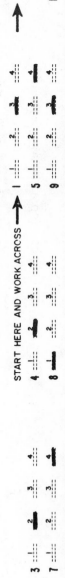

PART III   Unit 1.   Chemistry and Physics   (pp. 15 to 24)

START HERE AND WORK ACROSS

Unit 1.   Chemistry and Physics   (pp. 15 to 24)   (continued)

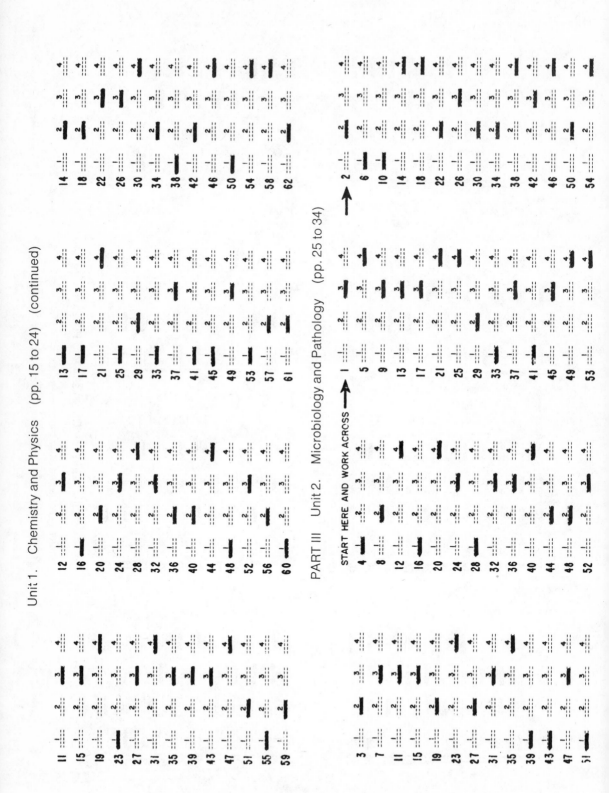

PART III   Unit 2.   Microbiology and Pathology   (pp. 25 to 34)

START HERE AND WORK ACROSS

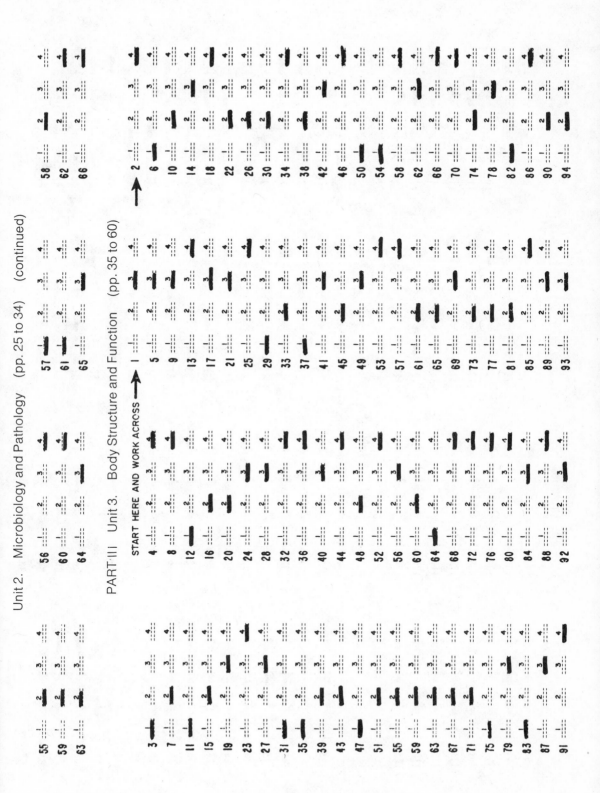

Unit 3.   Body Structure and Function   (pp. 35 to 60)   (continued)

PART IV   Nutrition   (pp. 61 to 76)

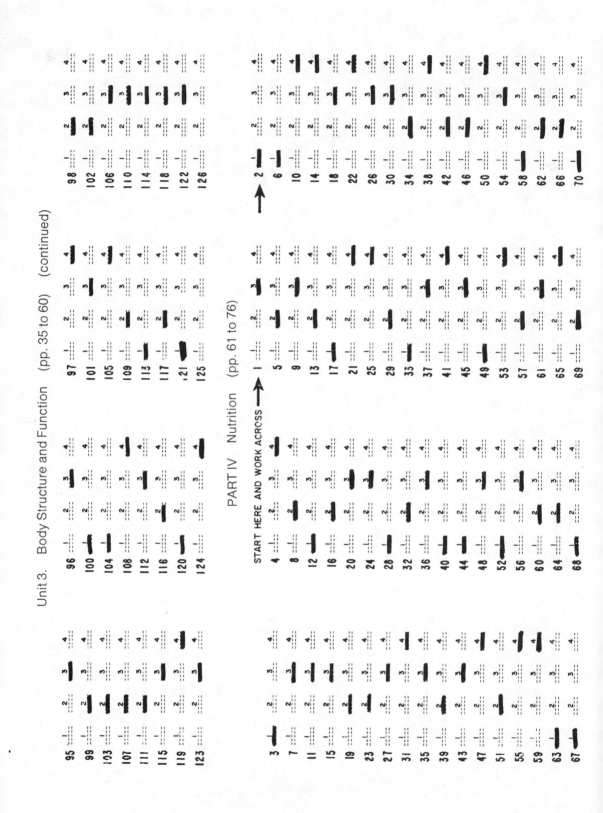

START HERE AND WORK ACROSS

Nutrition (pp. 61 to 76) (continued)

PART V Unit 1. Patient Care (pp. 77 to 100)

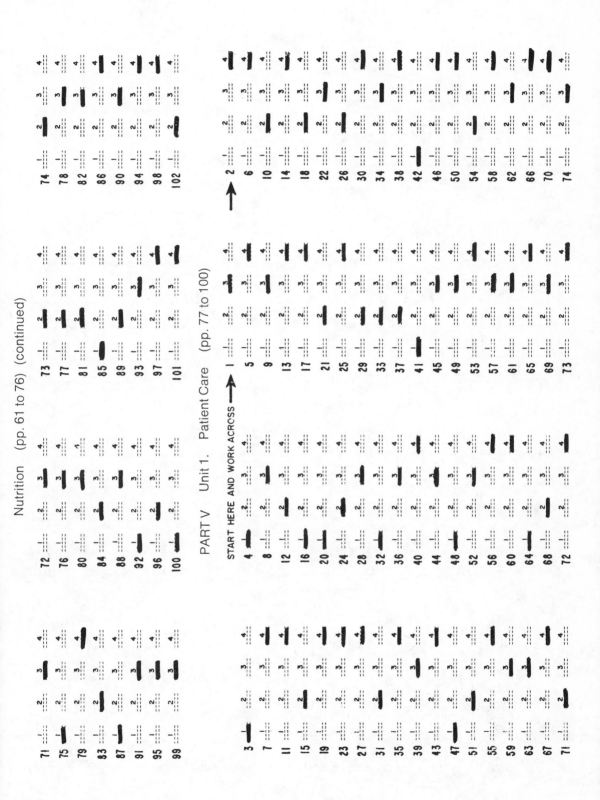

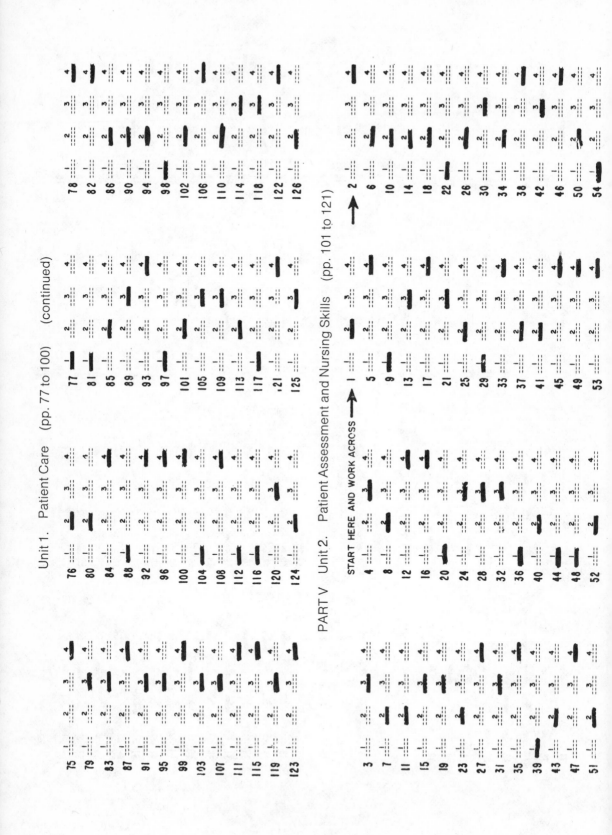

Unit 1. Patient Care (pp. 77 to 100) (continued)

PART V Unit 2. Patient Assessment and Nursing Skills (pp. 101 to 121)

START HERE AND WORK ACROSS →

Unit 2. Patient Assessment and Nursing Skills (pp. 101 to 121) (continued)

Question	Answer	Question	Answer	Question	Answer	Question	Answer
55	3	56	1	57	3	58	2
59	2	60	3	61	1	62	4
63	2	64	4	65	3	66	1
67	4	68	4	69	1	70	4
71	3	72	1	73	2	74	1
75	3	76	4	77	3	78	1
79	1	80	4	81	3	82	1
83	2	84	3	85	1	86	4
87	2	88	3	89	2	90	1
91	4	92	3	93	1	94	2
95	4	96	3	97	1	98	3
99	2	100	1	101	3	102	3
103	4	104	2	105	3	106	1
107	2	108	4	109	2	110	4
111	3	112	4	113	4	114	1
115	3	116	3	117	3	118	1
119	4	120	1	121	3	122	1
123	2	124	3	125	2	126	1
127	3	128	4	129	2	130	

PART VI Drugs and Their Administration (pp. 123 to 144)

START HERE AND WORK ACROSS →

Question	Answer	Question	Answer	Question	Answer	Question	Answer
				1	4	2	2
3	4	4	2	5	2	6	1
7	2	8	4	9	1	10	1
11	2	12	3	13	4	14	2
15	1	16	3	17	2	18	2
19	1	20	4	21	3	22	3
23	3	24	1	25	4	26	3
27	1	28	4	29	3	30	2

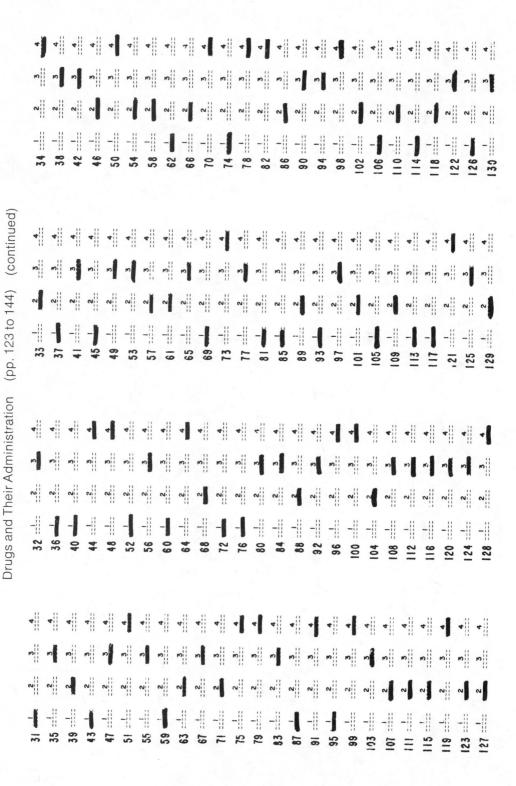

Drugs and Their Administration   (pp. 123 to 144)   (continued)

PART VII   Unit 1.   The Surgical Patient   (pp. 145 to 149)

START HERE AND WORK ACROSS →

PART VII   Unit 2.   The Patient with Cancer   (pp. 150 to 153)

START HERE AND WORK ACROSS →

PART VII   Unit 3.   The Aged and Chronically Ill   (pp. 154 to 161)

START HERE AND WORK ACROSS →

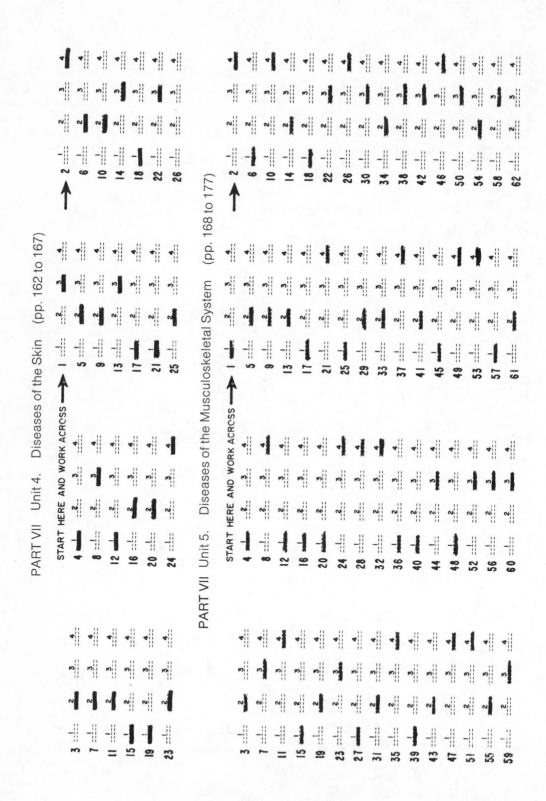

PART VII   Unit 4.   Diseases of the Skin   (pp. 162 to 167)

START HERE AND WORK ACROSS →

PART VII   Unit 5.   Diseases of the Musculoskeletal System   (pp. 168 to 177)

START HERE AND WORK ACROSS →

PART VII

Unit 6. Diseases of the Digestive Tract (pp. 178 to 182)

Unit 7. Diseases of the Accessory Organs of Digestion (pp. 183 to 193)

START HERE AND WORK ACROSS

PART VII Unit 8. Diseases of the Cardiovascular System (pp. 194 to 213)

START HERE AND WORK ACROSS

Unit 8.   Diseases of the Cardiovascular System   (pp. 194 to 213)   (continued)

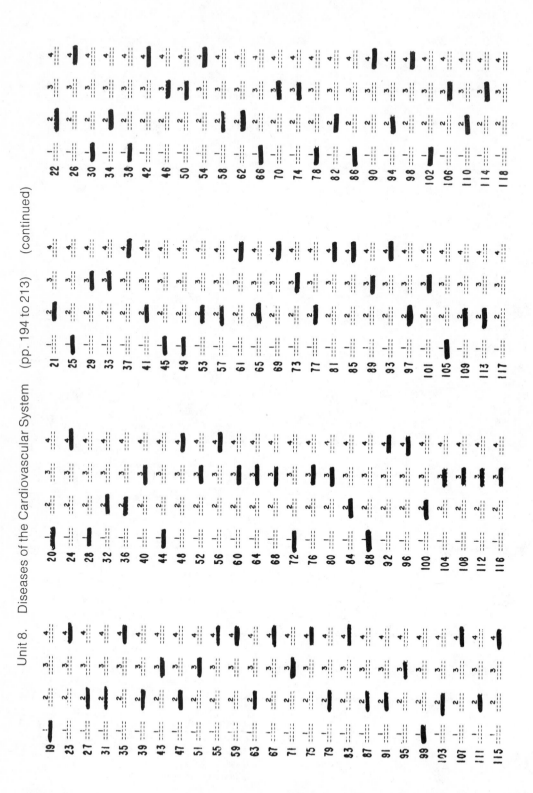

PART VII   Unit 9.   Diseases of the Respiratory System   (pp. 214 to 226)

PART VII   Unit 10.   The Urinary System   (pp. 227 to 233)

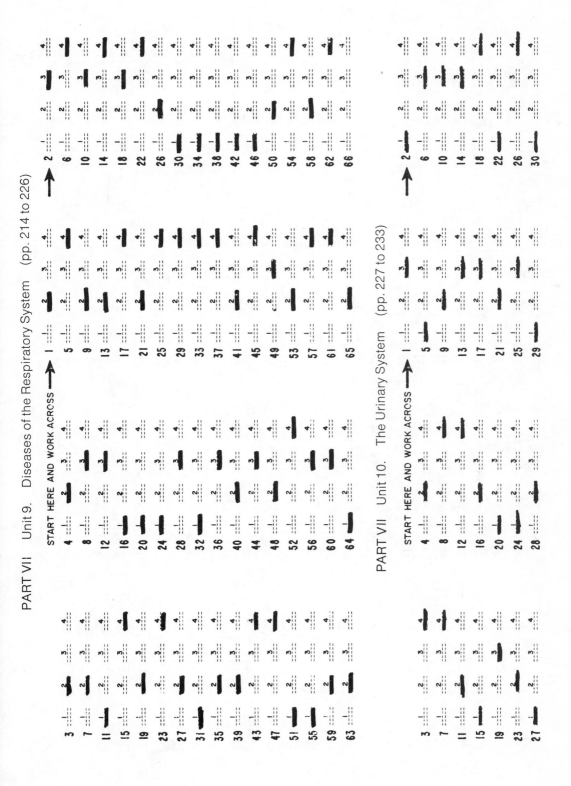

PART VII Unit 11. The Endocrine System (pp. 234 to 240)

START HERE AND WORK ACROSS →

PART VII Unit 12. The Female and Male Reproductive Systems (pp. 241 to 248)

START HERE AND WORK ACROSS →

PART VII Unit 13. Diseases of the Nervous System (pp. 249 to 254)

START HERE AND WORK ACROSS →

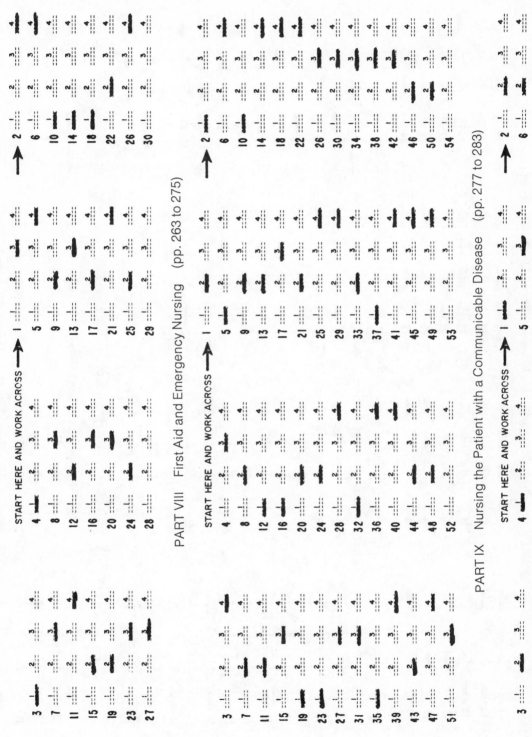

PART VII Unit 14. Disorders of the Eyes, Ears, and Throat (pp. 255 to 261)

PART VIII First Aid and Emergency Nursing (pp. 263 to 275)

PART IX Nursing the Patient with a Communicable Disease (pp. 277 to 283)

Nursing the Patient with a Communicable Disease   (pp. 277 to 283)   (continued)

PART X   Nursing the Emotionally Disturbed and the Mentally III   (pp. 285 to 294)

START HERE AND WORK ACROSS →

PART XI   Unit 1.   Human Reproduction and Pregnancy   (pp. 295 to 304)

START HERE AND WORK ACROSS →

Unit 1. Human Reproduction and Pregnancy (pp. 295 to 304) (continued)

PART XI Unit 2. Labor and Delivery (pp. 305 to 313)

START HERE AND WORK ACROSS →

PART XI Unit 3. The Puerperium (pp. 314 to 320)

START HERE AND WORK ACROSS →

PART XI   Unit 4.   The Newborn   (pp. 321 to 336)

START HERE AND WORK ACROSS →

PART XII   Unit 1.   The Infant and the Toddler   (pp. 337 to 362)

START HERE AND WORK ACROSS →

Unit 1.   The Infant and the Toddler   (pp. 337 to 362)   (continued)

PART XII   Unit 2.   The Preschool Child   (pp. 363 to 371)

START HERE AND WORK ACROSS

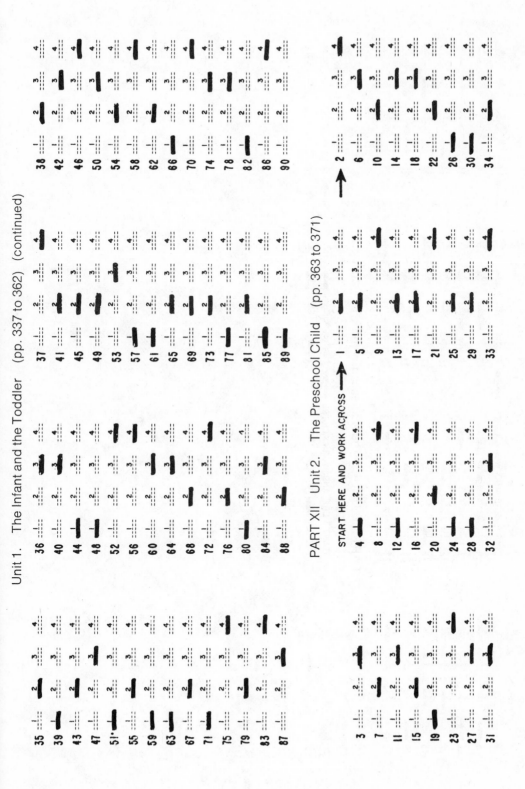

PART XII   Unit 3.   The School Age Child   (pp. 372 to 375)

START HERE AND WORK ACROSS →

PART XII   Unit 4.   The Adolescent   (pp. 376 to 378)

START HERE AND WORK ACROSS →